Brain2Brain

Brain2Brain

JOHN B. ARDEN

Brain2Brain

Enacting Client Change
Through the Persuasive Power of
NEUROSCIENCE

WILEY

Library of Congress Cataloging-in-Publication Data:

Arden, John Boghosian, author.
  Brain2Brain : enacting client change through the persuasive power of neuroscience / John Arden.
    p. ; cm.
  Includes index.
  ISBN 978-1-118-75688-1 (pbk)   ISBN 978-1-118-75667-6 (pdf)   ISBN 978-1-118-75689-8 (epub)
  I. Title.   II. Title: Brain 2 brain.   III. Title: Brain to brain.   IV. Title: Brain two brain.
  [DNLM: 1. Nervous System Physiological Phenomena.   2. Counseling–methods.   3. Mental
Disorders–pathology.   4. Neurosciences–methods.   5. Psychotherapy–methods. WL 102]
  RC480.5
  616.89'14—dc23

                                                                                          2014031893

Printed in the United States of America

10 9 8 7 6 5 4 3 2 1

CONTENTS

PREFACE

A sea change is beginning to occur in the mental health system. An international movement to break down the boundaries among the different schools of psychotherapy to find common denominators is occurring. These common denominators are brain based. The new integrative model subsumes the relevant contributions of the past and discards the purely theory driven cul-de-sacs based only on the tight confines of a particular school.

During my last 40 years working as a mental health administrator, training director, and psychologist, I have seen many phases, fads, and theories burst on the scene only to fade away a few years later. Many of these phases and theories conflicted with one another. People seeking help from one therapist may hear a completely different perspective about their problem than they would from another well-meaning therapist from a different theoretical school.

The focus of this book is to provide you, the therapist, with suggestions on how to integrate all the domains of research, including neuroscience, in a down-to-earth manner to help clients understand and deal with depression and anxiety. The techniques that I will describe are supported by a broad body of research and consistent with what we know about how the brain works. Going beyond what has been called evidence-based practices (EBPs), these methods are ones shown by research to be most efficacious for helping people who suffer from various psychological problems. I explain which brain systems are either over- or under-activated when clients are anxious or depressed. The methods I describe to help clients with these problems bring together all areas of psychological research and neuroscience that are relevant to psychotherapy. I offer suggestions on how to help clients learn to activate areas of their brains that have been underactivated and how to quiet down those areas that have been overactivated, so that they can enjoy life without being plagued by anxiety and/or depression. By learning more about the brain, clients understand what they need to do to neutralize excessive anxiety or lift depression.

Consider this book a user manual for the brain. New cars and DVD players come with user manuals. Our brains do not. Clients can learn to use their brains more effectively. Today we know quite a bit about which brain networks are overactivated and which are underactivated with anxiety and depression. Thanks to brain imaging techniques developed in the last 20-30 years, such as functional magnetic resonance imaging (fMRI), we can not only identify those neural firing patterns but also see how certain psychotherapeutic techniques can calm down overactivated areas while activating those areas that need to be activated. Essentially, we can teach our clients how to tune up their brains.

This book attempts to normalize psychological disorders and their resolution so that you can explain and make more tangible recommendations to your clients. We must leave behind those countertrends that pathologize normal human reactions to life stressors.

LETTING GO OF THE 20TH CENTURY

To gain an understanding of where we are going, it is important to use a bird's-eye perspective of where we have been. During the 20th century, as psychotherapy became a healthcare profession, the various schools of psychotherapy had little in common. This was because theorists of each school possessed very little understanding of how the brain worked. Some theorists even thought that brain activity was irrelevant. Freud and James did consider the brain important. However, Freud could only hypothesize about what the future might bring, saying "We must recollect that all of our provisional ideas in psychology will presumably one day be based on an organic substructure" (Freud, 1914). The father of American psychology, William James, speculated that "The act of will activates neural circuits" (James, 1890). Because they and others could not base their theories on the operation of the brain, a disparate range of theories emerged, from radical behaviorists to primal scream. We could refer to this era as the Cartesian Era, a brainless period with no common denominator.

The theoretical schools of the Cartesian Era became walled-off silos with self-reinforcing concepts relevant only within each school. Each built-in infrastructure of presumed competency and proficiency using the jargon of that theoretical school. Conferences are still held for devotees of those schools of thought where esoteric lectures are given and understood only by those with higher levels of acculturation within those schools. Many schools issue certificates. I once had dinner in Brisbane, Australia, with a group of "Level 4" eye movement desensitization and reprocessing (EMDR) practitioners. During a break in a lecture I was giving in Wellington, New Zealand, a woman approached me identifying herself as "one of the 24 masters of emotionally focused therapy (EFT)."

If a person from one of the many incarnations of the psychodynamic schools were to attend a conference of cognitive-behavioral therapy (CBT) or vice versa, even the most basic presentations would sound like a discussion among extraterrestrials. More troubling is the effect on people with psychological problems that we are trying to serve. As they go from a therapist of one school to a therapist of another school, they become increasingly confused by what they hear and what they are asked to do to recover from their psychological problems.

Turf battles among professional disciplines have left clients even more confused. Not surprisingly, the psychotherapy efficacy studies during the Cartesian

Era were bleak. For example, in 1952 Hans Eysenck published a study that showed that the mere passage of time was as effective as psychotherapy for many people. In the late 1950s, Timothy Leary, before his Harvard professorship and his devolution into a psychedelic haze, did a study in the Kaiser Permanente system that showed that people on a wait list for therapy did as well as people in psychotherapy.

In 1980, Smith, Glass, and Miller published the results of a large meta-analysis of multiple studies on the efficacy of psychotherapy. At the time, there were already in place many of the elements of a major change which served to obscure the insights that could be derived from the study's results. Their book, *The Benefits of Psychotherapy*, showed that psychotherapy in its generic form actually did work to help people with psychological problems find relief. But it was too little too late. Around 1980, a variety of factors combined to bring most mental health professionals to partially agree on a unifying model to embrace. The first factor was the publication of the third edition of the *Diagnostic and Statistical Manual of Mental Disorders* (*DSM-III*), which served as a more valuable contribution to our field than *DSM-I* and *II*, which contained far more theory than science. *DSM-III* was three times the size of *DSM-II* and contained science, albeit light, supporting its concepts. For example, there was a more coherent conceptualization of trauma, and the term "posttraumatic stress disorder" was born.

Simultaneous with the publication of *DSM-III* were the inventions of the selective serotonin reuptake inhibitors (SSRIs) and an opportunity to prescribe antidepressant medications that could not be used in a suicidal overdose. Prior to that time, the tricyclic antidepressants (TCAs) then in use often were associated with intentional or even accidental overdose. I was a community mental health administrator during that period, and I lost three clients who attended my programs to TCA overdoses in one year.

Occurring in the 1980s was the increasing dominance of CBT and the research demonstrating particular CBT techniques that eventually became known as EBPs. By 1990, economic forces converged with the *DSM-III*, medication, and evidence-based therapy developments to form the elements of managed care (which some call "managed dollar"). Last but not least, licensing laws were being refined, and practitioners within the system were required to attend accredited academic programs and internships to practice.

All these developments combined led Lloyd Linford and me to call the era beginning in 1980 Pax Medica (Arden & Linford, 2010; Linford & Arden, 2009). The term "Pax Medica" is, of course, a play on words, taken as a metaphor to mean the medical model. Similar to the concept of the Pax Romana (Roman peace), where 2,000 years ago Roman citizens could travel anywhere in the Roman world without problem and expect to be relatively safe, mental health providers who operated within the context of Pax Medica need not feel their competence was threatened. The medical model of Pax Medica dictated a pecking order of professionals. Since medication was considered one of the principal treatments for people with psychological problems, and psychiatrists, not psychologists, are licensed to prescribe these medications, psychiatrists are at the top of the pecking order.

Pax Medica has led to multiple cultural side effects that include regressive changes in the way mental health disciplines are conceptualized. Medications removed psychology from psychiatry and moved psychology toward the medical model. Since medication was seen as the first-line treatment and because it was presumed that the patients suffered from "chemical imbalances," psychiatrists retained their top position in the pecking order of mental health professionals.

Pax Medica is essentially a one-dimensional medical model that shaped economic forces to solidify around an emphasis on medication and less psychotherapy. Mental health professionals quickly fell in line and even began to speak "clinicalese." We referred to ourselves as "clinicians." When we sat in "treatment planning meetings," one might say "Okay, what's the diagnosis?" In response, another clinician would say, "Well, clinically speaking...." Another clinician would say, "Well, what's medically necessary?" Everyone sat there quite smug feeling like they knew what they were talking about.

Consistent with the Pax Medica concept of missing brain chemicals, biological psychiatry envisions psychological disorders as having a genetic etiology. The fact that the environment can contribute to changes in genetic expression and the brain changes with experience through neuroplasticity was not part of the intellectual landscape.

Pax Medica envisions discrete psychiatric disorders, similar to different medical diseases, such as diabetes, multiple sclerosis, and heart disease; so depression, anxiety, posttraumatic stress disorder (PTSD), dissociative disorders, and now, according to DSM-5, even bereavement is considered a medical problem. When two or more symptom clusters satisfy the diagnosis of two categories, the "clinician" notes "comorbidities." One of the many problems with this one-dimensional model is that often there is considerable overlap in many syndromes and often similar neural circuits are implicated, especially in anxiety disorders. As Bremner (2005) stated, PTSD and acute stress disorder (ASD) are better thought of as part of trauma spectrum disorders than as discrete disorders.

Many clients and unfortunately too many mental health professionals bought into the simplistic idea of genetic determinism that developed in the Pax Medica era. As such, they subscribed to the belief that some people, despite their best efforts, are genetically determined to develop "major depressive illness" for which the only cure is the "right medicine." This archaic belief does not emphasize that clients do anything to improve their mood. Believing that they are predestined to be depressed, they argue, "Why try?" They feel helpless and hopeless, which only increases their depression.

Clients need to be told that the field of epigenetics has shown that genes can be either expressed or suppressed by many factors that can lead to or away from depression. Some behaviors turn on genes; some turn them off. For example, psychosocial factors, including lack of social support as well as traumatic interpersonal events, such as intimate partner abuse, add to the risk of genetic vulnerability for depression.

The brain can be rewired to develop a habit. You can explain this to clients by describing how prior depressive episodes increase the chances of becoming depressed again. The severity of the depression increases the risk for more depression. Prior suicide attempts increase not only the risk of subsequent suicide attempts but also more episodes of severe depression.

Until approximately the year 2000, all the mental health professionals were aligned behind Pax Medica. Then the cracks in the alliance began to show in a steady stream of psychopharmacology efficacy studies published in highly esteemed journals, such as the *New England Journal of Medicine* and the *Journal of the Medical Association*, which seemed to dissolve the very foundation of the medical model. Indeed, during the first two decades of the 21st century, numerous articles detailing well-crafted studies have shown that the efficacy of antidepressant medication has been greatly overestimated and the long-term use of antianxiety medications is countertherapeutic.

One study, based in part on information derived through the use of the Freedom of Information Act, found that over the past 30 years, studies showing positive effects for antidepressant medications were 12 times more likely to be published than studies showing no efficacy (Turner, Matthews, Linardatos, Tell, & Rosenthal, 2008). It would be far too simplistic to assume that this disparity is due only to the mammoth power of big pharma. The culture of Pax Medica had a zeitgeist that psychological disorders can be cured, or at least managed by medication, the principal mode of treatment.

In an article published in *Scientific American* aptly entitled "Antidepressants: Good Drugs or Good Marketing?" it was suggested that due to the power of the simplistic model of what causes depression, only 50% of all drug trials over the past century were published or reported (Dobbs, 2006).

The early and widely touted success of SSRIs was based on faulty methodology as well as selective reporting. A large scale reanalysis of the studies of the efficacy of SSRIs indicate positive results fall between 56 to 60% (Taylor et. al., 2006). The fact that over half of patients taking SSRIs did become less depressed is respectable, but when compared to the percentage of people responding to a placebo, the hype related to the serotonin effect loses its luster. According to a meta-analysis of studies of people who are depressed, between 42% and 47% respond positively to a placebo (Arroll et al., 2005). That is roughly 10% less than the numbers of patients who responded to SSRIs, but how many of those responding favorably in the SSRI group actually experienced a placebo effect in response to the side effects of medications? Perhaps they may think, "Well, my stomach doesn't feel right, but I guess that is the price you pay for medicine to work."

Thanks again to the Freedom of Information Act, researchers from the University of Connecticut and George Washington University obtained efficacy data submitted to the Food and Drug Administration (FDA) for six SSRIs (Kirsch,

Scoboria, Moore, 2002). They found that 60% of the SSRI studies failed to show that they worked better than placebos. Roughly 80% of the patients' responses were duplicated in the placebo group. And when each group took a depression inventory after treatment, the score differed by only 10%.

The research literature has presented a growing body of criticism of the popularly assumed "truth" that low levels of serotonin cause depression. For example, although there is no direct way to measure the amount of serotonin in a person's brain, some researchers have attempted to lower the body's production of serotonin. Neurotransmitters are synthesized in the body from precursor amino acids. Serotonin is synthesized from tryptophan. Researchers at Arizona State University subjected people to a tryptophan-free diet to reduce their serotonin levels. While healthy people without a family history of depression showed no effects, one-third of healthy people with a family history of depression became depressed. The immediate question in regard to this finding is: What about the other 66% who did not get depressed? If serotonin is the sole culprit, these findings question that theory (Delgado, 2000). What is most striking is that two-thirds of people being treated with antidepressants became depressed after a mere five hours . But antidepressants usually take up to four weeks to be effective. This finding seems to suggest that the SSRIs do indeed affect serotonin systems, but how? Another study, from a completely different angle, showed that the drug called tianeptine (brand names Stablon, Coaxil, Tatinol, and Tianeurax) reduces depression; but it also acts to *reduce* serotonin levels (Fuchs et al., 2002). Tianeptine is the most popular antidepressant in France.

The brain is far too complex for linear Pax Medica explanations that depression is the result of low serotonin levels. Neurotransmitters do not operate independently. A change in one neurotransmitter will result in a nonlinear change in other neurotransmitters. Indeed, as Dunlap and Nemeroff (2009) pointed out, "It is now generally believed that disrupted signaling of no one single neurotransmitter is the etiologic agent for major depressive disorder because the monoamine systems interact extensively, both in the brain stem at the level of cell bodies and in the terminal projection regions" (p. 1069).

Researchers at Vanderbilt University found that 81% of those taking an SSRI relapsed in the year following treatment, while only 25% of those receiving CBT relapsed (Arroll et al., 2005). Similarly Sonia Dimidijian and colleagues from the University of Washington randomly assigned 240 people with major depression to a medication (paroxetine [Paxil]), a placebo, CBT, or behavior activation groups for 16 weeks. They found comparable results between behavior activation and medication. But in a subgroup of severely depressed people, behavior activation outperformed medication, CBT, and the placebo. Four times as many people dropped out of the medication treatment group than the CBT or behavior activation group. Behavior activation reaps rewards in behaviors that continue well after therapy. Such benefits do not accrue to patients taking medication, even when there is a positive response to the drugs.

In his book *Anatomy of an Epidemic*, Robert Whitaker (2010) meticulously detailed the alarming rise of people diagnosed with bipolar disorder and attention-deficit hyperactivity disorder (ADHD). There have been many factors contributing to the trend. The rise of big pharma represents only one part of the converging forces that have led to more diagnoses resulting from more disorders to treat with medication. The number of contributors to the development of *DSM-5* with affiliation to big pharma companies increased significantly over the number contributing to *DSM-IV*. It is well known that a significant number of psychiatrists receive their continuing medical education (CME) credits at luncheons and dinners sponsored by drug companies. More psychiatric medications are available than ever before, and with *DSM-5* more diagnostic disorders to "treat" with medications. This alarming trend is consistent with the general attitude of the large portion of the population that wants easy answers for complicated problems.

I do not mean to say that Pax Medica has not served a purpose. It has brought us all on one page from the confusion of the Cartesian Era. However, it offered a very limited understanding of brain function, with its focus on missing brain chemicals and its principal treatment, medication.

While I am not proposing that psychiatric medications should be avoided, minimizing their use until other approaches are employed is far more prudent than the excessive prescriptions inherent to the Pax Medica era. Before making a referral for a med evaluation or reaching for the prescription pad, mental health professionals should have clients try exercise and diet, which actually up-regulate neurotransmitter systems instead of down-regulating them.

Psychiatric medications certainly have a place in treatment. However, mental professionals, including primary care physicians who write 60% to 80% of the antidepressant and antianxiety prescriptions, go there far too quickly. Far too many people who do not need medications are prescribed medications.

Medications should be prescribed based on client genome, age, gender, and situation in life rather than a generic one medication per diagnosis. There are numerous reasons why the maxim "less is more" represents more than simply a sensible caution. Older adults cannot metabolize medications as easily as younger ones, and thus they require careful monitoring. To assume that the increasingly overburdened prescribing physicians have time to watch for synergistic reactions to other medications is hopeful thinking at best. Monitoring all the medical conditions and changing life situations of each patient is hard enough within managed care. Therapists should assume the responsibility of communicating details about each patient to the prescriber, given their higher frequency of contact and duration of the sessions.

EMBRACING THE 21ST CENTURY INTEGRATIVE APPROACH

The fragmented Cartesian and one-dimensional model Pax Medica trends of the 20th century are being replaced by an integrated multidimensional model of the 21st century. Brain-based therapy integrates the common factors. Thanks to major developments in psychotherapy research, neuropsychology, epigenetics, psycho-neuroimmunology, and nutritional neuroscience, we know far more about what contributes to brain health. The contributions from these fields are now being combined with psychological research on such areas as development, memory, cognition, and attachment (Arden & Linford, 2009a,b; Cozolino, 2010). A robust and multidimensional approach is synthesizing knowledge gained in all these areas. Contributions from this large body of research contribute to a coherent and integrated whole, like pieces of the puzzle in the next figure.

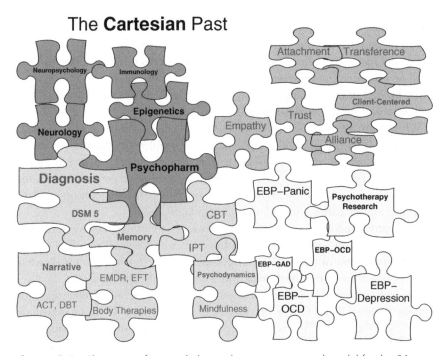

Figure 0.1   The areas of research that make up an integrated model for the 21st century. These include the neuroscience cluster, the focus on the alliance, the systems of psychological theory (including diagnosis), and evidence-based practices.

Psychotherapy researchers who have pioneered outcome management studies and those who have contributed to EBPs are looking for common factors among therapies (Barlow & Craske, 2007; Lambert, 2008). To do so, research in neuroscience, memory, attention, cognition, and developmental psychology, such as attachment research, is needed.

The emerging brain-based common-factor approach must include client education. We are now in a far better position to make sense of anxiety and depression and how to help people overcome these problems. The more clients know about what they are experiencing from a science-driven rather than a theory-driven perspective, the more tangible are the remedies. The sea change in psychotherapy, therefore, should include a strong effort to depathologize psychological problems. If clients are given actual information that includes a description of what the scientific literature says about anxiety, depression, and the brain in layman's terms, their experience is demystified and relies less on confusing circular descriptions.

If clients are not given coherent practical information, they run the risk of thinking that they have some kind of incurable illness that only a mental health professional understands and that the prognosis may not be hopeful. Labeling a psychological disorder without explaining it is not only disrespectful but tends to make clients feel less hopeful that something can be done about it. Not providing a coherent and understandable road map about what to do to achieve relief, beyond taking medication, perpetuates the false hope of Pax Medica. Like most people, they probably want to understand why they are having a difficult time recovering from excessive anxiety or depression and want to know what to do about it.

A brain-based description of clients' psychological problems can offer tangible road maps for constructive steps to be taken with you in therapy. It is similar to the narrative therapy concept of externalizing the problem so that the problem is the problem, not clients themselves. Ironically, clients' brains are central to their problems. Explain that their anxiety is partly connected to the overactivity of the amygdala and the right prefrontal cortex (R-PFC) relative to the left. Then explain that avoidance kindles even more activity in the R-PFC, which serves only to increase anxiety. Alternatively, incremental exposure to what makes them anxious activates the left PFC and eventually increases positive emotions and calms amygdala overactivity. This knowledge can increase clients' motivation to engage more and avoid less.

The changes happening in the 21st century will dissolve the separate schools of psychotherapy and their special languages accessed only by members. The alphabet soup of special clubs—CBT, ACT, IPT, DBT, EMDR, EFT, RET, and so on—needs to discarded in favor of one model focused on brain-based common factors. The new model is not eclectic, as if therapists pick and choose tricks from each of the clubs. Instead, it discards beliefs that make sense only within a particular belief system.

Brain-based therapy discriminates between what is therapeutic and what is not. It requires techniques consistent with how the brain works. Like all client-centered oriented therapies, it relies on the therapist's alliance with the client, while at the same time it employs common methods from a wide range of theoretical perspectives.

The change requires no gurus. In fact, gurus of the Cartesian schools, or brand names, distract at best and derail at worst the effort to find common factors to serve those in need of psychological services. The future is more open sourced than proprietary; no one group, or brand, will own it. Conferences of the future will feature speakers who explore the common factors. The focus on the stature or popularity of the individual speakers will fade while the focus shifts to the topics and interrelationships they explore.

Moving beyond the separate schools of psychotherapy necessitates shedding one of the lingering effects of the Cartesian Era: a brainless psychology. Yet a word of caution about the recent development of merely tacking on the words "neuroscience" and "mindfulness" to conferences and publications. Sometimes they are only window dressing, ways to flow with the latest fad. To ensure that these efforts actually contribute to the change, they must be grounded in science.

Brain-based therapy is not a new type of therapy but an integrative approach that finds common denominators among schools of psychotherapy. A brain-based approach moves us beyond pure theory and combines many fields of research. For example, psychotherapy research has illuminated what factors are important to the psychotherapeutic relationship. In particular, outcome management studies have confirmed Carl Rogers's insights into the importance of enhancing the therapeutic alliance.

Attachment studies have revealed how various types of attachment styles play out in relationships through the life span, the potential to develop anxiety and/ or depression, and brain activation patterns associated with the various attachment styles. Developmental psychology has shed light on how early adversity can impair psychological development and the brain as well as what factors lead to resiliency through the life cycle.

Evidence-supported practices have matured significantly since being introduced over the last 30 years. In fact, some of the early pioneers of EBPs have now moved to find common factors among approaches.

Memory research in many ways forms the foundation for understanding the human experience. When memory systems become deregulated, psychological problems result. Memory research has also shown how adequate integration of memory systems increases mental health.

Neuroscience is the relatively new area. Thanks to research using fMRI, positron emission tomography (PET), single photon emission computed tomography (SPECT), and many other tools, we have an operational understanding of those brain systems involved in anxiety disorders and depression.

The truly integrated model of psychotherapy in the 21st century must not perpetuate dualism of the Cartesian Era. Instead, it should incorporate how the mind, brain, and immune system interact as people adapt to their particular interpersonal and cultural environment. Too often in the past, psychotherapeutic efforts have focused single aspects of clients' lives and disregard other parts. Until recently, Western medicine has taken the same disjointed path. Integrative and functional medicine attempt to take into account the multiple physiological systems in the human body and how they interrelate dynamically. Why wouldn't psychotherapy do the same thing?

The immune system, for example, is not only affected by the mind but affects the brain and the mind in a bidirectional relationship. Excess inflammatory cytokines can result in more susceptibility to develop PTSD posttrauma (see Chapter 7) and "sickness behavior," resulting in depression (see Chapter 9). Similarly, type 2 diabetes increases depression, and depression increases the vulnerability to develop diabetes. Even the multiple systemic effects of the gastrointestinal (GI) tract affect the mood and cognition, while mood affects the GI tract. Approximately 80% of the serotonin in the body is found in the GI tract, not in the brain, which means that serotoninergic activity in the GI tract affects the brain. The vagus nerve system that extends to most of the organs in the thoracic cavity, including the heart, comes down from the brain, but activity goes back up as well. A person's vagal tone contributes to better or worse affect regulation and to anxiety and irritability accordingly. These are but a few of the many domains relevant to psychotherapy. We need to account for their interactions in therapy and inform clients about how their mental health and physical health are connected and can be enhanced.

BASE

BASE is a mnemonic that incorporates the main elements of an integrated brain-based therapy.

  B—for brain. Because we now know much more about how anxiety and depression occur in the brain, you can feel more confident that the therapeutic plans you develop make sense. For example, since clients with anxiety tend to have a hyperactivated R-PFC with hypoactivity in the L-PFC, you need to be watchful to balance the activation of the two hemispheres.
  A—for alliance. Without the "safe" part of the safe emergency, you may not address the challenge aspect successfully. The alliance is built by kindling

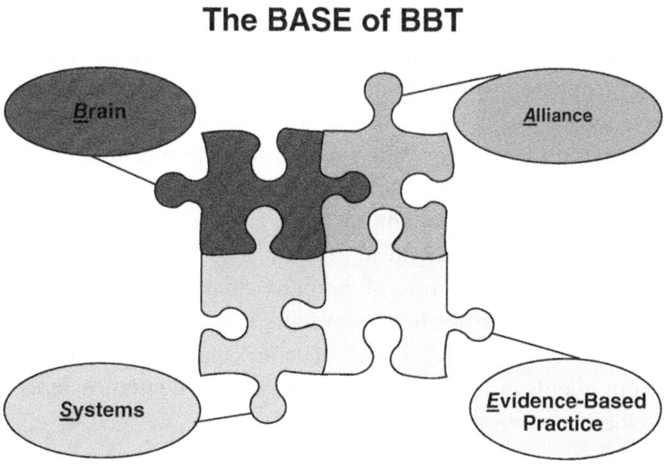

The BASE of BBT

Figure 0.2 The BASE mnemonic puzzle representing the brain (neuroscience), the alliance, system of psychological theories, and evidence-based practice.

the social brain networks. You can help clients gain a stronger sense of "earned" security.

S—for systems of psychological theories and intervention. These systems include the diagnostic paradigm as well as research in memory and cognition. Also relevant are the cross-validated aspects of the psychotherapeutic schools. Here again, the challenge is to find concepts and therapeutic approaches that provide a common denominator.

E—for evidenced-based practices. There is not an EBP for every psychological problem, but there is a rich literature base for anxiety disorders and depression.

PLAN FOR THIS BOOK

This book describes how you can boil all the factors that account for the complexity of effective psychotherapy down to coherent descriptions to convey to your clients. The brain serves as the common denominator for all relevant and efficacious approaches. Talking about the brain in the context of anxiety and depression combined with EBPs explains what is going on as well as giving a road map for recovery.

The integrated brain-based psychoeducational approach does not preclude other aspects of psychotherapy, it encompasses them. Since one of the principal aspects of effective psychotherapy is the enhancement of the therapeutic alliance, this approach builds credibility and trust by providing coherent information and clear, constructive suggestions. So often in the past, clients not only were confused but did not fully trust that their therapists knew how or why they felt so badly. Many well-meaning therapists did convey empathy, but empathy alone without credibility provides little more than support from a friend.

Marshaling therapeutic change requires boosting clients' knowledge of their situations and what they can do about it. This knowledge kindles motivation to do what it takes to resolve the situation. Without client motivation, you do all the work for no apparent gain. Clients deserve to know what the therapist knows about their conditions; otherwise, the information is locked away, as if it were esoteric and sacred knowledge. When such information is kept from clients, it becomes a secret that creates a paradoxical effect: Clients potentially feel worse, and fears that the problem is something really complicated beyond their understanding" fuel more anxiety and dread.

This book offers three levels of narrative that describe the brain-based common denominators of psychotherapy. The main narrative is supplemented by two sidebar boxes. One sidebar offers specific suggestions regarding what you can say to your clients in session. The other describes the neuroscience research backing up the main narrative.

ACKNOWLEDGMENTS

I would like to give credit to Ashley Taggert for coming up with the title *Brain2Brain* for this book. Not only does it convey the intent of teaching clients about their brains, but it also highlights the brain-to-brain interaction.

I also want to thank Rachel Livsey, my editor at John Wiley & Sons, for her openness, suggestions, and graciousness during our conversations leading up to the publication. She and her assistant, Melinda Noack, have been very flexible and supportive during the process. It was a great pleasure working with them.

ABOUT THE AUTHOR

JOHN ARDEN, PhD, is the author or coauthor of 13 books, translated into 16 languages, including *Brain-Based Therapy with Adults* and *Brain-Based Therapy with Children and Adolescents*; *Conquering Post Traumatic Stress Disorder*; *Consciousness, Dreams and Self: A Transdisciplinary Approach*; *Science, Theology, and Consciousness*; *The Brain-Based Anxiety Workbook*; *The Brain-Based OCD Workbook*; *Rewire Your Brain*; and *The Brain Bible*. He is director of training in mental health for the Kaiser Permanente Medical Centers for Northern California. He oversees training programs in 24 medical centers, where over 130 postdoctoral psychology residents and social workers, counselors, and psychology interns are trained each year.

Chapter 1

APPLYING NEUROSCIENCE

A client in the 20th century said, "I quit seeing my analyst because he was doing therapy behind my back." Therapy of the 21st century can foster a greater alliance by lifting the veil of esoteric knowledge and sharing it with a client. By gaining a practical understanding of how the brain operates during therapy, clients can gain confidence in you and the motivation to do those things that make their brains operate at optimum levels to avoid needless anxiety and depression.

This book describes the brain-based common ground of psychological research and psychotherapeutic approaches. From this vantage point we can shed useless and purely theory-based approaches while retaining the common-factor ones that are supported by research. In other words, we are not looking to put old wine in new skins. Rather, it's time to get rid of the vinegar while retaining the good wine. This effort requires that we replace the wineskins with clear glass to lift the veil revealing true knowledge.

Throughout this book, I offer suggestions on how to use the practical information from neuroscience to help your clients understand and deal with depression and anxiety. In doing so, I describe a robust body of neuroscience research that is consistent with evidence-based practices (EBPs) that can form the basis of therapy. The new developments in neuroscience have revealed what brain systems are over- or under-activated in people with various psychological disorders. The methods described in this book describe how to bring this information into the dialogue with clients.

Clients can learn to activate areas of their brains that have been underactivated and how to quiet down those areas that have been overactivated, so that they can live without being plagued by anxiety and/or depression. By learning more about their brains from you, clients can make better sense of the things they need to do to deal with excessive anxiety or depression. Therapy can offer a "brain tune-up" facilitated by information about the brain and research-tested approaches to resolving anxiety as well as depression.

Consider this book a multilevel user manual for the brain. On one level I describe how to help clients learn more about the brain in general, so that they can use their brains more effectively to ameliorate excessive anxiety and/or depression. On another level, I give suggestions on what you can literally say to clients in sidebars titled "Client Education." In sidebars labeled "Neuroscience," I describe in more detail research underlying the running text.

TEACHING PRACTICAL NEUROSCIENCE

A variety of new developments in neuroscience are significantly relevant to psychotherapy. These factors can be explained to clients and used to provide the context for suggestions that you make for behavioral change. Each of the next factors can be considered part of the wide body of information that can help guide therapy:

- Epigenetics
- Neuroplasticity
- Neurogenesis
- Affect asymmetry
- Prefrontal cortex, striatum, and habit formation
- Default mode network
- Psychoneuroimmunology

Genes Need Not Be Destiny

I have encountered many clients over the last 40 years who are convinced that they are genetically determined to have an anxiety disorder or depression. They believed that their genes hardwired them for mental illness. During the last 10 years, I have introduced such clients to revolutionary new discoveries in the field referred to as epigenetics, which reveals that genes are not always destiny.

NEUROSCIENCE

The rapidly evolving field of epigenetics, meaning "above the genome," studies the gene–environment interaction that brings about the expression of the genes (which make up an individual's phenotype). Epigenetics involves the study of the molecular process of methylation of cytosine bases in DNA and modifications of histones by acetylation.

There is a difference between the words "genotype" and "phenotype." What clients do, including what they eat and their environment, can either influence the activation of genes or suppress genes from activating. Clients have control over their destiny by influencing their biology. Thus, they are not doomed to suffer from anxiety or depression. Since clients can turn on and off genes by changing their behavior, they can certainly do those things that will rewire the brain—practicing the brain-based therapeutic techniques you teach—to diminish the amount of anxiety or depression they experience.

CLIENT EDUCATION

Genes are not destiny. What you do will have a profound effect on what genes are turned on or off. Even if you are genetically vulnerable to a particular illness or depression, you can do things to suppress the expression of those genes. In other words, your behavior can turn your genes on or off.

A wide variety of studies have shown that a person's biological parents can have less influence on her life than her adoptive parents. For example, children whose biological families had a history of violence were adopted into nonviolent families; as they grew up, only 13% of the adopted cohort expressed antisocial traits. In contrast, 45% of children from nonviolent biological origins adopted into families with aggressive histories became antisocial (Cadoret, Yates, Troughton, Woodworth, & Stewart, 1995).

The fact that behavior can have an effect on genetic structure occurs at the telomere level. Telomeres, which are the ends of the linear chromosomes, generally shorten with cell division and age. Their maintenance is fundamental to all healthy animals. The enzyme that adds nucleotides to telomere ends, called telomerase, has been linked to aging and aging-related diseases (Aubert & Lansdorp, 2008). Many growth hormones play important roles in telomerase activity while transforming growth factor beta (TGF-β) inhibits telomerase. Stress and depression have been associated with shorter telomere length; exercise has been associated with longer telomere length (Cherkas et al., 2008). In Chapter 2, I describe five fundamental lifestyle practices that, when not practiced on a regular basis, lead not only to anxiety and depression but also to the shortening of telomeres.

Building New Neurons

One of the most exciting areas of neuroscience to share with clients is the brain's potential to grow new cells. The discovery of neurogenesis reversed what we thought we knew as recently as the 1980s. It had been assumed that we are all born with as many new brain cells as we will ever have and that healthy living protects those that we had not lost due to fever, head injury, or toxic assaults, such as alcohol and aging. We now know that it actually is possible to grow new neurons in specific areas of the brain throughout our lives. For example, new neurons arise in the olfactory bulbs in pregnant women, and neurogenesis can occur in the hippocampus, specifically in the dentate gyrus, as well as the prefronted cortex.

Neurogenesis is facilitated by various growth factors, referred to as neurotropic factors. Chief among them is brain-derived neurotropic factor (BDNF), which plays a crucial role in reinforcing neuroplasticity and neurogenesis. BDNF is like organic fertilizer; it helps consolidate the connections between neurons, promotes the growth of myelin to make neurons fire more efficiently, and acts on stem cells in the hippocampus to grow into new neurons.

The factors that can decrease neurogenesis include aging and chronically high cortisol due to chronic stress or recurrent depression. It is no accident that one theory ascribes the development of depression to blocked neurogenesis. Major assaults to brain cells, such as radiation and traumatic brain injury, also decrease neurogenesis.

As described in later chapters, the integrity of the hippocampus is of supreme importance to mental health. The hippocampus contains many cortisol receptors. When there is a moderate increase of cortisol, in effect the hippocampus acts as a negative feedback mechanism, tamping down release of additional cortisol. Unfortunately, when it is flooded with excessive amounts of cortisol, the hippocampus can atrophy. The hippocampus is key to the acquisition of explicit memory (as discussed in Chapter 3). Since damage to the hippocampus impairs explicit memory, building new neurons there is vital to cognition, as well as for retaining the negative feedback function.

Clients can increase neurogenesis through aerobic exercise, fasting, consuming fewer calories than in the typical Western diet, and increasing consumption of omega-3 fatty acids. The most powerful method is aerobic exercise; its fundamental importance is discussed in Chapter 2.

CLIENT EDUCATION

You can grow new neurons in the area of your brain that lays down new memories, called the hippocampus, to improve your memory capacity. New neurons develop by engaging in aerobic exercise and maintaining a healthy diet.

Rewiring the Brain

Psychologists have long known that people who are plagued by psychological disorders, such as anxiety and depression, can learn to overcome these problems and go on to lead happy and productive lives. What we did not know until relatively recently was how those changes took place in the brain. A process known as neuroplasticity illustrates how the brain is not hardwired but rather soft-wired by experience.

The mere fact that neuroplasticity is possible can give hope to clients suffering from depression and/or anxiety. Perhaps they believed that their brains were hardwired to suffer from anxiety or that they will be depressed until they die. Learning that the brain can change so that they will no longer suffer can serve to motivate clients in therapy. The trick is how you explain that this can happen and what clients must do to make it happen. Since most clients have a hard time remembering the cumbersome term "neuroplasticity," I use the phrase "rewire your brain" (Arden, 2010).

CLIENT EDUCATION

Your brain is not hardwired but soft-wired. Our job together is to rewire you brain so that you no longer suffer from anxiety and depression.

Clients often are surprised to learn of the sheer complexity of the brain, which contains roughly 100 billion neurons. Since neurons are social, they maintain, on average, 10,000 connections to other neurons. Neuroplasticity, as the name implies, means that neurons are malleable and plastic, in that they change based on learning experiences. Each of the connections between neurons actually consists of microscopic gaps called synapses, and learning establishes and strengthens synaptic relationships. Neurons communicate with one another by sending chemical messengers, of approximately 100 different types, including neurotransmitters, neuromodulators, and neurohormones, across the synapses. This rich cornucopia is partially dependent on a balanced diet. An impoverished diet produces impoverished neurochemistry and probably more anxiety and depressive symptoms. Although the subject of diet is taken up in more detail in Chapter 2, it is important to make clear that healthy brain chemistry is dependent on a healthy diet. Neuroplasticity requires soft and pliable cells that can change shape to facilitate new synaptic connections. A diet consisting of excessive bad fats and simple carbohydrates can result in rigid cell membranes that impair neuroplasticity.

NEUROSCIENCE

A piece of brain tissue the size of a match tip contains approximately 1 billion synapses. The neurochemical activity between synapses potentiates neurons to fire; this is referred to as an action potential. Those neurons involved in perception fire up to 300 impulses per second. The two main neurotransmitters in the brain are glutamate and gamma-aminobutyric acid (GABA). They are the workhorses in the brain, and their effects take place in milliseconds. While glutamate is primarily activating, GABA is inhibiting.

The so-called white matter, composed of glial cells, is much more abundant; there is up to 10 to 15 times more white matter than neurons. Once thought to be nothing more than fat cells that glue the brain together, we now know that glial cells perform many critical functions in the brain, including communicating among themselves through calcium waves.

Explaining to clients how they acquire a new memory can serve as a good example of neuroplasticity. When they learn something new and practice recalling it, the more easily they can recall that information in the future. That is what studying is all about. When they practice the new skill, such as speaking in a foreign language, they are wiring their brains to remember that language's vocabulary and intonation and to conjugate verbs. The more they practice speaking the language, the greater the synaptic connections between groups of neurons that make those language skills possible.

CLIENT EDUCATION

Rewiring your brain means that the more you practice a new skill, the more your brain changes to make that skill come easily.

Similarly, the brain-based solution to overcoming anxiety and depression involves neuroplasticity. Just as they can learn to speak a foreign language, clients can learn to not feel anxiety in situations that are not dangerous. Neuroplasticity makes it possible to learn to feel calm and enjoy life despite previously believing it was impossible.

The concept of "neuroplasticity" stems back to one of the field's founding fathers, Donald O. Hebb (1904–1985), who demonstrated that mental stimulation results in actual structural change to the brain. Hebb brought lab rats home for his children to play with and found that when those rats were back at the lab, they learned more quickly than cage-bound rats. They had developed bigger and heavier brains. A paraphrase from Hebb that has become a sort of mantra is "Neurons that fire together wire together." In other words, once you get neurons to fire together to support a new behavior and perform that behavior repeatedly, those neurons will link together to make that behavior an enduring habit.

To understand how to ensure that their brains can rewire, clients should be informed that they need a moderate degree of discomfort. This means that they should not wait until they feel no anxiety before making changes. In fact, if they wait until they feel no anxiety before they make changes, the wait will be endless. A useful analogy is to old vinyl records, where a needle detected microscopic changes in the grooves on the record as it spun on a turntable. If the record was damaged, the needle would get stuck in the same groove and repeat the same phrase in the song over and over again. To get the needle to jump out of the too-deep groove, the listener had to get up off the couch and bump the needle. So too is it with the bad habits of anxiety and depression. Clients need to do what they do not feel comfortable doing in order to establish the new habit. In other words, they need to expose themselves to relatively safe but anxiety-provoking situations in order to feel calm and positive when in the same situation later.

Over 100 years ago, two psychologists, Robert M. Yerkes and John D. Dodson (1908) developed what has since been referred to as the Yerkes-Dodson law, which dictates that performance increases with physiological and mental arousal up to a point. When the arousal is too high or too low, performance decreases. This concept is best illustrated in what has been referred to as the inverted U-shape curve, which increases with moderate levels of arousal.

CLIENT EDUCATION

To feel better, your job is to do what you don't feel like doing so that eventually you feel like doing it.

There are many ways to describe how the brain rewires with a moderate level of arousal. Consider explaining that it is always more difficult in the beginning. Then practice the mantra "Cells that fire together wire together" until it becomes truth. Making the rewiring possible requires that clients understand the need to get out of their comfort zones, much like bumping that needle on the record player. This process requires intensive, repetitive behavioral change.

Therapy based on the neuroplasticity of the brain does not emphasize prolonged focus on the identification and overactivation of sad memories; repetition of the same story with its associated negative emotions for the assumed benefit of catharsis is countertherapeutic. In fact, reliving the same sad memories over and over again makes stronger those sad memories and the feelings associated with them. The identification and activation of neural circuits is productive only to the degree that it enables later change-oriented interventions (Grawe, 2007). The goal is to facilitate positive change, altering the problem, and to establish neural circuits that construct a solution with repetition, new thoughts, behavioral patterns, and emotions.

NEUROSCIENCE

Neuroplasticity involves several changes in the brain that result from learning, including the development of new synaptic connections, strengthening of connections through what has been called long-term potentiation (LTP), the growth of new dendrites (dendritogenesis), and neurogenesis (Buonomano & Merzenich, 1998). The changes in synaptic efficacy and LTP result from increases in receptor density, up-regulating their activity, greater glial cell availability, and changes in the shape and structure of synapses.

(continued)

(*continued*)

> Neuroplasticity involves raising the levels of a variety of neurotransmitters. For example, the activating neurotransmitter glutamate, which is the brain's workhorse, needs a moderate boost to reach the specialized glutamate receptors the N-methyl-D-aspartate (NMDA) receptors to develop LTP so as to ensure that the neurons will fire together easily again later. Accessing the NMDA glutamate receptors is critical to kick off secondary messengers, facilitating LTP.
>
> The opposite of LTP is long-term depression (LTD), not to be confused with the psychological disorder of depression. It refers to the fact that with no use, there is depressed activity among those synapses where there was previous activity. LTD of neural circuits associated with anxiety and depression is our goal in therapy. One way of framing LTD is to say "Neurons that fire out of sync lose their link."

The concept of "dosing" has long been discussed in the psychotherapy research literature in regard to how many sessions and what frequency of sessions therapists must provide to achieve efficacy. This discussion also includes the exposure paradigm, which relates to how many exposure sessions and what degree of intensity are needed. The Subjective Units of Distress Scale (SUDS) has been used to measure appropriate gradients of intensity. The issues of dosing and exposure can be understood within the context of neuroplasticity.

During the mid-20th century, Fritz Perls and colleagues introduced the concept of a "safe emergency" to describe feeling safe in the therapeutic relationship while being challenged to go beyond what feels safe (Perls, Hefferine, & Goodwin, 1951). Despite the importance of this concept, therapists have a rich tradition of cultivating only the safety part; the emergency side needs to be utilized in therapy. Of course, the safety of therapeutic alliance is paramount, but we also want to produce change.

CLIENT EDUCATION

You need to get out of your comfort zone to rewire your brain. But don't worry: You can do it incrementally. Instead of diving off the high dive when you don't know how to swim, try jumping off the edge of the pool into the deep water, which is out of your comfort zone.

When clients tell you that they want to wait until they feel totally confident and calm before facing the challenge of dealing with anxiety, you can say that actually a moderate degree of anxiety and discomfort can work to rewire the brain so that they will no longer suffer from excessive anxiety. Of course, you will be there to walk clients through it as their partner. Together you will work through incremental exposure exercises; although they will never feel totally ready to face the challenge, with sustained effort and practice, they will be able to master it eventually.

You can describe many provocative and well-known illustrations of neuro-plasticity to clients to help them understand that practice is key. For example, London cabdrivers go through a rigorous training program called "the Knowl-edge" that can take up to four years. Researchers at University College London examined the brains of these cabbies and found that the longer they were on the job, the larger the size of their posterior right hippocampus, which lays down spatial-based memories (Maguire et al., 2000). Because cabbies must learn the highly complicated map of London, the posterior right hippocampus helps them develop a sort of GPS system in their brains. The point of this illustration is that when a particular area of the brain gets used in a use-it-or-lose-it manner, that part becomes larger due to neuroplasticity.

A variety of other example may resonate with clients. Adults who juggled three balls for three months were found to have increased gray matter in the brain areas making this type of agility possible (specifically the midtemporal area and left posterior intraparietal sulcus). Then, after months of little or no juggling, the gray matter in the area decreased and approached baseline values (Draginski et al., 2004). The critical point raised by this study is that not only does the area necessary to develop the specified skill get larger with practice, but when it is not used, it goes back to its earlier size. In other words, the lose-it factor of the use-it-or-lose-it concept occurs with a lack of consistent exercise. Other skills also have illustrated specific neuroplastic changes to the brain. Musicians such as vio-linists who use specific fingers to play their instruments showed enlarged areas of their somatosensory strips associated with those fingers (Pantev, Roberts, Schulz, Engelien, & Ross, 2001). Blind Braille readers showed enlarged cortical areas associated with their reading finger compared to blind non-Braille readers and to sighted people (Pascual-Leone & Torres, 1993).

Clients often need practical descriptions of how to get started and what degree of rigor is necessary to make neuroplasticity work for them. To increase neuroplasticity, clients must challenge themselves with tasks that are of sufficient difficulty and of increasing difficulty as they master each level. To make the tasks of sufficient intensity, clients can engage in a few learning sessions each day, with at least three learning sessions each week for several weeks. This degree of rigor is very much like when people are bodybuilding: They need to lift more weight than they can easily lift, with three reps of 10, three times per week, over the course of several weeks. Only then are recognizable changes apparent in muscle mass.

Another point to highlight regarding how to produce neuroplasticity concerns a heightened degree of attention. Attention and maintaining alertness involves a variety of neurotransmitters. For example, moderate activation of the neurotrans-mitter norepinephrine (NE) is optimal at moderate levels, as illustrated by the inverse U. Too little or too much NE impairs new learning. NE is one of the many neurotransmitters involved in anxiety disorders and, in the extreme, panic attacks. However, a moderate level of NE keeps people focused, and capable of challenging themselves to deal with the bad habits of anxiety so that they can rewire their brains.

NEUROSCIENCE

Not enough NE fails to activate the prefrontal cortex (PFC); too much turns it off. In fact, different types of NE receptors are involved in turning the PFC on and off. In a panic attack, as occurs when the brain gets flooded with an excess amount of NE, the alpha 1 receptors are turned on while the PFC is turned off. In this case, the amygdala hijacks the PFC, promoting anxiety-laced decisions without adequate prefrontal activity. A moderate degree of NE hitting the alpha 2A receptors is optimum to keep clients alert, in command of their mood, and able to benefit from neuroplasticity. Clients need to learn to get out of their comfort zone, which will raise their levels of NE, turn on their PFCs, and rewire their brains.

Emotion and the Hemispheres

Most clients are surprised to learn that the two brain hemispheres process emotion differently. Some people are already aware that their right hemisphere includes talents in seeing the big picture, the general gist of a situation, visuo-spatial perceptions, and the ability to locate where they are in space. They also may know that their left hemisphere is talented at details, routinized behaviors, and language.

NEUROSCIENCE

Both hemispheres of the brain contain all four lobes of the cortex: frontal, temporal, parietal, and occipital. For example, the primary areas in both frontal lobes are involved in movement. The parietal lobe is specialized for spatial and sensory skills; the temporal lobe is specialized in auditory skills; the frontal lobe with movement, and the occipital lobe is specialized in vision skills. Although each lobe is specialized in certain functions, each also is part of the right or the left hemisphere, which reflect the general talents of each hemisphere.

Although the two hemispheres represent functional asymmetries, some of their functions have been overgeneralized in popular culture. The truth is that both hemispheres, when working together, play vital roles in adaptive life. The role of the right hemisphere in the perception of the big picture is facilitated by long myelinated axons linking distant regions of the brain. The right hemisphere is involved in early stages of learning. The left hemisphere is involved in routinization and activates once information is learned. When a person is faced with problems to solve, the left hemisphere makes it more likely for him or her to arrive at known solutions that worked in the past.

Psychologist Richard Davidson, of the University of Wisconsin, Madison, has shown that a person's affective style is related to his or her set point, which is the ratio of activity between the right and left PFC. Davidson has proposed that the set point represents the range of our default emotional tone. The set point is represented by the ratio of neural activity between the right and left hemispheres, which is slightly skewed to the right or left (Davidson & Irwin, 1999). Whether a person suffers a great injury that results in paralysis or wins the lottery, within a year or two the person's emotional tone will settle back to the set point that existed before, to hover around being generally positive if skewed to the left or negative if skewed to the right.

Particular neural activation patterns are associated with a particular mood status, so that when people are anxious or distressed, their amygdala and right PFC (R-PFC) activate more than the left. In contrast, when they are in a positive mood, those areas are relatively inactive while the left PFC (L-PFC) activates. In general, more activation of the left prefrontal area is associated with upbeat mood states and positive emotional set points while more right-side activity is associated with being easily upset and suffering from periodic anxiety and/or depression.

CLIENT EDUCATION

Your right and left front part of your brain process emotion differently. When there is more activity in your right front part than your left, you tend to experience more anxiety and depression.

Clients who are overly anxious tend to have hyperactivity in the right PFC relative to the left (Davidson, Pizzagalli, Nitschke, & Putnam, 2002). Accordingly, such clients have a shortage of positive feelings and little behavior directed toward the attainment of positive goals. In fact, research has consistently shown that people who suffer from anxiety disorders and depression have overactive

R-PFCs and underactive L-PFCs. To make these distinctions relevant to behavior and practical, explain that the R-PFC is involved in avoidant and withdrawal behaviors while the L-PFC is involved in "approach" behaviors. These contrasting tendencies reveal important information about anxiety and depression as well as what to do about them. The immediate paradox to address is that when clients avoid what makes them anxious, they make their already overactive R-PFCs even more overactive, which ironically makes them even more anxious and depressed. When people approach what makes them anxious, they activate their L-PFCs, which are better able to control the amygdala's overactivity.

Another way to explain the functional differences between the right and left PFC is to stress that since the R-PFC is oriented toward the big picture, when it is overactivated, people may feel overwhelmed by everything. The L-PFC, in contrast, focuses on the details—the small picture. When the L-PFC is activated, people are approaching life and engaged in behaviors to accomplish goals and experience positive feelings.

CLIENT EDUCATION

When you are overwhelmed with anxiety or depression, it is best to shift from the big picture to the small and do something that approaches a goal in a piecemeal, incremental manner.

NEUROSCIENCE

The right dorsolateral prefrontal cortex (R-DLPFC) is associated with avoidance/withdrawal behaviors while the left dorsolateral prefrontal cortex (L-DLPFC) is associated with approach behaviors. The left orbitofrontal cortex (L-OFC) is associated with positive emotions while the right OFC (R-OFC) is associated with negative emotions.

There are also significant functional affect asymmetries associated with the amygdala. For example, greater activation of the left amygdala is associated with pleasant stimuli and reduced depression (Davidson et al., 2002). In contrast, greater activation of the right amygdala or an enlarged right amygdala is associated with anxiety disorders. Criminals who have committed affectively charged violent crimes have increased activity in the right amygdala and right hemispheres in general. As an illustration of the role of the right hemisphere in social perception as well as anxiety, surgical removal of the right amygdala has been shown to decrease a person's ability to recognize fear in faces.

Although the effect asymmetry distinction generally applies to most people, there are some gender-related differences. It is noteworthy that the two hemispheres are not exactly symmetrical. A degree of asymmetry is evident, especially in men. Where the R-PFC is wider, thicker, and protrudes over the L-PFC while the left occipital lobe is wider than and protrudes over the right occipital lobe.

Even the representation of reward and punishment shows affective asymmetry, with the left medial region of the PFC responding more strongly to rewards and the right one to punishment (O'Doherty, Kringelbach, Rolls, Hornak, & Andrews, 2001). Approaching goals is associated with the DLPFC. Hyperactivity of the R-PFC appears to be a negative prognostic indicator for responding to a selective serotonin reuptake inhibitor (Bruder et al., 2001). Patients who respond better have less right-side dominance.

There are neurochemical asymmetries as well. For example, while dopamine (DA) appears relatively more active in the left hemisphere, NE appears to be more active in the right hemisphere. This is particularly relevant in clients seeking help with anxiety. Increases in NE are associated with anxiety disorders and posttraumatic stress disorder (PTSD), consistent with right-hemisphere overactivation. There are other asymmetries, including in estrogen receptors, which are more prevalent in the right hemisphere.

Activating the Brain's Brain

Every discussion with clients about the brain requires a major focus on the PFC. The PFC represents the apex of brain evolution and allows our species to ask questions such as "What is thought?" Effective psychotherapy by necessity involves the PFC. It functions as the "executive" brain or executive control center, the brain's brain. Without the PFC, there would be no civilization. People would be totally, instead of partially, ruled by their emotions.

One way to illustrate the central importance of the PFC in affect regulation is to highlight how teenagers struggle to contain their emotions. Because the PFC is the last brain structure to myelinate, teens are in the process of developing identity, insight, and a sense of self as competent and independent individuals. Since many adult clients have difficulty with the same challenges, teaching them about PFC development can be an effective way to hone in on the skills that need practice.

The skills of two parts of the PFC that are important to describe are the DLPFC and the OFC (see Figure 1.1). When the OFC is working well, it provides affect regulation and is enhanced by the social skills of empathy, attachment, warmth, and love. As discussed in Chapter 2, clients who were abused or had insecure attachment tend to lack these talents. Fortunately, therapy and very positive intimate relationships can rebuild the OFC. The OFC plays a major role in the affect regulation because of its connections with the amygdala. It is more involved in

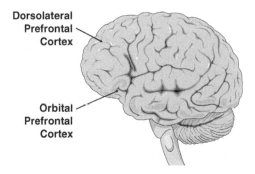

Dorsolateral
Prefrontal
Cortex

Orbital
Prefrontal
Cortex

Figure 1.1 Two key areas of the prefrontal cortex, the dorsolateral prefrontal cortex and the orbital frontal cortex.

emotion than some other areas traditionally considered part of the so-called limbic system. For that reason, I agree with neuroscientist Joseph LeDoux (LeDoux, & Schiller, 2009) that it is best to discard the term "limbic system." The amygdala, which is discussed in greater detail in Chapter 4, plays a major role in stress and the development of anxiety. Since the OFC maintains significant connections to the amygdala, it can neutralize needless anxiety if the client's descending connections are strong. If the OFC is undeveloped and the ascending connections dominate, the amygdala can hijack the PFC and generate anxiety-laced thoughts.

CLIENT EDUCATION

With sustained practice, you can train the more advanced part of your brain to neutralize irrational anxiety generated by the more primitive part of your brain.

The DLPFC is the most advanced part of the brain evolutionarily. It does not fully myelinate until approximately age 25. It is involved in many executive functions including attention, problem solving, and working memory. The eminent psychologist George Miller noted that an individual can hold in mind 7, plus or minus 2, pieces of information for 20 to 30 seconds (Miller, 1956). The DLPFC is involved in working memory, which keeps thoughts and plans in mind while following through with the task. One way to describe working memory is to say "When you walk into a room and forget what you had in mind to do in there, your DLPFC was not doing its job." The DLPFC also plays an important role in regulating follow-through on anxiety and depression, reducing behaviors.

When the PFC in general is impaired, executive functions falter. When specific areas of the PFC falter, such as when there are deficits in the OFC and DLPFC, different types of executive functions can be impaired. This was first illustrated by the most famous neurology patient in history, Phineas Gage, who lost his OFC when a steel rod shot into his right eye and through it. Once well-mannered and polite, he became disinhibited and rude. When he saw a woman he wanted, he grabbed her, and he said what he felt like saying, with no fore-thought or concern about the consequences. Many people with OFC deficits are in the criminal justice system, convicted of assault and other violent offenses. An OFC deficit that is highlighted in Chapter 5 includes being insensitive to ambiguity. The picture is quite different with DLPFC deficits, which include pseudodepression, marked by a lack of spontaneity and of affect rather than nega-tive affect. In other words, people with DLPFC deficits look depressed but deny depression when asked.

One way to assess whether and in what way clients suffer from PFC deficits is to assess their types of attention problems. OFC impairments often result in attention-deficit/hyperactivity disorder (ADHD), where the problem involves dif-ficulty with affect regulation. Because the DLPFC is highly involved in working memory, deficits result in a higher incidence of attention-deficit disorder (ADD). Here the difficulty is in maintaining attention and following through on the exe-cution and the completion of goals.

ADD and ADHD are overdiagnosed and do not represent discrete disorders but rather a spectrum of executive function problems. Brown (2005) identified six executive functions that, when impaired, can result in attention problems. They include:

1. Activation—organizing, prioritizing, and activating to work (versus impul-sive or procrastinating);
2. Focus—sustaining and shifting attention to tasks
3. Regulating alertness—sustaining effort and processing speed (versus drowsiness and running out of energy);
4. Managing frustration—affect regulation and modulating emotions (versus affective labiality);
5. Memory—utilizing working memory and accessing recall; and
6. Action—monitoring and self-regulating action (acting without sufficient forethought).

NEUROSCIENCE

The far front portion of the PFC, referred to as the anterior PFC, is critical for juggling more than one concurrent behavioral task or mental plan. The anterior PFC has more dendritic spines per cell and rich spine density, making it able to integrate a broad range of inputs (Ramnani & Owen, 2004). It is bidirectionally interconnected with the heteromodal association regions of the posterior cortex. These interconnections makes the anterior PFC adept at integrating outcomes of several cognitive operations in the context of a superordinate goal.

Habits: Developing Good Ones and Breaking Bad Ones

Habits are by nature automatic behaviors that we perform repeatedly without engaging conscious awareness. Many habits help us navigate through the day and accomplish goals, such as driving a car to work or typing an email. As such, they are part of our procedural memory, discussed in Chapter 2. Habits are driven by the striatum, a subcortical area in the basal ganglia. A variety of habits are not practical, including those that are extremely disturbing, such as the compulsive behaviors associated with obsessive-compulsive disorder (OCD), which are described in Chapter 8.

Many clients state that they derive enjoyment from only a limited number of activities. They report feeling stuck in bad habits because of assumed hardwired limitations. You can help them understand that the development of a habit is actually soft wired and part of the reward circuit. Because the reward circuits can drive behavior faster decisions made by an impaired PFC, it can be very difficult to inhibit a habit behavior driven by the reward circuits, once they have been triggered. These circuits are activated when presented with opportunities for immediate reward. One of the goals of therapy, therefore, is to help clients increase the range of positive habits that they can employ to reap rewards.

CLIENT EDUCATION

Your bad habits are not hardwired into your brain but are soft wired because you have repeated them over and over again. If you practice, you can develop new, positive habits.

Clients can develop new habits by first kindling activity in the PFC through deciding to do something different, which serves to break them out of autopilot. However, since clients may have great difficulty changing their behavior merely from gaining insight and "knowing better," they need to be motivated to change. To set the conditions so that they can develop the motivation to modify their behavior, they need to make changes to the daily environment to support the new behavior pattern. Clients can be informed that the neural infrastructure for motivation includes the nucleus accumbens, which represents a key part of the reward circuit. When the ventral tegmental area (VTA) signals the availability and expected value of opportunities to obtain immediate rewards, it provides DA to the nucleus accumbens. When medium spiny (MS) neurons in the nucleus accumbens receive increased levels of DA, they become stronger and can restrain the automatic (habit) activity of the striatum. However, when MS neurons are weak, the striatum becomes uninhibited and behaves automatically so that it is harder to restrain habits. With conscious and sustained attention, the PFC can block habit behaviors generated by the striatal autopilot system.

Productive behaviors that are also enjoyable increase the strength of MS neurons. These circuits underlie ability to inhibit old habits and motivate clients to continue to engage in new behaviors. However, when opportunities for gratification are slim, MS neurons become weak, and old habits are difficult to inhibit. When clients' lives are enriched with the opportunity to take care of immediate needs and solve problems, so that they cultivate a greater range of pleasurable activities, their MS neurons become powerful enough to inhibit the drive toward immediate gratification to old habits by engaging in new productive behaviors.

Since much of the success of psychotherapy is dependent on client motivation, it is interesting to note that the nucleus accumbens and the amygdala are in close proximity and comprise a significant part of the motivational system underlying positive and negative reinforcement. The nucleus accumbens integrates incoming sensory information, evaluates emotional memory coming from the amygdala, influences decisions made by the PFC regarding motivated behavior, and results in either "go" or "stop" behavior (Hoebel, Rada, Mark, & Pothos, 1999). If clients feel that the result of their behavior will be positive, those synapses mediated by DA strengthen, and the associated motivation to engage in that behavior again increases.

With your guidance, clients can build the motivation to develop a wider range of gratifying experiences. Since the reward system in the brain uses DA as one of its neurotransmitters, DA neurons encode the expected value of an opportunity. The greater clients' expectations about the opportunity, the faster the neurons fire. The intensity is commensurate to the expected benefits. Clients may benefit from learning that these DA-containing VTA neurons fire when tempted by the possibility of quick pleasures. This means that clients run the risk of acting on those cravings even though they may be self-destructive in the long term, as is the case of many addictive behaviors.

NEUROSCIENCE

The speed of firing of DA neurons varies. Slow, constant firing allows them to damp down expectations when the opportunity was overestimated. Firing speeds up if the promise of rewards is high or if the situation is particularly tempting, especially based on prior rewards. How much neurons in the nucleus accumbens fire at the time of engaging in an activity predicts whether clients will repeat the activity. The firing rate of the VTA's DA neurons indicates the value of reward opportunities; the faster the rate of firing, the greater the anticipated reward. The amount of DA the VTA neurons release provides a measure of the number and value of opportunities clients encountered recently. The sum total of rewarding experiences modifies clients' MS neurons and general vulnerability to opportunities to succumb to immediate gratification.

(continued)

(*continued*)

> The MS neurons have special dynamic receptors, referred to as D2 receptors, that fire more readily and are harder to turn off when DA hits them (Dong et al., 2006). The total value of the recently experienced opportunity gets translated into the strength or excitability of the MS neurons (Trafton & Gifford, 2008). As clients push themselves to encounter more rewarding opportunities, turning off the MS neurons becomes more difficult. As these MS neurons inhibit the enactment of habitual immediate gratification-seeking behaviors, strengthening MS neurons reduce impulsivity and enactment of shortsighted habits. This means that it becomes easier for clients to avoid repeating bad habits and to try more varied, pleasurable, or productive activities.
>
> By strengthening the MS neurons through increasing the variety of pleasurable behaviors, clients are better able to break bad habits. This is because the MS neurons are inhibitory; they turn off the striatum circuits. The end result is that the automatic habits that the striatum memorized are inhibited in favor of the acquisition of new behaviors. This process represents a viable method to break bad habits.

You can inform clients that they can rewire their brains to expand the range of activities that give them a sense of satisfaction and pleasure by trying out and behaving as if new activities were indeed fun. Tell them that the more they practice these behaviors, the easier it will be to break the bad habit of deriving pleasure from only one behavior. As new healthy and pleasurable behaviors are trained into the habit circuits, they will become easier to do and will be triggered more frequently than unhealthful behaviors.

CLIENT EDUCATION

> The Alcoholics Anonymous and Narcotics Anonymous sayings "Fake it until you make it" and "Act as if" carry the wisdom that to acquire a new positive habit by doing it when you don't feel like it, you will eventually feel like it.

With habits, good and bad, there exists a dynamic neurochemistry. For the destructive habits such as addiction, a variety of neurotransmitters are at play. The addictive process, whether in regard to drugs and alcohol or a behavior, such as gambling, involves an increase in the firing rate of DA neurons. The brain looks for cues to predict the availability of the reward and increases its estimation of how pleasurable taking the drug or engaging in the behavior will be. The firing rate of the DA circuits increases each time clients take the drug or engage in the behavior until eventually their DA neurons cannot fire any faster. To keep comparisons between natural rewards and drug rewards to scale, their brains are forced to start reducing DA neuron firing in response to natural rewards. Eventually, every association with the drug or behavior will serve as a craving cue. A burst of DA neurons fire, fueling clients' anticipation of a reward and the greater likelihood that they will behave in some way to achieve the reward.

NEUROSCIENCE

DA is one of the most widely studied neurotransmitters associated with addiction and has been implicated in many mood-altering substances. The DA hypothesis states that drugs of abuse involve the release of DA in the mesolimbic DA system, especially to the nucleus accumbens. For this reason, DA has been overgeneralized as the pleasure neurotransmitter and more appropriately understood as associated with the anticipation of pleasure. It is at the heart of all reinforcing behaviors and has been called the currency of reward. It signals survival importance as well because of its role in motivation.

Addiction to drugs such as cocaine relies on glutamate as well as DA. For example, mice that had been genetically altered to lack glutamate receptors do not addictively use cocaine, even though it has the same effect on their dopaminergic systems as it does with mice that are not genetically altered. For all these reasons, glutamate may be related to drug seeking (motivation) and drug memories, and may be implicated in relapse.

As noted earlier, glutamate is the principal activating neurotransmitter in the brain and is considered the brain's workhorse. It is associated with learning, memory, and motivation through its critical role in neuroplasticity. The NMDA receptors are glutamate receptors that are activated by a moderate burst of glutamate, which facilitates LTP. Glutamate, therefore, helps the brain to adapt to the environment; often referred to as key in neuroadaptation. The glutamate system maintains projections to the orbitofrontal cortex (OFC) and therefore plays a role in executive functions, especially affect regulation.

One confusing experience, for both client and therapist, occurs when symptoms get worse instead of better after a period of intense psychotherapeutic work. Because most behaviors, whether good or bad, are reinforced in some way, when the reward does not occur, there often is an "extinction burst" where the bad behavior escalates the first few times the reward is not received. Clients need to be informed that the extinction burst is just that, a burst, a last gasp of a habit soon to be broken. If clients hang on and do not fall back into what had been too easy in the past, they can break the pull of the bad habit.

CLIENT EDUCATION

Rewiring your brain to change bad habits into good habits often includes the confusing experience of briefly feeling worse before you feel better. To feel better on a regular basis, you must ride through a brief period of feeling worse.

Default Mode Network

Although many therapists hate to admit it, occasionally they space out and day-dream during sessions. Clients fade off too, but their tendency generates more concern and all sorts of interpretations, such as "Is he resistant to interpreta-tion?" or "Has she shut down?" While these interpretations may be spot on, a variety of other factors are operative that do not necessarily involve resistance. The truth is that all humans spend a great deal of time spacing out. This ten-dency has been associated with a pattern of brain activity known as the default mode network (DMN). Up to 30% of our waking hours are spent in the DMN, daydreaming, ruminating and in self-referential thought. To illustrate how much energy is being used in the DMN, only 5% more brain energy is used to pay attention above the baseline (DMN) when something in the present environ-ment captures your attention. The DMN increases activity when the DLPFC is not engaged, and you and/or clients may be stressed, bored, not experiencing novelty, or simply tired.

NEUROSCIENCE

The areas of the brain identified as active in the DMN include the medial parietal area with the posterior cingulate and adjacent precuneus, which are involved in remembering events in our lives. Also involved is the medial PFC (mPFC), including the ventral ACC, which is involved in imagining what others are thinking as well as our own emotional state. Collectively this network is critical to our sense of self.

A variety of DMN patterns of neural activity have been associated with various psychological disorders. One of the malfunctions in the DMN includes schizo-phrenia, which includes a defective mPFC resulting in impaired self-reflection, whereby clients may not be sure where their own thoughts come from. With depressed clients, the DMN may generate obsessive ruminations about negative experiences that occurred in the past.

The DMN also can be the source of creative thought or insights, such as put-ting together concepts generated by discussions in therapy. Therapists have long asked such questions as "Where did you just go?" or "What are you reflecting on right now?" Accordingly, you can help clients make their DMNs useful by encouraging them to reflect on what they just imagined or ruminated about or what ideas were just generated. In this way, you can teach clients to use the DLPFC to focus on what the present moment has to do with where they had been.

Rewiring the brain requires stepping out of the DMN and activating the PFC to direct the desired behavioral change. Since it can be difficult to remember how to make changes that rewire the brain, you can teach clients a mnemonic recipe for feeding the brain, namely FEED.

F—for focus. This involves turning on the PFC, a part of the brain critical for learning anything new. When clients focus on the here and now, they engage working memory and DLPFC connections with the hippocampus for the acquisition of long-term memory.

E—for effort. Clients must make the effort to do what they do not feel like doing. If they continue to do what they felt like doing, they would do what they have always done out of habit. Like an old record player, if the record is damaged, the same record track is repeated over and over again. Clients must "bump the needle."

E—for effortlessness. Effortlessness occurs after a new habit has been developed. Not only will clients repeat the new skill, behavior, mood, and/or memory, but their brains will require less work to repeat it.

D—for determination. Determination to stay in practice is critical, because if the acquired skill is not practiced, the brain too loses the connections, just like muscles that atrophy with too little use.

Therapeutic Brain Networks

Introducing the systems of the social brain provides the context for describing the importance of relationships, including the therapeutic relationship. More than half a century ago, Carl Rogers astutely described many of the characteristics of building an effective alliance. He highlighted the importance of active listening, pacing, and reflection, which led the way to generations of therapists, including even Heinz Kohut from the psychoanalytic perspective (who did not give Rogers the credit he deserved). In chemical dependency treatment programs, Bill Miller used a Rogerian-inspired motivational interviewing technique to work around resistance and generate motivation. Outcome management studies are now called evidence-based outcomes to highlight the importance of the alliance.

Although he did not know about the social brain networks in the brain that make the alliance possible, Rogers argued that clients naturally get better with the corrective influence of positive relationships. We may conceptualize the neural networks that makes the alliance possible as the therapeutic brain. These networks comprise the safe part of the safe emergency.

Since much of the thrust of this book is to lift the veil of esoteric knowledge and discard useless theory so that therapy can be transparent, understandable to clients, and effective, describing the therapeutic brain will add yet another point of clarification. This description highlights the therapeutic relationship between you and your clients but also sensitizes clients to their relationships with other people.

Consistent with the focus on the dynamic qualities of the therapeutic relationship, in recent years there has been an increased interest in attachment throughout the life cycle. The therapeutic relationship taps into the unique ways each of us have learned to engage in relationships. The manner in which we engage one another depends on the therapeutic brain networks, those same networks that also make therapy possible.

The neural circuits making up the therapeutic brain system include the cingulate cortex, the OFC, the amygdala, the insula, and facial expression modules. Let us start with the cingulate cortex, which is the gyrus just above the corpus coallosum. The very front part is called the anterior cingulate cortex (ACC); it integrates cognitive and emotional information from the cortex (Bush, Luu, & Posner, 2000).

CLIENT EDUCATION

Your anterior cingulate cortex makes it possible for you to feel the pain of another person and express authentic empathy.

Our ancestors traveled in bands where members had to work together for survival; rejection or ostracism could result in death. The ACC evolved with physical and social pain functions because banishment could result in pain and ultimate death (Eisenberger & Lieberman, 2004). Feeling rejected, excluded, or ostracized activates the ACC, which acts as a sort of alarm system for both emotional and physical pain.

NEUROSCIENCE

The cingulate cortex, so named because of its ringlike shape, circles around the corpus callosum. The ACC is involved in emotions, in executive behaviors, and in concentration and inhibition of competing responses that would make concentration and executive behaviors difficult. Impairment in the ACC has been correlated with traumatic disorders.

The ACC is active when detecting emotional signals from self and others (Critchley et al., 2004). The dorsal (top) ACC activates when fear of rejection occurs (Eisenberger & Lieberman, 2004). It is also activated when someone we love experiences pain or social ridicule. Overall, the ACC serves as part of the neural basis for cooperation. Damage to it results in reduced empathy and/or maternal behavior.

One way to introduce the insula is to ask clients if they ever had gut feelings about the emotional state of another person. The reason that they have these feelings is because the insula serves as a conduit between subcortical areas and the cortex. The insula draws on information from body areas, as well as from the amygdala and hippocampus. As an illustration of how the insula can be sensitive to internal body states, a series of studies examined the brains of Tibetan meditators. The longer the monks practiced meditation, the larger their insulas, due to neuroplasticity. It also links the mirror neuron system (discussed below) with body states. Based on all of these socially focused skills, some researchers have developed an insula hypothesis of empathy (Carr, Iacoboni, Dubeau, Mazziotta, & Lenzi, 2003). Accordingly, the insula is one of the brain areas associated with empathy (Iacoboni & Lenzi, 2002). It is a key intersection in the brain, positioned between the frontal cortex and other limbic areas (Iacoboni, 2003). The insula also works with the PFC to interpret and regulate emotional experiences.

CLIENT EDUCATION

Have you ever had a gut feeling about what another person might be feeling? That intuition is made possible by a part of your brain called the insula.

Mirror neurons were initially discovered in macaque monkeys when researchers learned that specific neurons fire to replicate what another individual is doing (Rizzolatti & Arbib, 1998). For example, when a person observes someone move her arm but does not more her arm herself, neurons in her own brain fire as if she were moving her arm. One theory suggests that mirror neurons have garnered considerable attention in the mainstream press as well as in pop psychological models. It is important, however, to focus on what science can support. Mirror neurons were critical for our evolutionary development, because they helped one individual predict the goal-directed behavior of another. This skill provided an adaptive advantage to stay safe from potential danger if an observed individual meant harm. When perceiving positive emotion, mirror neurons are associated with the capacity to experience empathy (Iacobini, 2003; Miller, 2005). Mirror neurons are found in various areas of the PFC, posterior parietal lobe, superior temporal sulcus, insula, and cingulate cortex, all areas that are associated with social brain networks.

Like mirror neurons, another type of socially sensitive neuron is found in abundance in humans but largely absent in most other species. Named for its spindly shape, so-called spindle cells were first identified by Constantin von Economo (1929), who noted that their long axons allow them to communicate with other neurons over relatively long distances. They are found in the OFC, insula, and ACC, especially in the right hemisphere, and are rich in serotonin and DA receptors. Spindle cells respond extremely quickly to socially and emotionally evocative interactions, providing for greater behavioral flexibility to deal with complex social environments. They are involved in making snap judgments and solving complex problems in emotionally charged social situations.

Spindle cells start their migration to portions of the OFC and ACC when people are about 4 months of age. How richly and where they connect with other cells depends on the interpersonal environment the child experiences. A warm and loving family atmosphere promotes strong and healthy connections while family stress with poor bonding results in weak connections (Allman, Erwin, Nimchimsky, & Hof, 2001). During development, they are vulnerable to neglect, abuse, and trauma, which results in deficits in subsequent social intuition.

NEUROSCIENCE

There also appears to be hemispheric asymmetry in talent for detecting emotions. The right hemisphere is adept at intuiting emotions of other people, independent of the personal significance of those other people (Etcoff, 1989). In fact, the right hemisphere is so perceptive at detecting emotion that some researchers have considered patients with aphasia as having an edge at lie detection (Etcoff, Ekman, Frank, Magee, & Torreano, 1992). This point is based on the fact that aphasia is generally associated with damage in the left hemisphere, leaving the right hemisphere dominant.

Since information from the right ear is processed by the left hemisphere and information from the left ear is processed by the right hemisphere, listening to someone speak with the right ear is associated with decoding the meaning of the words. In contrast, listening with the left ear decodes information and the emotional inflection in the speaker's voice. Those who respond well to cognitive-behavioral therapy (CBT) to alleviate depression tend to favor right-ear processing relative to those who do not respond to CBT and do not respond to right-ear processing (Bruder et al., 1997).

The mirror neuron system (MNS) contributes to the feeling of emotional empathy. In contrast, the area at the junction of the temporal and parietal lobes, called the temporoparietal junction (TPJ), contributes to feeling cognitive empathy. Cognitive empathy involves knowing intellectually what another person is enduring.

As therapists, we need to balance our MNS and TPJ empathy systems. While our MNS allows us to "feel" what our clients feel emotionally, through monitoring our own gut reactions to clients, we can convey emotional empathy. We also can "understand" our clients through our TPJ system by maintaining cognitive empathy without being engulfed in feelings of rage or hopelessness.

When putting many of these skills together, psychologists have described the socially intuitive skill referred to as the theory of mind (TOM), which represents the ability to look at another individual and develop a hypothesis about what he or she might be thinking. This ability is largely absent in people with autism spectrum disorders (ASD).

The social brain systems that contribute to the TOM include the amygdala, the insula, the right temporal parietal junction, and the anterior cingulate (Siegal & Varley, 2002). It appears that there is some asymmetry, with the R-OFC involved in decoding mental states and the L-OFC involved in reasoning about those states (Sabbagh, 2004). Finally, there are three major brain areas associated with the TOM, including the mPFC for self-related mental states, the superior temporal sulcus for goals and outcome, and the inferior frontal area for actions and goals (Frith & Frith, 2001). The TOM is particularly important when looking at an individual whose expression is neutral or somewhat ambiguous.

Working with Facial Expressions

Paul Eckman (1990), expanding on the pioneering work of Charles Darwin a century earlier on emotional expression as seen in the face, meticulously developed a cross-culture taxonomy of facial expressions. The subtleties of facial expressions are quite significant in an integrative approach to psychotherapy. Facial expressions represent a window through which you and clients communicate on a nonconscious level, utilizing many of the therapeutic brain networks.

We view objects and faces with different brain systems. The facial-reading systems include the amygdala, fusiform gyrus, and supertemporal gyrus (Gauthier, Skudlarski, Gore, & Anderson, 2000). We can read faces when they are right-side up but not when they are are upside-down (Kilts, Egan, Gideon, Ely, & Hoffman, 2003). When we view faces upside-down, we view them as objects and are unable to read their emotional content. ASD clients read faces as if they were viewing objects.

By using your facial expressions, you can model and influence client facial expressions and mood and change their mood through their MNS. Your expression of emotion occurs through the laterality of affect in the brain as well as the face. The feedback system is bidirectional: within you, within a client, and between the two of you.

Let us break this down level by level. Since the right field of vision for both eyes sends information to the left hemisphere of the brain and the left field of vision sends information to the right hemisphere of the brain, when looking at a client's face, your left field of vision is looking at the right side of the face, which is controlled by the client's left hemisphere. Since the client's left hemisphere is associated with positive emotion, your right hemisphere (which is more talented than your left at reading emotions) is picking up on whether the client may be experiencing positive emotion. Since the client is doing the same thing with you, both of you are sharing a significant amount of emotional information below conscious awareness. In other words, you are nonconsciously sharing one another's mood.

Contracting muscles on the left side of the face activates right-hemisphere and negative bias, such as with a smirk. Researchers have attempted to identify all the factors associated with an authentic smile and have noted that bilateral smiles elevate L-PFC and positive moods. In addition to the symmetry in the lower part of the face, researchers have focused on the area around the eyes. Guillaume Duchenne (1806–1875) identified the orbicularis oculi muscle around the eyes. An authentic smile, or what has been dubbed a D smile (with a bow to Duchenne), involves crinkling or crow's feet around the eyes. Non-D smiles (no crinkling around the eyes) possibly mask negative states and are more likely to be asymmetrical in the lower part of the face. While D smiles are associated with left-PFC activation and involve positive emotion, non-D smiles involve R-PFC activation and negative emotion (Ekman, 2007).

Smiling kindles positive moods, both when expressed and when witnessed. Perceiving the smiles of others triggers the release of DA (Depue & Morrone-Strupinsky, 2005). Even presenting smiles for a fraction of a second followed by neutral stimulus increases the positive reaction to that stimulus (Dimburg & Ohman, 1996). In the past, it was assumed that if a person smiles or even laughs during a stressful situation, it is reflected as incongruence in the psyche. Yet smiling during periods of stress decreases cardiovascular arousal back to baseline levels (Fredrickson & Levenson, 1998).

Ekman and his colleagues (1990) have shown that a variety of facial expressions have been identified across cultures, and these expressions cannot be totally inhibited. Dubbed "microexpressions," they essentially leak out for a fraction of a second. Therapists can be trained to detect microexpressions consciously. You and your clients are already detecting many of these microexpressions on a nonconscious level. Pulling the information into conscious awareness can enhance your detection of client moods.

Laughter is indeed good medicine, not only in general but also in therapy. Laughing triggers multiple physiological benefits. Breathing out, as is the case with laughter, triggers the vagal nerve and the parasympathetic nervous system, increasing relaxation. One way to explain the benefit of laughing to clients is to note that when they laugh, it is all exhaling, which accesses the parasympathetic nervous system. This is in contrast to breathing in, which is more like a gasp and accesses the sympathetic nervous system. Laughing also exercises and relaxes the muscles and lowers overall heart rate and blood pressure (Kuhn, 1994; Pearce, 2004). Laughter decreases overall stress by a variety of routes, by lowering cortisol levels and by providing a boost to the immune system, such as through increasing natural killer cell activity (Berk et al., 1988; Takahashi et al., 2001). From an epigenetic perspective, laughter has been shown to alter gene expression as well as increase longevity and improve cognitive function (Hayashi et al., 2006; Yoder & Haude, 1995). Not surprisingly, laughter stimulates the DA reward system (Mobbs, Greicius, Abdel-Azim, Menon, & Reiss, 2003). When clients do not feel like laughing because they are too anxious or depressed, motivate them to "fake it to make it" by practicing with them and by suggesting that they practice through watching funny movies with friends.

CLIENT EDUCATION

The saying "laughter is good medicine" is true. It *is* good medicine. The more you practice laughing, the more likely you will feel like laughing, and the more likely you will feel good.

Kindling laughter circuits activates the supplementary motor area (SMA). From the SMA to the insula and then to the amygdala, this network of neural activity together enhances overall well-being. When sharing a laugh with clients, both of you experience mirth and shared understanding as well as a psychological boost from humor. Sharing humor has been shown to aid in reducing anxiety, stress, and depression (Deaner & McConatha, 1993; Wooten, 1996; Yovetich, Alexander, & Hudak, 1990). Humor has been shown to boost self-esteem, energy, hope, and sense of empowerment (Bellert, 1989; Martin, Kuiper, Olinger, & Dance, 1993; Wooten, 1996).

Pulling Practical Neuroscience Together

Kindling all the therapeutic brain networks just described not only enhances the alliance, reduces anxiety and depression, and boosts the immune system, it also enhances the placebo effect. Significant literature has accumulated on the benefits of the placebo effect in the amelioration of medical problems. Maximizing the placebo effect includes combining good listening skills, empathetic attention, gaze attunement, appropriate touch, communication style (language and prosody), welcoming physical appearance, physical proximity, and asymmetrical power dynamics between therapist–client (Kradin, 2008).

Effective therapy taps into all the social brain networks by enhancing close and trusting relationships, the same networks that drive secure attachment. Neuroplasticity can be optimized through the activation of the therapeutic brain networks with moderate states of arousal that clients experience when challenged. When you provide this multimodal input, clients enhance neuroplasticity, including glutamate and its NMDA receptors. Insights that you offer in therapy are best if they provide a means for the activation of affect and cognition. Traditionally, therapy has focused on the co-construction of new narratives, which has worked to reconsolidate memories that code in meaning and factor in a sense of self-confidence and resiliency.

Understanding the importance of activating their social brain networks helps motivate clients to expand their social support system networks, even when they do not want to do so. These networks are intricately entwined with those underlying a positive sense of well-being. Social support, including therapy, kindles not only the social brain networks but also the reward systems in the brain. Specifically, the empathetic networks involving the ACC, insula, and MNS work together with DA neurons which are associated within the circuit involving the nucleus accumbens to code the feeling of and the anticipation of pleasure. Clients often strive to please their therapists, in part to activate the social brain networks. The same social brain networks are operative for clients in groups when they feel supported and understood by peers and strive to repeat the experience by coming back to the next group session.

Unfortunately, this system works to reinforce negative behaviors as well. Secondary gain can be powerful when clients receive a great deal of support and attention for being depressed or anxious. This type of reward encourages client brains to repeat the state that preceded getting the reward. Essentially, when they receive rewards when they feel bad, they will be paradoxically and implicitly encouraged to feel bad again, even if those feelings or behaviors hurt them over the long term.

Informing clients that these activity-defendant social brain networks must be continually kindled to maximize mental health can increase their motivation to engage in social activity. These social brain networks can be introduced as critical parts of the mental health system. The polyvagal system includes not only nerves that extend to many of the organs in the thoracic cavity but also the muscles in the lower part of the face. By engaging in mutually supportive relationships, clients can regulate their heart rates. This social engagement system allows both clients and their companions, engaged in a conversation, to read the gut feelings of the other by intuiting the other's emotional state through mirror neurons and spindle cells. By practicing empathy and emotional intuition, attachment skills can be maximized, earning clients a greater sense of internal security. The safe emergency allows the client to transform old, maladaptive habits into adaptive behavior, positive moods, and resiliency. Because psychotherapy requires neuroplasticity, the introduction of safe states of mind and new behaviors that are sufficiently practiced enough entrain the brain to establish enduring traits.

The challenge is to keep clients' brain bias toward their PFCs and hippocampal networks instead of amygdala-dominated states. Dynamic stability, resiliency, and affect regulation involves "self"-organization, borrowing a term from complexity theory to facilitate a leap to a higher level of mastery. Considering the affect asymmetry and the ratio of activity in each hemisphere, therapy involves bumping the set point so that clients' R-PFCs do not dominate. Finally, given that clients, like most people, can spend 30% of waking hours in DMN, helping them make this network useful involves teaching them to engage their PFCs to bring to consciousness those thoughts, daydreams, and ruminations and to develop insight into how they relate to solutions in the current circumstances.

The neurodynamics of the brain cannot be coherently modeled after the simplistic and outdated Pax Medica perspective. While Pax Medica employs linear causes and effects, it is clear that the brain is a complex system characterized by nonlinear change. As complex self-organizing systems, humans tend toward increasing complexity. Optimally, we maintain continuity and flexibility while we need new inputs to expand, just as a lake maintains fresh water, unlike a stagnant pond. Our brains exist in chaotic but stable states. In far-from-equilibrium conditions, as when a person's life is in flux, there is sensitive receptivity to small changes in life that can later result in large changes. In other words, clients are more receptive to making changes when their lives are in upheaval.

Since clients need a safe emergency to change, they need the support and sense of safety that the therapeutic relationship provides through the social brain networks while at the same time the encouragement to step out of their comfort zone so that they can produce neuroplastic change in the brain. Changes in clients' experience create changes in their brain biology, while the inverse is also true: Changes in their brain biology affect experience.

Following a rich, initially philosophical and now scientific tradition beginning with Heraclitus (550 BCE) who pronounced "Everything flows and nothing stays. . . . You cannot step in the same river twice," complexity theory has emerged as a multidisciplinary field of inquiry that examines how complex systems change. Humans are certainly complex systems, and for that reason, change in humans occurs nonlinearly. After a period of far-from-equilibrium conditions—essentially a period of turbulence in clients' lives—they can leap to a higher level of organization.

NEUROSCIENCE

Psychology can borrow the term "attractors" from complexity and chaos theory to represent how emotions act as attractors because they "motivate" clients to act. While strong attractors require little energy, weak attractors require energy and effort. Similarly, neural networks that require the smallest energy expenditure occur effortlessly. Lasting psychological change usually occurs after a new habit has been learned, such as feeling confident in the face of stress.

After a client achieves good coping skills, he uses less energy to deal with a stressful situation. Durable affect regulation can be seen as a type of "self"-organization. This means that the client can grow and adapt to

(continued)

(*continued*)

more complex situations. Therapy is potentially most advantageous as you look for and find periods of flux (readiness for change). When those "far-from-equilibrium" conditions occur, you can introduce a thought or stir a feeling that can trigger a ripple effect, leading to a change of plans. States of mind (in Complexity Theory weak attractors) can become enduring traits (strong attractors) through practice and neuroplasticity. Brain-based therapy strives to induce repeated states (weak attractors) such as positive moods, which, when repeated often enough through neuroplasticity, become traits (or strong attractors).

Meaning is biopsychosocial. It comes from the relative compatibility of biological and psychological states, and the interpersonal experience. Because these states co-exist in varying degrees in the flow of time, meaning too varies. While there is a general degree of continuity, there is a natural tension between stability and change. Ideally, through development of "self"-organization, the client's sense of self-identity, there is a nonlinear progression in meaning to leaps to higher levels of organization in the client's sense of self-identity.

You can assist clients to disinhibit the expression of adaptive patterns that have already been developed but are rarely implemented (Aleksandrowicz & Levine, 2005). In other words, you can help strengthen those neural networks that support adaptive behaviors and weaken those that inhibit those behaviors.

NEUROSCIENCE

During the last 25 years, evidence has been building that psychotherapy changes the brain. For example, psychotherapy and its effects on the brain show:

- Reduced amygdalar activity in treated clients with phobias (Straube, Glauer, Dilger, Mentzel, & Miltner, 2006), panic (Prasko et al., 2004), and social phobias (Furmark et al., 2002).
- Reduced frontal activity in treated clients with depression (Goldapple et al., 2004).
- Increased ACC activation in clients with PTSD (Felmingham et al., 2007).
- Increased hippocampal activity in people with depression (Goldapple et al., 2004).
- Decreased caudate activity in clients with OCD (Baxter et al., 1992).

One of the main conceptual shifts offered by brain-based therapy includes teaching people about their brains to boost their confidence in therapy. No longer does therapy need to rely solely on clients' trust in therapists. This trust can be built on by adding science instead of merely theory in the rationale for promoting insight and behavioral change. By explaining the brain networks involved in anxiety and depression, as well as how to remediate dysregulation of these networks, you can foster greater trust and confidence. This approach is similar in one respect to narrative therapy, where the therapist helps clients externalize the problem to reduce stigma while it encourages the alliance and discourages resistance.

Like a brain tune-up led by you, the therapist, you can say, "This is our common project." Clients can be encouraged to make specific behavioral changes to rewire their brains. When they invariably note that they are feeling not quite ready and fully confident that they can face the challenge of making the behavioral change, you may note: "To rewire your brain, you will need to do some things you don't feel like doing." If clients request delaying the changes until they feel less anxiety, you may respond by saying "Moderate anxiety is a good thing. It helps neuroplasticity." Then, to provide the "safe" part of the safe emergency, you may say, "Don't worry, I'll be there with you as your partner."

Chapter 2

PROMOTING BRAIN HEALTH

Just as it is foolish to build a house on sand, so is it equally foolish to try to engage in therapy clients who are behaving in ways that impair their brain. Helping clients build and maintain a firm and healthy foundation of brain health is a prerequisite for effective psychotherapy.

Five factors have consistently received robust research support for the health and longevity of the brain (Arden, 2014). Clients can remember each factor by using the mnemonic SEEDS and using it in the phrase "Planting and cultivating SEEDS reaps a harvest of clear thinking and the capability of positive moods." This chapter describes each of the SEEDS factors and its fundamental importance to brain health.

FIRST *S* OF PLANTING SEEDS

Our forebears evolved socially through working together for mutual survival and developing keen social skills. These interpersonal sensitivities permitted our ancestors to sense possible rejection because they would have been dead meat, literally, if they were kicked out of the band. As described in Chapter 1, the regulatory networks of the social brain are responsible for many aspects of interpersonal connectivity. They support enhanced bonding, attachment, affiliation with others, fear regulation, the sense of safety, and affect regulation.

Motivating clients to expand their social support system networks when they feel least motivated to do so can be a challenge. Clients may regard the poor quality of relationships only as a symptom, not also a cause of a poor sense of well-being. Clients may be more motivated if they can understand the importance of activating their social brain networks and how they are intricately entwined with those that underlie positive relationships and a positive sense of well-being.

Social isolation is one of the most common causes as well as symptoms of anxiety and depression. Social support buffers anxiety and depression. To address that factor, therapists have long encouraged clients to boost and cultivate their social support system, only to hear that clients do not feel up to it and perhaps will do so when they feel better. The irony is that they would feel better with social support. Because they are generally not convinced that social support will help, I describe how their brains thrive on social interaction. Then they become curious enough, take initial steps to verify the truth.

First I note that social skills have been central to the evolution and survival of our species. Specific regions of the brain working together made complicated interpersonal relationships possible during our long evolutionary existence as hunter-gatherers. Not only did our ancestors work together to gain access to food, but they developed keen sensitivities to the potential of being rejected by the group. If they were rejected, they could lose access to food or a mate and lose the protection that being in a group offers. Those highly sensitive brain systems are still with us today to make human communication possible. Often clients are astonished by how sophisticated these social brain networks are. They are also alarmed to hear that when these systems are not activated regularly, people are vulnerable to multiple health problems.

There have been consistent reports that loneliness and/or poor-quality relationships are associated with psychological disorders. From the perspective of affect asymmetry research described in Chapter 1, withdrawal and avoidance are associated with the over-activation of the right prefrontal cortex (R-PFC), which is also associated with anxiety and depression. Thus, poor relationships and/or loneliness are associated with depression (Russell & Cutrona, 1991).

CLIENT EDUCATION

Your brain has neural circuits that thrive on positive social interaction. When they are not activated, your health suffers.

The social brain networks play a critical role in almost every aspect of health. To explain how fundamental social experiences and the social brain networks that make them possible are connected to almost every aspect of health, you may want to point out that the absence of social support leads to changes in cognition, emotional stability, susceptibility to illness, dementia, and the pace of aging. People who are lonely late in life have been found to develop dementia symptoms more quickly and in general to suffer from cognitive decline (Bassuk, Glass, & Berkman, 1999).

NEUROSCIENCE

Relationship quality is also correlated with the integrity of the cardiovascular system. Healthy relationships boost the immune system; scanty or poor relationships undermine the immune system. For example, strong associations have been found between relationships and cardiovascular reactivity (Lepore, Allen, & Evans, 1993), blood pressure (Spitzer, Llabre, Ironson, Gellman, & Schneiderman, 1992), cortisol levels (Kiecolt-Glaser et al., 1984), serum cholesterol (Thomas, Goodwin, & Goodwin, 1985), vulnerability to catching a cold (Cohen et al., 2003), anxiety (Cohen et al., 2003), natural killer cells (Kiecolt-Glaser et al., 1984), and sleep (Cohen et al., 2003). Social support or its lack even affects chromosomes; loneliness can lead to cell aging through the shortening of telomere length. Telomeres are the caps on the ends of chromosomes that protect them like tassels on the ends of shoe laces. Shorter telomeres lead to greater damage to the chromosomes as occurs in aging.

By simultaneously cultivating secure attachment dynamics through the social brain networks and enhancing therapeutic alliance, clients gain confidence and motivation to practice the behaviors you recommend. This shift to a strong approach orientation from a withdrawal/avoidance orientation also helps change the neurodynamic set point from the R-PFC to the left prefrontal cortex (L-PFC), with an associated increase in positive feelings.

NEUROSCIENCE

Telomeres are noncoding sequences at the ends of chromosomes that serve as senescence clocks. They serve as psychobiomarkers linked to social status, perceived stress, and depression, and are predictive of mortality (Epel, 2009).

Telomerase, which is an enzyme that prevents telomere shortening, promotes cell resilience and is also a psychobiomarker linked to social status, perceived stress, and depression and is predictive of mortality (Epel, 2009).

Social support, including therapy, kindles not only the social brain networks but also the brain's reward systems. Specifically, the networks underlying the capacity for empathy, including the anterior cingulate cortex (ACC), insula, and mirror neuron system, work together with dopaminergic neuron circuits to target the nucleus accumbens to code the feeling of recurring empathy and associated pleasure. Even clients who are not aware of these networks often strive for approval of others and for your approval, which activates the social brain networks. The same social brain networks are operative for clients in a group when they feel understood by peers and strive to repeat the experience by coming back to the next group session.

The neural correlates of emotional processing in response to facial expressions reveal how the social brain networks contribute to implicit communication. The amygdala has been associated with processing fearful and sad faces; the cingulate gyrus tends to be activated in response to happy faces. The orbitofrontal cortex (OFC) tends to be activated by angry faces, while disgust preferentially activates the insula and the basal ganglia (Batty & Taylor, 2003). This social brain system can work to reinforce negative behaviors as well. Secondary gain can be powerful when clients receive a great deal of support and attention for being depressed or anxious. These rewards encourage clients' social brain networks to repeat the state that preceded getting the reward. Essentially, when clients receive rewards when they feel or act badly, they will be encouraged to feel or act badly again, even if those feelings or behaviors hurt them over the long term.

The social interactions that transform a neutral or even a stressful situation into an exhilarating one are indeed social medicine.

FIRST *E* OF SEEDS

Most of our evolutionary history was spent as hunter-gatherers, with our ancestors moving some 10 miles per day. Even after the advent of agriculture, farming caused people to expend a great deal of physical energy. Only relatively recently have people failed to use a healthy amount of physical energy commensurate with the bodies we have inherited. The lack of movement bogs down the entire body, resulting in chronic illness and psychological problems.

Aerobic exercise contributes to multiple brain-building processes. Accordingly, it has been associated with longevity and reduced vulnerability to dementia. Exercise optimizes neuroplasticity and neurogenesis, which as I described in Chapter 1, involves the birth of new neurons in the hippocampus and the prefrontal cortex (PFC). Neurogenesis is, in part, facilitated by the release of brain-derived neurotrophic factor (BDNF), euphemistically called "Miracle Grow" because of its facility to spur brain growth.

Mechanism	Impact
Gene Expression	Neuroplasticity (Cottman & Blanchard, 2002)
Brain-Derived Neurotrophic Factor (BDNF)	Neurogenesis (Adlard et al., 2005)
Insulin-like Growth Factor (IGF-1)	Glucose usage (Carro et al., 200)
Nerve Growth Factor	Enhanced Neuroplasticity (Neeper et al., 1996)
Vascular Endothelial Growth Factor (VEGF)	Enhanced blood vessel support (Fabel et al., 2003)

Figure 2.1 The multiple effects of exercise on the brain.

NEUROSCIENCE

Exercise also spurs vascular endothelial growth factor (VEGF) by creating an infrastructure to provide fuel to the cells by helping to construct and enhance the blood vessels. VEGF comes to the rescue of wear and tear on the body by building more capillaries in the body and the brain.

VEGF increases the permeability of the blood–brain barrier, which allows substances vital to neurogenesis into the brain during exercise. Exercise also promotes fibroblast growth factor (FGF-2), which is critical for neurogenesis. It helps tissues to grow, and while it is in the brain, it aids in neuroplasticity.

Up to 19% of chronically depressed clients endure a shrinkage in the size of their hippocampus. Slowing or even reversing this tendency has major significance for mental health, both cognitively and emotionally. Exercise optimizes mood by boosting a wide range of metabolic reactions, including the neurotransmitters serotonin, dopamine (DA), and norepinephrine (NE). Not surprisingly, exercise optimizes cognition by increasing alertness, attention, motivation, and cognitive flexibility.

It has long been known that exercise can alleviate depression. Many studies have clearly shown that aerobic exercise provides powerful therapeutic effects. For example, in the San Francisco Bay Area study of 8,023 people who were tracked for 26 years, researchers found that those who did not exercise were 1.5 times more likely to be depressed. A Finnish study of 3,403 people found that those that exercised two to three times per week were less depressed, angry, stressed, and cynical. A Dutch study of 19,288 twins and their families found that those who exercised were less anxious, depressed, and neurotic and were more socially outgoing. A Columbia University study of 8,098 people also found a positive relationship between exercise and depression (reviewed in Ratey, 2008).

Clients often want to know what type of exercise yields the best antidepressant results. An Ohio State study found that 45 minutes of walking per day at least 5 days per week with a heart rate at 60% to 70% of maximum lowered Beck Depression Inventory mean scores from 14.81 to 3.27 compared to no change for controls who were depressed nonwalkers. A University of Wisconsin study found that jogging was as effective as psychotherapy for moderate depression. While after one year 90% of the exercise group were no longer depressed, only 50% of the psychotherapy group were not depressed. A Duke University study found that exercise was as effective as sertraline (Zoloft). At 6-month follow-up, exercise was 50% more effective in preventing relapse. Combining exercise and sertraline added no benefit in terms of relapse (Babyak et al., 2000). Based on these and other studies, a National Institute of Mental Health panel concluded that long-term exercise is effective in reducing moderate depression.

CLIENT EDUCATION

Exercise is the best antidepressant, and there are good side effects, not bad side effects!

As noted in Chapter 3, the psychoneuroimmunological intersection will increasingly represent an important focus in psychotherapy. Exercise plays a crucial role in keeping inflammation in check. High levels of cytokines also contribute to inflammation. Cytokine levels rise in response to poor diet, no exercise, and considerable stress. Also, elevations are typically seen after surgery or when clients carry extra weight, especially if that weight is belly fat. Inflammation represents a major causal factor in the development of many psychological disorders, including depression, as discussed in Chapter 9. Exercise helps lower inflammation as measured by its effect on lowering C-reactive protein.

Exercise has long been associated with minimizing and shrinking fat cells. Excessive fat cells have become increasingly associated with contributing physiologically to psychological problems. It had been well established that obesity contributes to cardiovascular problems and the development of type 2 diabetes. But recent research shows that carrying excess fat cells also is associated with multiple cognitive and emotional deficits. Where those fat cells are positioned on the body also makes a difference. In contrast to fat carried in the thighs and buttocks, belly fat is especially destructive to organ systems because of its proximity to the organs in the thoracic cavity. Visceral fat, or fat closer to these organs, is more dangerous than subcutaneous fat, which is, as the name implies, just below the skin. Belly fat generates inflammation by releasing inflammatory cytokines, which lower BDNF and increase the potential for dementia.

CLIENT EDUCATION

If carrying extra weight, be especially concerned if you have the apple shape. Better yet, lose the body fat for the sake of your brain. Exercise is one of the best ways to do it.

Not only is exercise a powerful antidepressant, but it is also a very effective anxiolytic. Aerobic exercise can lower anxiety by, among others things, reducing muscle tension, building brain resources (neuroplasticity and neurogenesis), increasing gamma-aminobutyric acid (GABA) and serotonin, improving resilience and self-mastery, and freeing up energy that had been immobilized by inaction.

CLIENT EDUCATION

When you're stressed and feeling anxious, a quick dose of exercise can help calm you down.

EDUCATION

The education factor represents the second E of SEEDS because there is a foundational importance of ongoing learning throughout the life cycle. Although acquiring advanced degrees is a method by which education can be structured, ongoing learning need not result in a degree. By ongoing learning, clients build the neural networks by which to view their lives realistically. Clients who do not apply and expand their cognitive capacity through ongoing learning may be prone to fall back on a default mode of rumination, along with negative mood states. Education, which can be considered cognitive exercise, provides people with the capacity to look ahead to possibilities in the future rather than imperfections in the past.

CLIENT EDUCATION

Through ongoing learning, you can expand yourself to possibilities rather than contract yourself to lamenting the imperfections of the past. Ongoing learning is but one of the many ways in which education works as an antidepressant.

Education also provides a means through which clients can develop the cognitive reserves to increase brain longevity and health. The Whitehall studies in the United Kingdom and the Nuns Study as well as numerous other studies have clearly shown that those with higher levels of education are generally happier and less likely to develop dementia symptoms than those with lower levels of education (Marmot, 1994; Snowdon,1997).

CLIENT EDUCATION

Ongoing learning will build in a reserve of neural circuits that will increase the longevity of your brain. In other words, later in life the more you can lose without looking like you lost neural circuits because you have a greater number in reserve.

NEUROSCIENCE

Learning can be either enhanced or dulled by various neurochemicals that add to or blunt the consolidation of different aspects of memory. For example, estrogen improves memory. Alcohol, tetrahydrocannabinol (THC), and cocaine impair memory. Oxytocin release occurs with strong feelings of social connectiveness and with physical touch. Elevated levels of oxytocin inhibit some negative memory consolidation and enhance encoding of positive social memory, such as the effects of therapy.

People who are highly stressed and or depressed have elevated levels of cortisol. High levels of cortisol inhibit learning, and sustained high levels lead to hippocampal atrophy. With the sustained release of cortisol, the dendritic spines in the hippocampus retract. High and low NE levels also impair memory function. Last but not least, the neurotransmitter DA is required for normal working memory. This is one of the reasons why drugs like methylphenidate (Ritalin) and amphetamines and dextroamphetamines (Adderal) are used to treat attention-deficit hyperactivity disorder. But the simple anticipation of pleasure elevates the release of DA.

Given that memory is not a single skill but rather a spectrum of learning skills, helping clients improve their memory involves helping them to orchestrate those skills. With the baby boomer generation entering their senior years, increasing numbers of people will be seeking psychological help to improve their memory.

D OF SEEDS

One of the most neglected yet fundamentally critical parts of each client's life is diet. What clients eat and do not eat, and how consistently clients consume nutritious foods, can determine their capacity for attention, their ability to learn from psychotherapy, their mood, and eventually their likelihood to develop dementia.

For example, Claire illustrated the health-related cost of not providing herself with a balanced diet. She was a petite young woman who smiled apologetically as I called out her name in the waiting room. I did my best to make her feel welcome so that she would have no need to feel embarrassed. Yet, from the first few moments of sitting down, she showed me why she had asked for the appointment, as her breath quickened and her voice sped up in an anxiety spiral out of control. Pretty soon the words came out so fast that I was having difficulty following what she was trying to say. Her initial description of free-floating anxiety was logical, but soon she jumped around from subject to subject without a coherent flow to connect each idea. Then she abruptly became silent, with her eyes looking terrified.

"Have these nervous episodes occurred often?" I asked.

She nodded nervously, her eyes searching mine for an answer to her fear. She held a paper coffee cup in her hand. Fortunately it had a plastic lid snugly in place. Otherwise there would have been coffee all over my carpet.

I pointed to the cup.

"A tall skinny latte," she said matter-of-factly.

"What did you have for breakfast?"

"Just a croissant. I'm on a diet," she answered, as if I were wasting time with irrelevant questions.

After some gentle prodding, she revealed that she often skipped lunch and drank coffee the rest of the afternoon so as to avoid "constant fatigue." In the evening she had a glass "or two" of wine "because of the stress of the day." Not surprisingly, she had insomnia.

Doing my best to not sound pedantic, I described the importance of a balanced diet to create the brain chemistry necessary to keep her calm and energized through the day. I cautioned her about her excess consumption of coffee and simple carbohydrates, also describing their adverse consequences on her mood, cognition, and sleep. Also, I described the dysregulation of her neurochemistry that resulted from her use of alcohol to chill out.

CLIENT EDUCATION

The foods you eat provide the raw materials to build the neurochemicals that make brains function efficiently. If that raw material is in short supply or if it is composed of simple carbohydrates, trans-fatty acids, or other forms of phony food, your capacity to make use of therapy can be in vain because your brain cannot work properly.

Assessing the contents and the frequency of client meals is critical, as balanced meals should be evenly spaced in time. Some clients report that they try to get all their nutrition in one large meal per day while they skip the other meals. They should be informed that evenly spaced small meals are optimum. Smaller meals three to four times per day provide better support for memory and stable moods. In contrast, large meals stress the gastrointestinal (GI) tract and create adverse systemic effects resulting in rapid rises in triglycerides and blood sugar. Not surprisingly, large meals increase the risk factors for cardiovascular disease and diabetes.

The meal that "breaks a fast" is so named because it comes after the longest period of time without food. Breakfast is the foundational meal for the day. Despite the critical importance of that meal, I have encountered countless people who state matter-of-factly that they are not breakfast people and skip breakfast or, like Claire, eat a poor breakfast only to suffer multiple emotional and cognitive deficits. Skipping breakfast contributes to cognitive deficits in areas such as problem solving, working memory, concentration, and attention. Clients who skip breakfast also suffer from affect regulatory deficits, such as mood swings, depression, and decreased energy, while simultaneously having increased stress reactivity and anxiety.

Maintaining a balanced diet is particularly critical for older adults. Skipping a meal or consuming foods with poor nutrients contributes to greater health-related costs for the brain because aging slows the production of antioxidants, making older brains more vulnerable to oxidative free-radical attacks, eventually resulting in cell loss. Aging makes us less resistant to inflammation overall, which is particularly relevant because inflammation contributes to dementia. Many older adults unwittingly contribute to inflammation through the consumption of sugar and other simple carbohydrates. It is recommended that older adults—and people of all ages—eliminate sugar and simple carbohydrates entirely.

CLIENT EDUCATION

Balanced nutrition contributes to balanced neurochemistry and a healthy brain. The normal and healthy spectrum of neurochemistry is dependent on a balance of nutrients, including amino acids, from the foods you consume.

The neurochemical orchestra involves these steps: After eating, the food is absorbed in the GI tract. Amino acids and other nutrients, including vitamins and minerals, are carried through the bloodstream to the brain. Then enzymes convert the amino acid precursors into neurotransmitters. This conversion can also take place indirectly when insulin is released from the pancreas, which draws amino acids from the blood and tissues. An inadequate balance of these nutrients results in deficits in emotional stability and the clarity of thought.

After neurotransmitters are synthesized from amino acids in the diet, they are stored in the synaptic vesicles in the presynaptic membranes. When a neuron fires, it releases the neurotransmitter from the presynaptic membrane into the synapses. The neurotransmitter then finds the right receptor, like a key fits into a lock, on a postsynaptic membrane. If enough of the neurotransmitter reaches the right receptors, the neuron will fire, which is called an action potential. In an effort to conserve the unused neurotransmitters they are reabsorbed back into the presynaptic membrane for use later. This process is technically called "reuptake."

NEUROSCIENCE

One of the many dietary aspects of the neurochemistry of stress associated with the amygdala and serotonin involves the level of tryptophan in the diet. Because tryptophan is converted into serotonin, when there is less of it in our diet it has a direct effect on the level of serotonin in the body. Decreased levels of serotonin in the amygdala are associated with increased firing and a decreased threshold for firing. Serotonin acts through GABAnergic interneurons in the amygdala, which modulate glutamatergic input (Morgan, Krystal, & Southwick, 2008). Increases in the level of serotonin are associated with an increased threshold for activating the amygdala. In other words, much more stress is needed to trigger its activity.

One way to point out how a poor diet can impair brain function is to describe the relationship between the OFC and serotonin. There are large numbers of serotonin receptors in the OFC. When there is a drop in the serotonin level in the OFC, it is less able to inhibit the overactivity of the amygdala. Point out that the body makes serotonin when people consume foods containing a specific amino acid, tryptophan. Tryptophan depletion impairs reverse learning tasks, which includes the ability to evaluate, integrate, and act on environmental cues, and to stop responding to something when it becomes unhealthy and shift back to something healthier (Robbins & Everitt, 1995).

CLIENT EDUCATION

A vivid and dramatic example of how your diet affects your brain and your ability to think clearly occurs when the food you eat does not include the amino acid tryptophan. It is converted into the neurotransmitter serotonin, and your OFC needs it to help you control your emotions and learn from your mistakes.

Officer Mike's Muffins

Mike felt tense all the time and wondered if he really had what it took to be a police officer. The area of the city that comprised his beat was a low-crime area compared to others. It was rare for him to have to respond to a murder scene or armed robbery. Yet he was hypervigilant and felt that the area would soon erupt in a crime spree.

By the time he came to see me, his wife was complaining that he was irritable at home, reclusive, and rolled around in his sleep during the night. He told me that he was trying to be healthier than many of his peers. When they met at a coffee shop, they ordered doughnuts while he ordered banana nut muffins. They ordered coffee with sugar, but he drank his black. Despite these "efforts," he wasn't sure why his belly was so large.

Lunch typically included "Something quick that I can eat while driving." When I asked for him to be more specific, he gave me a look that said "Shut up!" With a loud sigh he responded, "What is it with you and all these food questions? Didn't you hear me say I feel stressed all the time?"

"I'm asking about your blood chemistry because, when it is out of balance, it can contribute to irritability."

"Look, I am no drug user and I rarely drink. All I need is some medication to straighten out my brain chemistry."

When I told him about how diet can either build or deplete the body's neuro-transmitters, neurohormones, and neuromodulators and have a direct effect on brain structure, he shrugged.

"Lunch?" I repeated.

"Usually an egg roll at this take-out Chinese place and a Diet Coke or three."

"Are they fried and is the Coke caffeinated?"

He nodded.

"Dinner?"

"I eat a good dinner, usually pasta and a Coke. So what's the problem?"

"Your meals and your beverages explain at least partly why you are feeling tense, irritable, and unable to concentrate and why you are uneasy while sleeping."

When I explained the effect of the simple carbohydrates and trans-fatty acids on his brain and mood, Mike shook his head. "Wait a minute! The muffin has nuts and bananas in it and is advertised as natural."

"Typically those muffins contain white flour as their main ingredient, and the banana is probably flavoring. They are also loaded with trans-fatty acids. That maybe 400-calorie muffin gives you the illusion of breaking a fast."

Brains are dependent on glucose, which is their principal fuel. When glucose levels are either too high or too low, multiple cognitive, behavioral, and affect regu-latory problems occur that appear like anxiety and depression. When blood sugar drops below 50 milligrams per milliliter, symptoms include free-floating anxiety and irritability, which are similar to the symptoms of generalized anxiety disorder. In addition, the symptoms of panic may occur, such as shakiness, light-headedness, rapid heartbeat, difficulty concentrating, and short-term memory problems.

NEUROSCIENCE

Too much glucose resulting from the consumption of large quantities of simple carbohydrates, especially sugar, can be quite damaging to the structure and function of the brain. Glycation (excess glucose) results in multiple long-term adverse metabolic processes, including blocking protein from moving freely and impairing the actual structure of cells. The body's membranes become gunked up from the excess glucose, slowing down neural communication. This can result in interference with synaptic transmission between neurons; structural damage to the mitochondria, which are the cells' energy factories; cellular damage from free radicals; and inflammation, a death sentence to cells.

Researchers have long attempted to measure the adverse effects of accumulated glucose in the body. The glycemic index measures the amount of glucose in food. The higher the glycemic content of the food, the higher the glycemic index. A more complete measure of the effect of glycerin on the body is referred to as glycemic load (GL), which is a measure of rise in blood sugar. The higher a food's GL, the greater the adverse insulin effects. These adverse effects lead to the development of the plague of the 21st century, metabolic syndrome, and long-term devastating consequences, heart disease, stroke, and type 2 diabetes. Many neurologists are now calling Alzheimer's disease type 3 diabetes. Therefore, long-term consumption of foods with a high GL leads to a great risk of cardiovascular disorders, obesity, diabetes, inflammation, and Alzheimer's disease.

CLIENT EDUCATION

Inflammation results in many adverse consequences and ultimately contributes to dementia. There are several causes of inflammation, and glycation is one of them. Glycation as measured by GL can damage essential fatty acids in the brain and lead to a form of free-radical damage called malondialdehyde(MDA). The higher the GL, the higher the MDA. Another form of free-radical damage to fatty acids is called isoprostane. Even mild elevations of isoprostane are associated with Alzheimer's disease.

High levels of glucose in the brain cause cells to prematurely age. One of the many ways that GL causes brain aging is by creating advanced glycation end products (AGEs). Acting like a chemical glue, AGEs then attach molecules to one another, causing them to cross-link. Cross-linking causes cells in the brain to become stiff and rigid, resulting in a diminished ability to produce neuroplasticity. In other words, AGEs dampen learning ability.

CLIENT EDUCATION

If you eat a lot of food with simple carbohydrates, especially sugar, your brain cells age prematurely. They become stiff and rigid, and render you less capable of rewiring your brain to learn new things, such as feeling calm in the face of anxiety and lifting yourself out of depression.

There are good fats and bad fats. If clients eat too much of the bad fats, their brains are less capable of functioning adequately. Some generally good fats, such as EFAs, can become bad fats if they are not balanced with other essential fatty acids. During the last 40 years, the relative amount of omega-3 fatty acids to omega-6 and 9 fatty acids in the standard Western diet has become extremely lopsided. The vast reduction in omega-3 fatty acid consumption is due to the reduction of cereal germ (which contains EFAs) by current milling practices and decreased fish consumption, among other factors.

The increase in bad fats in the mainstream Western diet is also due to the way foods are prepared, especially when they are fried. Trans-fatty acids are formed when vegetable oil is heated for a long time in a metal container, as occurs with deep frying. Trans-fatty acids tend to be solid at body temperature and act like saturated fat in the body. Trans-fatty acids are also quite destructive to the brain and result in multiple cognitive and affect regulatory deficits. Over the past 30 years there has also been a 2,500% increase in trans-fatty acid consumption, which interferes with EFA synthesis. Simultaneously, there has been a 250% increase in sugar intake, which interferes with the enzymes of EFA synthesis. Meanwhile, there has been a significant increase in the consumption of linoleic acid (LA) oils, including corn, sesame, safflower, and sunflower oils. The hydrogenation of most oils in commercial processing has also diminished their quality.

Trans-fatty acids can:

- Be absorbed directly by the nerve membranes.
- Block the body's ability to make its own EFAs.
- Alter the synthesis of neurotransmitters, such as DA.
- Negatively affect the brain's blood supply.
- Increase bad (LDL) cholesterol while decreasing good (HDL) cholesterol.
- Increase plaque in the blood vessels.
- Increase blood clots.
- Increase triglycerides, which causes the blood to be sluggish and reduces the amount of oxygen to the brain.
- Cause excess body fat, which can have a destructive effect on the brain (i.e., through the release of inflammatory cytokines).
- Make nerve cell membranes rigid and inflexible, interfering with their functioning.

Increased triglycerides from vegetable oil and animal fat are correlated with depression.

CLIENT EDUCATION

Fried foods and the trans-fatty acids they contain are quite destructive to your brain and result in multiple deficits in your ability to think clearly and control your emotions. Trans-fatty acids are found in many foods, including cookies, doughnuts, potato chips, candy, mayonnaise, vegetable shortening, crackers, cake, deep-fried foods, cheese puffs, and margarine.

Besides being caused by dietary impoverishment, EFA depletion can be due to a variety of the other factors that can cascade exponentially. Like a dietary impoverishment of EFAs, chronic stress can result in a loss of EFA seven if client diets are healthy. You can look for the symptoms of stress related to loss of EFAs if clients have dry eyes, soft nails, increased thirst, attention problems, and weakness. Ask clients about these symptoms as well as frequent infections and poor wound healing.

NEUROSCIENCE

Omega-3 inhibits cytokine synthesis. Cytokines are proteins, peptides (a derivative of amino acids), and glycoproteins (proteins with carbohydrates). The presence of high levels of inflammatory cytokines can wreak havoc in the human body, especially on the brain. EFAs balance the influences of cytokine activity. When EFAs are not balanced, cytokines such as IL-1 and IL-6 can cause inflammation and turn the immune system against cells, attacking and killing them. An increase in cytokines has been associated with depression, anxiety, and cognitive problems, including poor memory.

The essential fatty acid omega-3 has structural importance and many critical functions. Up to 20% of the brain is composed of EFAs, and one-third of myelin is composed of EFAs. Yet although the international recommended daily amount consumed is 650 milligrams (mg), current American average consumption of omega-3 is only 130 mg. The imbalanced ratio between omega-3 and omega-6 has been correlated with depression.

NEUROSCIENCE

There are many different forms of omega-3 fatty acids, including alpha-linolenic acid, docosahexaenoic acid (DHA), docosapentaenoic acid, eicosapentaenoic acid (EPA), eicosatrienoic acid, eicosatetraenoic acid, stearidonic acid, tetracosahexaenoic acid (nisinic acid), and tetracosapentaenoic acid.

The omega-3 EFAs EPA and DHA have received considerable research attention because of their critical functions in maintaining a healthy brain. EPA effects receptor functioning. It is used to manufacture more synapses critical for neuroplasticity. EPA is involved in the conversion of L-tryptophan to serotonin and the control of its breakdown. This is one of the main reasons why many mental health professionals recommend that depressed patients take an omega-3 supplement as an adjunct to treatment for depression, including with antidepressant medication. EPA also helps to reduce the risk of blood clots and the amount of arterial plaque. Among its other brain-protecting benefits are its anti-inflammatory effects. EPA also helps lower triglycerides (fats in the blood) and blood pressure.

DHA contributes to the structural integrity of neurons. High concentrations of DHA are found in synaptic membranes and mitochondria. DHA is critical for synaptic transmission and membrane fluidity. It is also critical in keeping cell membranes soft and flexible; without this flexibility, the potential for neuroplasticity is significantly impaired. In other words, clients would find it difficult to learn from therapy. Last but not least, DHA is important for holding receptors in place. Soft and flexible membranes are capable of altering the shapes of the receptors.

There are also many different omega-6 fatty acids. These include gamma-linoleic acid, eicosadienoic acid, dihomo-gamma-linoleic acid, docosadienoic acid, arachidonic acid (AA), and LA. The two that have received considerable research attention are AA and LA, which is used in the biosynthesis of AA and thus some prostaglandins. LA is found in the lipids of cell membranes. Abundant in many vegetable oils, especially in poppy seed, safflower, and sunflower oils, LA competes with omega-3s for positions in cell membranes.

AA is one of the most abundant fatty acids in the brain and is present in similar quantities to the omega-3 EFA DHA. The two account for approximately 20% of fatty acid content in the brain. AA helps to maintain hippocampal cell membrane fluidity and protects the brain from oxidative stress by activating peroxisomal proliferator-activated receptors. It also activates syntaxin-3, a protein involved in the growth and repair of neurons. Overexpression or disturbances in the AA enzyme cascade may be associated with neurological disorders such as Alzheimer's disease and bipolar disorder, while a higher level of AA is implicated in depression.

Like the plastic covering electrical wires to ensure that they do not short out, myelin covers the axons to ensure that there is healthy and efficient conductivity. A brain becomes significantly impaired when myelin is degraded in any way. For example, demyelinating diseases, such as multiple sclerosis, are devastating.

In the fast-paced and too often superficial context of managed care, more appropriately referred to as "managed dollar," healthcare professionals have little time to perform a comprehensive health assessment of their clients. One part any assessment should include concerns EFA deficiencies. You are well advised to assess the type of client fat intake by not only doing inventories of what they consume but also assessing symptoms of deficiency. The symptoms of fatty acid imbalance might include the presence of dandruff, dry skin, dry and unmanageable hair, brittle and easily broken nails, excessive thirst, depression, and/or cognitive fog and memory problems.

Vitamin D has recently gained the spotlight, not only for older adults but for all adults, due to its importance for the immune system and its many effects on the brain. Clients with little sun exposure during the winter months, especially those living in the far North (or the far South in the Southern Hemisphere) in winter, are susceptible to low vitamin D levels. Many people are now taking supplements because their primary care physicians are measuring vitamin D levels.

NEUROSCIENCE

Vitamin D receptors are located in the cortex, hippocampus, and cerebellum, making this vitamin important in cognition, memory, and movement. Vitamin D deficiency is common in older adults and is implicated in various neurological disorders. It is also associated with depression. With regard to its neuroprotective effects, vitamin D is associated with brain-derived neurotrophic factor (BDNF), glial cell line–derived neurotrophic factor (GDNF), and nerve growth factor (NGF).

The importance of adequate hydration cannot be overstated. Considering that approximately 60% of the body is water, dehydration is a syndrome too often experienced by many clients, especially older adults. Dehydration can contribute to significant brain impairment. A person can survive a few weeks without food but only 3 days without water.

Dehydration contributes to structural brain deficits. Brain cells shrivel up, enlarging ventricles (the spaces within the brain containing cerebrospinal fluid [CSF]). Dehydrated brains work harder with poor results. Some of the early and most obvious symptoms include impaired cognition, including forgetfulness, speech problems, and deficits in attention. Many clients assume they are staying adequately hydrated although they consume diuretic drinks and soft drinks loaded with sugar.

SECOND *S* OF PLANTING SEEDS

The final S of SEEDS is for sleep. The importance of sleep for the brain cannot be overstated. Sleep represents one of the foundational healthy behaviors that needs to be established and maintained on a regular basis. For this reason, it is one of the foundational SEEDS factors. Sleep represents approximately one-third of our lives; as such, it plays a critical role in the restorative and revitalizing functions of the brain.

All too often, a well-meaning therapist attempts to help a client with insomnia by making a medication referral to a prescriber for medication. Yet William Dement, the dean of sleep researchers, found that physicians get not much more than 15 to 20 minutes in education about sleep. Typically, what they do learn is about what medications promote sleep. Unfortunately, most medications that they prescribe impair sleep architecture. Specifically, many medications, especially benzodiazepines, reduce slow-wave sleep, which is the most restorative to the immune system and actually provides the body with rest. Healthy sleep architecture is critical for cognition, emotional stability, and metabolic processes.

NEUROSCIENCE

Sleep is involved in the actual structure and repair of cells through its role in protein synthesis (Ding et al., 2004; see Figure 2.2). Sleep also is involved in the critical synthesis and transport of cholesterol. The balance between HDL and LDL, in favor of HDL, is critical for not only overall health but specifically brain health. Sleep is involved in memory consolidation and the movement and transformation of molecules associated with synaptic plasticity (Taishi et al., 2001). Not surprisingly, therefore, good quality sleep is associated with LTP, and even down to the genetic level, healthy sleep is associated with gene expression.

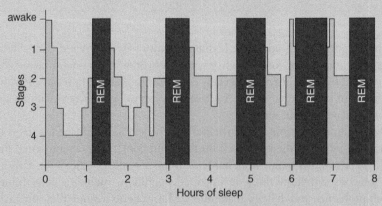

Figure 2.2 The stages of sleep.

Sleep is critical for the maintenance of the brain. It serves many functions, and without an adequate amount of regular sleep, multiple health deficits arise. For example, sleep has been shown to be crucial for gene transcription involving synaptic consolidation, protein synthesis, and myelin formation. Sleep is critical for the synthesis and transportation of cholesterol, and cholesterol makes up a significant proportion of myelin.

NEUROSCIENCE

Sleep has been identified as critical for memory consolidation. While non–rapid eye movement (NREM) sleep has been shown to be important for the strengthening of hippocampal memories, REM sleep has been shown to be important for cortical memory (Plihal & Born, 1997). During NREM sleep, information flows out of the hippocampus and into the cortex. During REM sleep, information flows from the cortex to the hippocampus (Buzsáki, 1996).

During dreaming (REM sleep), there is a lack of input from the hippocampus to the cortex and dorsolateral PFC (DLPFC) activity. This means that attention and cohesive memories take the back seat during dreaming. During dreaming the cortex receives little spatial and temporal coherence from the hippocampus. Accordingly, it produces dreams and images that include weak associations, unpredictable juxtapositions of barely related objects, locations, and characters in often illogical sequences. Dream images and plotlines float free from associations in time and space.

In contrast to REM sleep, during NREM sleep there is a flow of information from the hippocampus to the cortex, although still without DLPFC involvement. This outflow of hippocampal information to the cortex may serve to reinforce old memories. In contrast, the blocking of hippocampal outflow during REM sleep helps prevent semantic associations from falling back into predictable, overlearned patterns and aids in the formation of new memories (Stickgold, 2002).

Many memory consolidation processes also occur during sleep. For this reason, disrupted or shallow sleep can impair memory. Specific types of memory are associated with specific stages of sleep. REM sleep improves implicit procedural memory. NREM sleep improves explicit (declarative) memory. Some sleep medications as well as caffeine and alcohol can contribute to shallow sleep. For this reason, you should check whether clients are consuming these substances and consider their impact not only on sleep architecture but also on specific types of memory.

Sleeping after learning leads to better memory consolidation than during wakefulness. For this reason, the concept of "sleeping on something" actually works. A single night of sleep deprivation causes a significant deficit in hippocampal activity and impairs episodic memory encoding, resulting in worse subsequent memory recall.

(continued)

(continued)

> Only after more than 6 hours of sleep does memory improve over the 24 hours following learning something new (Stickgold, 2002). Sleep improves and stabilizes memory, making it more robust and resistant to interference the next day. During sleep, the brain dissects memories, retaining only the most salient details that play a crucial role in retaining emotional memories. For this reason, the belief that one should never go to sleep angry makes sense. Sleep selectively enhances episodic memories that are emotionally salient and enhances emotional memories, creating a long-lasting representation of distressing experiences.
>
> Semantic memory activates weak associations in REM sleep but strong associations in NREM sleep. REM and NREM sleep differ as well in neurotransmitter activation. Serotonin, dominates in NREM sleep (Portas et al., 1998); acetylcholine (ACh) dominates during REM sleep (Kametani & Kawamura, 1990). The shift to REM and processing memories in the cortex is dependent on turning off release of serontonin and NE. An excess amount of NE during this shift plays a larger role in producing a dysfunctional system and nightmares.

Sleep disruption in people with major depression is common. People with depression take longer to fall asleep and then experience fragmented sleep. They spend less time in deep (slow-wave) sleep and more time in REM sleep (Peterson & Benca, 2006). The increase in REM sleep is associated with unipolar, not bipolar, depression (Rao et al., 2002). Healthy sleep habits, also referred to as sleep hygiene, is critical; if clients sleep fewer than 7 hours a night, there will be an increase in cortisol and adrenaline, which increase anxiety while also increasing depression.

Too often in the past, mental health professionals considered the sleep problems of depressed clients as symptoms rather than as causes. The truth is that there is a bidirectional relationship between sleep loss and depression. The alterations in sleep architecture include insomnia or hypersomnia, early-morning awakening, loss of slow-wave sleep, and abnormalities in REM sleep. Depressed clients often enter REM sleep abnormally early relative to other stages and spend more time in REM sleep.

Sleep deprivation has many adverse consequences (McEwen, 2006), including these:

- Decreased parasympathetic tone.
- Increased blood pressure.
- Elevated evening cortisol, glucose, and insulin
- Elevated inflammatory cytokines.
- Increased appetite and caloric load, which contributes further to increased blood pressure, cortisol, and inflammatory cytokines.
- Abnormal fat deposition.
- Depressed and solidus or impaired mood.

NEUROSCIENCE

The lateral hypothalamus contains hypocretin (also called orexin) and melanin-concentrating hormone (MCH) neurons. The hypocretin neurons reinforce arousal by sending excitatory projections back to the various nuclei in the ascending reticular activating system (Pack & Pien, 2011). Hypocretin neurons discharge exclusively during wakefulness and are silent during NREM and REM sleep. They have also been implicated in the sleep disorder narcolepsy. Adenosine, a breakdown product of adenosine triphosphate (ATP), is an inhibitory neuromodulator that functions as a sleep-inducing factor. Adenosine promotes NREM sleep in part through its inhibitory effects on cholinergic activity neurons.

As therapists seeing people who report problems with insomnia, our job is to help screen out factors contributing to the problem that clients and physicians have not yet identified. Many medications have side effects that include insomnia. These include: appetite suppressants, asthma medications, corticosteroids, decongestants, diuretics, heart medications, kidney medications, and Parkinson's medications.

CLIENT EDUCATION

Medical Conditions That Contribute to Insomnia
- Cancer
- Epilepsy
- Fibromyalgia
- Huntington's disease
- Hypertension
- Hyperthyroidism
- Kidney disease
- Parkinson's disease

Medications with Side Effects That Include Insomnia
- Appetite suppressants
- Asthma medications
- Corticosteroids
- Decongestants
- Diuretics
- Heart medications
- Parkinson's medications
- Kidney medications

Sleep deprivation increases the hormone ghrelin, which promotes appetite and food intake. It is well established that there is a relationship between insufficient sleep and the development of obesity and diabetes. For example, in just 5 days during which time in bed is limited to 4 hours, glucose tolerance (rate of decrease of glucose from the blood) is 40% lower than normal, reaching a range consistent with the prediabetic state (Knutson et al., 2009). Even 1 week of sleep deprivation can lead to weight gain because of an increase in production of ghrelin, which promotes appetite. Simultaneously, there is a decline in the production of the hormone leptin, which curbs appetite. To make matters worse, increased appetite related to sleep loss is associated with the consumption of starchy, high-carbohydrate foods, sweets, and other high-calorie foods. Sleep-deprived people tend to consume 33% to 45% more of these foods than do non-sleep-deprived people. Unfortunately, the increase in appetite does not include hunger for fruits, vegetables, and high-protein foods.

Promoting Sleep Hygiene

Clients can be taught a variety of sleep hygiene techniques to get the deepest and most efficient sleep. To get the best night's sleep possible, clients must follow all the guidelines simultaneously. One of the easiest suggestions to understand is to suggest that clients cut their caffeine intake to none in the afternoon and no caffeine on an empty stomach, even in the morning. A suggestion requiring a little more explanation is to maintain a balanced and regular intake of nutritious food, without which neurochemistry is unbalanced. Three meals a day should be the minimum, and they should be evenly spread throughout the day. Certain foods, such as sugar and other simple carbohydrates, can exacerbate insomnia, as they cause a rapid rise in glucose and anxious alertness.

They may try eating a light snack with complex carbohydrates before bed. Foods rich with L-tryptophan are advisable. They should avoid protein snacks at night because protein blocks the synthesis of serotonin and, as a result, promotes alertness.

Many clients are unaware that their diet has a major effect on sleep. Information about neurochemistry and diet can be quite helpful. For example, consuming foods rich in tryptophan in the evening will help people become sleepy. Tryptophan is an amino acid that converts to serotonin and melatonin, both of which calm as well as sedate. Some complex carbohydrates contain tryptophan. Complex carbohydrates, such as whole grains, including wheat bread, contain tryptophan, which converts to serotonin on a long-term basis, promoting a slow and sustained rise in glucose. This is the concept behind the folk remedy of a warm glass of milk to promote sleepiness; milk contains both tryptophan and calcium. Vitamins can also influence sleep. Deficiencies of B vitamins, calcium, and magnesium may inhibit sleep.

CLIENT EDUCATION

Follow these guidelines for a good night's sleep:

- Avoid drinking large quantities of liquid at night. Drinking too much lowers the sleep threshold and causes people to wake up to urinate.
- Avoid bright light at least a few hours before going to sleep. When the retina senses light, it signals the pineal gland to suppress the release of melatonin.
- Resist the temptation to work on the computer into the late evening (to avoid the light).
- Avoid all daytime naps. Naps steal sleep from the nighttime.
- Don't eat anything with sugar or salt before bed.

In sharp conflict to our biological predisposition, house lights are on many houses after it is dark outside, and people stare at computers and television screens in bed, disrupting their natural biological rhythms. The circadian rhythm is strongly affected by daylight and darkness. Daylight comes in through the eyes to the retina, then signals the superchiasmatic nucleus (SCN), to then signal the pineal gland of the hypothalamus, which is positioned in the middle of the brain and receives the signal that it is daylight. This information serves to suppress the release of melatonin, the hormone that regulates the circadian rhythm, signaling that it is daytime and not the time to become sedated. Alternately, when it's dark, the retina sends information to the pineal gland that it should produce melatonin.

NEUROSCIENCE

The SCN of the hypothalamus serves as the central circadian pacemaker. It is synchronized to the external environment by various signals, such as light. The SCN receives light information from the retinohypothalamic tract, geniculohypothalamic tract, and projections from the raphe nuclei. The photic information the SCN is transmitted to the pineal gland, which is responsible for the release of melatonin during a dark period. Melatonin influences the phases of the circadian clock.

Tell clients that because the amount of light they are exposed to during the day affects their sleep, they should maximize their exposure to bright light in the daytime to set their body clock to match the natural day/night cycle. At night, they should do the opposite and minimize their exposure to light, especially if they suffer from insomnia. For this reason, it is best to avoid using the computer in the late evening. When looking at the computer screen for extended periods of time, people are essentially looking at light. This light tricks the brain into adjusting to a daytime pattern and suppresses the pineal gland's secretion of melatonin.

Though I am not promoting computer use late at night, the program F.lux (https://justgetflux.com/) changes the type of light emitted from the screen, thus avoiding the melatonin suppression problem. Generally, however, the use of soft light during the few hours before going to sleep is recommended.

The circadian rhythm is tied not only to light exposure but also to body temperature. Insomnia can result in difficulty regulating body temperature, so a warm body temperature at night will lead to a light sleep, while a cool body temperature will promote deep sleep. Ideally, when people go to sleep at night, their body temperature should be in the process of dropping.

CLIENT EDUCATION

If you toss and turn for more than 1½ hours after going to bed, get up and go to another room. By getting out of bed, your body temperature will begin to drop. Once your body temperature cools down and you get sleepy, go back in bed and tell yourself that since you're lying in bed anyway, you might as well use the time to relax. Use relaxation methods to quiet your mind down. Use passive effort to promote sleep instead of trying too hard to get to sleep.

Just before we get up, our body temperature should be back on the rise. When clients get out of bed in the morning, they should expose themselves to the natural light and move their bodies; in this way, their body temperature will continue to rise to meet the demands of the day. Overall, clients may be relieved to learn that if they are sleep deprived, they probably will feel bad only just after waking up. Once they expose themselves to light and move around, they will feel better.

CLIENT EDUCATION

Your body temperature can actually increase at night if you fail to exercise during the day. By exercising during the late afternoon and early evening, you can promote a dip in your nighttime body temperature. For optimal sleep, exercise 3 to 6 hours before bedtime. Exercising in that window of time helps elevate your heart rate and body temperature while still leaving enough time for them to drop before sleep. If you exercise less than 3 hours before bed, your heart rate will still be up and your body temperature will be too high to promote good sleep.

> You can decrease your body temperature at night by keeping your bedroom cool. If the bedroom is stuffy and warm, you should open a window and make sure that you don't use too many blankets. If you find yourself sweating at all, throw off a blanket. The bottom line is to stay cool, not hot or cold.

Chronic anxiety up-regulates NE, epinephrine, and cortisol, which keeps clients tense and anxious, promoting shallow sleep at best and insomnia at worst. The less time clients spend in the deep stages of sleep, which help boost the immune system, the more vulnerable they will be to whatever viruses are prevalent.

Practicing relaxation techniques during the day and the evening provides an antidote to excessive activation of the sympathetic branch of the autonomic nervous system. Accordingly, clients can fade into sleep more easily at night, reducing the effects of stress, and also calm the body and brain for sleep. Easing into sleep through relaxation contrasts to what occurs when clients try too hard to fall asleep. When people lie in bed worrying about not sleeping, they promote fast brain waves and the release of epinephrine and NE, the activating neurotransmitters that increase muscle tension, heart rate, blood pressure, and other stress hormones.

Cognitive-behavioral therapy (CBT) approaches to help clients achieve sleep efficiency have been employed for good reason. Many clients adopt a variety of negative sleep thoughts, which serve to confound sleep problems. These thoughts can range from thinking "I'm not going to get to sleep tonight" if a client has trouble sleeping to thinking "I'm going to be ruined tomorrow if I don't get sleep soon!" Even the next day, thoughts about the loss of sleep add to daytime stress and insomnia the next night.

CLIENT EDUCATION

The way you think about insomnia can actually increase it. To develop alternative thoughts about sleep, try repeating these to yourself:

"This isn't great, but at least I've got my core sleep."
"If I don't get a good night's sleep tonight, I will tomorrow night."
"I may get back to sleep, I may not. Either way, it is not the end of the world."

One suggestion that clients may initially find difficult to understand is to not try too hard to go to sleep. Trying too hard will lead to frustration, a paradoxical effect, and an anxious state of mind. The harder people try to go to sleep, the harder it will be to induce sleep. Instead, suggest that clients tell themselves "It's okay if I just get a few hours of sleep tonight. I will sleep better the next night." This change in expectation will free clients up to be able to relax.

Describing a well-known study is a great way to explain the paradoxical effect of trying too hard to get to sleep. Twenty subjects were separated into two groups, then rated for how quickly they got to sleep. Ten subjects were told that they could win $100 if their group got to sleep the most quickly. The other 10 were told nothing of the kind, simply "Good night." Members of the group that thought they were competing took longer to get to sleep.

Context is important. With insomnia, the bed can become an enemy and a negative cue. Clients should be advised to not do anything in their beds other than sleep (except for sex). They should not watch television, balance a checkbook, discuss finances with a spouse, or argue in bed. Clients should make the bed carry only one association: sleep. If clients can't sleep and find themselves tossing and turning, they should get up and go to another room. They should do all planning for the next day before they get into bed. While in bed, if they think of something they need to remember, they should get up and write it down. Clients should tell themselves that they will postpone thinking or worrying about anything until the next day.

The relationship between emotions and sleep is dynamic. The mood people go to bed with tends to resonate throughout the night during sleep. The saying "never go to sleep angry" makes sense because sleep selectively enhances emotionally salient episodic memories so that emotional memories are long lasting. Because sleep typically enhances potentially traumatic representations of distressing experiences, sleep deprivation right after a traumatic event is actually beneficial.

Because the brain is wired to pay attention to novelty, encourage clients to try to ensure that there are few intermittent sounds to grab their attention while they are in bed. This is one of the several reasons to recommend avoiding keeping the television on at night; it can periodically grab their attention and wake them up. If the environment outside their bedroom is noisy, you can suggest using a white noise machine, such as a fan, which produces a monotonous and constant hum of background noise. Such devices can serve as good screens for other noises, such as barking dogs and passing traffic. Another way to muffle sound and place it into the distance is to use good-quality earplugs.

Clients should be encouraged to change the way they think about sleep. By using a CBT approach, you can help them identify anxious thoughts and replace them with accurate information about sleep. For example, if they wake up in the middle of the night, they should reframe their wakefulness by adopting realistic thoughts about sleep, such as that they will probably enjoy rebound sleep the next night. By doing so, they will be better able to get back to sleep when they wake up because the accurate thoughts will take needless pressure off them. Consequently they will probably relax enough to get to sleep.

It is quite common for clients to attempt to solve their insomnia by using remedies that actually exacerbate the problem. People with insomnia often attempt to self-medicate with alcohol. They drink in the evening only to find themselves awake a few hours later, unaware that the alcohol caused mid–sleep-cycle insomnia. Approximately 10% of all sleep-maintenance problems (middle insomnia) are caused by alcohol. Alcohol contributes to mid–sleep-cycle awakening because it wears off during sleep.

CLIENT EDUCATION

When you buy in to the medical model and take either prescribed or over-the-counter drugs for insomnia, you'll sink into quicksand. It is best to avoid using either over-the-counter sleep aids or prescribed medications, commonly called sleeping pills. People who use sleeping pills often find that, initially, they help them get to sleep. However, the presumed benefit wears off quickly, and the drug exacerbates sleep insomnia. Even when the drugs initially seem work, the quality of sleep is poor, and people wake up feeling less rested in the morning. Like alcohol, sleeping pills suppress important stages of sleep. They also lead to tolerance and withdrawal. In other words, over a short period of time, people "need" more of the drug to get to sleep. Then when they try to get to sleep without the medication, they find it harder to do so than had they not used the drug at all. Drug-associated sleep problems occur with prescribed medications as well as the over-the-counter types.

Determining the type of insomnia clients have can reveal information about its cause and remedy. There are two main types of insomnia: early insomnia and sleep-maintenance insomnia. Clients with early insomnia have difficulty getting to sleep. They may worry that they can't get to sleep as soon as they go to bed. It can be quite reassuring for people to learn that most people take between 15 and 20 minutes to get to sleep. If, however, it regularly takes clients a couple of hours to get to sleep, they have early insomnia.

With sleep-maintenance insomnia, clients have difficulty staying asleep. Although they might fall asleep easily, they wake up in the middle of the night and have trouble getting back to sleep. Clients benefit by recognizing that people tend to overestimate sleep-maintenance insomnia. Most people wake up from time to time in the middle of the night and go back to sleep relatively quickly. If it takes someone more than 1½ hours to get back to sleep on a regular basis, he or she probably has sleep-maintenance insomnia.

CLIENT EDUCATION

If you have early insomnia, expose yourself to bright light in the early morning. This ensures that your melatonin production stays low and your body temperature is high throughout the day. By nighttime, your body

(continued)

(*continued*)

temperature swings back to the lowest when it should be low, during the first part of the sleep cycle.

If you have sleep-maintenance insomnia, expose yourself to bright light in the late morning, so that your body temperature is lowest in the middle hours of your sleep cycle so you can stay asleep.

Many clients who suffer from both types of insomnia try to adjust to the sleep deprivation by doing precisely the wrong things in an effort to "catch up" on the lost sleep. They should be advised to avoid taking a nap during the day or sleeping longer in the morning to compensate for sleep loss. Those bad habits make it more difficult to adjust their circadian rhythm and sleep the next night.

Tell clients that chronic insomnia is a bad habit that can be broken by structuring sleep into a schedule. The sleep-scheduling technique requires that clients change their bedtime schedule. By adjusting the time they go to bed, they build up "sleep pressure," or sleepiness, and are able to go to sleep and stay asleep through the night. This technique works because people who are sleep deprived naturally fall asleep earlier the next night to catch up on lost sleep.

The sleep-scheduling technique requires that clients get up at the same time each morning, despite how long they slept the previous night. Here is the tricky part: Instead of going to bed earlier at the end of the next day, clients should go to bed *later*. They may think, "I'm sleep deprived. I need to allow myself as much chance to sleep as possible, even if I toss and turn!" However, stress that by using this technique, clients are working to build up sleep pressure.

When employing the sleep-scheduling technique, calculate how many hours on average clients actually sleep and add 1 more hour. This formula determines how much sleep time to allow clients. For example, if a client averaged 5½ hours of sleep per night in the past month, despite staying in bed for 8½ hours, he or she can allow 6½ hours of potential sleep time. A client whose normal wake-up time is 6:00 AM should go to bed at 11:30 PM.

The goal of this method is to fill up most of the time clients spend in bed with sleep by following this plan for at least 4 weeks. When the body temperature adjusts to the new bedtime and the sleep pressure builds, clients can add another hour, so that the clients go to bed one hour earlier, to give themselves 7½ hours to sleep. Next they allow themselves up to 8 hours.

The sleep-scheduling technique is useful for people with chronic insomnia, not for people who experience a night or two of poor sleep. But people with chronic insomnia will understand that they must rewire their brains to repair the sleep cycle. The sleep-scheduling technique provides the structure and repetition necessary to acquire a new healthy habit. The central concept for clients to grasp is that since their sleep cycle is out of sync, sleep scheduling helps it get back into sync to increase sleep efficiency.

CLIENT EDUCATION

Sleep Hygiene Guidelines

In summary follow all, not just a few, of these techniques simultaneously to get a better night's sleep.

- Cut caffeine intake, and avoid drinking caffeine during the afternoon and on an empty stomach.
- Be sure to eat three balanced meals a day.
- Avoid sugar and other simple carbohydrates.
- Don't try too hard to go to sleep. You will only be frustrated and work yourself into an anxious state of mind. Rather tell yourself, "It's okay if I get just a few hours of sleep tonight. I will sleep better the next night." This change in expectation will free you up enough to relax and get to sleep. The harder you try to go to sleep, the harder it will be to induce sleep.
- Don't use your bed for anything but sleep (and sex).
- If you can't sleep, get up and go to another room.
- Avoid drinking large quantities of liquid at night. Drinking a lot lowers the sleep threshold because you will be prone to wake up to urinate.
- Avoid bright light for at least a few hours before going to sleep. Don't work on the computer into the late evening.
- Do all your planning for the next day before you get into bed. If you think of something you need to remember, get up and write it down.
- Postpone thinking or worrying about anything until the next day.
- Avoid daytime napping. Naps steal sleep from the nighttime.
- Eat a light snack with complex carbohydrates before bed (such as foods rich in L-tryptophan).
- Avoid eating anything with sugar or salt before bed.
- Avoid protein snacks at night; protein blocks the synthesis of serotonin and promotes alertness.
- Exercise 3 to 6 hours before going to bed. A brisk walk before or after dinner is perfect.
- If noise bothers you, use earplugs or a white-noise machine.
- Avoid alcohol.
- If you are troubled by chronic insomnia, try the sleep-scheduling technique.
- Try relaxation exercises to help go to sleep or get back to sleep if you wake up during the night.

Chapter 3

DEVELOPING MEMORY SYSTEMS

Memory and development are intertwined as nurtured nature. This means that nature and nurture are two sides of the same coin and are coded into memory. Our personalities, even our psychopathology, form by how our brain adapts to interactions with family members and friends. Over time, the accumulated effects of these integrative adaptations of the brain form the dimensions of memory.

Explaining the memory systems is paramount to psychotherapy. Effective therapy changes memory through a dynamic interactive process, modified from the forever-changing vantage point of the present. The potential malleability of memory makes psychotherapy possible. Memory is not solely about the past; it also is the basis for reaching for the future to change our lives.

MEMORY SYSTEMS

When working well together, the multiple memory systems can create positive experiences and alleviate psychological problems. Therefore, learning about the memory systems and knowing how they work together or become dysregulated is a foundational competency of mental health professionals.

Let us start by taking a look at how experience is encoded in memory. Psychologists have long studied how short-term memory (STM) transfers to long-term memory (LTM). For its part, STM is intertwined with attention. Beyond a simple process of holding information in mind for brief periods of time, the capacity to sustain attention, despite distractions in the environment, requires a significant degree of executive control. The dorsolateral prefrontal cortex (DLPFC) and other neural networks provide the goal-directed executive skills that enable people to focus on tasks through completion.

Working memory represents the capacity to perform complex mental operations, such as mental arithmetic. Working memory load represents the limits of what we can hold in mind and "work on" at the same time with two or more streams of information. As tasks become more demanding, so does working memory load and the potential for the stimulus-driven attention system to take over. These limits can be dangerous as people attempt to multitask, such as driving while talking on cell phones. Each year 2,600 deaths and 330,000 injuries in the United States result from using cell phones while driving.

The capacity to engage in a conversation and screen out distractions is referred to as controlled attention. In contrast, stimulus-driven attention represents the tendency to become easily distracted by a stimulus in the environment. For example, the cocktail party effect illustrates how a person at a party becomes distracted from a conversation he is having with one person if he hears his name uttered by a different person engaged in another conversation. One-third of people are unable to avoid being distracted and to maintain attention on their conversation.

Unlike working memory, LTM requires actual structural change in the brain through neuroplasticity. LTM forms the fabric of our personality, dictating our habitual way of reacting to the world around us. Explaining how memory, developmental experience, and personality are interrelated can provide the context for you to help clients make sense of the therapeutic goals you set together.

LTM is composed of two broad systems, that which is nonconscious and that which is conscious. These two types of LTM also are referred to as nondeclarative and declarative. Whereas nondeclarative memory is nonconscious, it is difficult to declare with conscious effort. In other words, we can feel a certain way without knowing how or why. Declarative memory can be declared by conscious mind. Accordingly, nondeclarative memory represents activity in subcortical areas, such as the amygdala and basal ganglia (BG), associated with emotion and movement, respectively. In contrast, declarative memory is associated with the hippocampus and the cortex; accordingly, it is semantic, episodic, and context driven.

These two broad-based LTM systems have been referred to as implicit (nonconscious) and explicit (conscious) (see Figure 3.1). The implicit system is so named because it is implicit in what we do and how we feel without our conscious effort. The explicit memory system, being relatively easily declared, is available to our awareness. Clients may suffer from a dysregulation between the implicit and explicit systems. In other words, these two systems can be out of sync, as is the case with posttraumatic stress disorder (PTSD). One of the goals of therapy is to reintegrate the two systems.

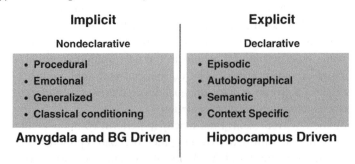

Figure 3.1   The two long-term memory systems, the Implicit and Explicit systems.

Explicit memory is dependent on conscious awareness and encoding of working memory. In fact, working memory can be thought of as the gateway to long-term explicit memory, as there is a neuroanatomical connection between the DLPFC and the hippocampus. As people code in an explicit memory, the feedback loop between the DLPFC and the hippocampus work together to ensure that the relevant content of working memory influences the consolidation of LTM. Thus, focused attention is needed to form explicit memories. The hippocampus does not go online until much later than the amygdala, and the explicit memory capacity generally begins after 3 years old.

Unlike implicit memory, which is dependent on subcortical modules, explicit memory is dependent on the hippocampus and cortex, parts of the brain that do not begin to mature until the second year of life. So-called infantile amnesia—the concept that we repress difficult early childhood experiences, as hypothesized by Freud—makes very little sense from a neuropsychological perspective. Taking the psychoanalytic concept of infantile amnesia to the ridiculous extreme, Otto Rank theorized early in the 20th century that we all suffer from "birth trauma." Accordingly, we all spend the rest of our lives trying to get over being born.

On a less absurd level, but still ignoring the complexities and limitations of memory, some therapists believe that the reason we do not remember events during the first few years is because we have repressed them. Many clients have asked me to perform hypnotic age regression so they can "discover" what their lives were like during their first year. I spent a fair amount of time during the 1980s and 1990s augmenting therapy with hypnosis. I know that I cannot provide a time machine to help people view explicit memories that were never encoded.

For example, one client, Brenda, stated that she never felt comfortable with her father. She asked that I put her in a trance to "take me back to my first year so that I can see how he held me. Maybe he wasn't as gentle as my mother." What was available for clear recollection in her explicit memory were the multiple memories of her father behaving in a grouchy and irritable manner at the dinner table. The entire family walked on eggshells around him.

I explained that explicit memory is generally not encoded until age 3 or 4. And even when recalling those memories, the vantage point of the present day determines and colors what is remembered. "Besides," I said, "why go looking for mice that may not be there when you have a big elephant in the room? Your memories are quite clear that your father made everyone tense."

CLIENT EDUCATION

You possess different types of memory, one for feeling states and another used for describing events. The brain systems for the memory system used to remember events does not go online until age 3 or 4. For that reason, you cannot go back to capture memories that were never encoded.

Many well-meaning therapists who have little knowledge about the memory systems have done a great deal of damage to their clients by attempting to uncover so-called repressed memories. In the late 1980s and 1990s, several articles were published in memory research literature following reports by therapists who claimed to uncover previously repressed memories from clients who were under hypnotic age regression or similar methods. In a study performed by Elizabeth Loftus of 183 claims of repressed memories of childhood abuse, 100% reported and/or torture or mutilation. However, there was no clear evidence that the events actually occurred. Apparently, in an effort to "treat" the residual effects of the assumed trauma, 100% of clients were in therapy 3 to 5 years after the first "memory" was "recovered." Of those people, 83% were employed before therapy, but only 37% remained employed after therapy. Because their families were traumatized by the news of these "recovered memories," 23% of the clients lost parental custody of their children, and 100% of the clients were estranged from their families. While 10% had suicidal ideation before therapy, 67% had suicidal ideation after therapy!

One way to understand the results of this and other studies of so-called repressed memories is that the subjects incurred trauma from therapy. In other words, what was assumed to be therapeutic actually was abusive. In the coming decades, therapists who base their efforts solely on theory without disregard to research will not only be considered lacking in competence but also committing malpractice. One person who attended one of my seminars in Auckland, New Zealand, asked, "But isn't there such a thing as bad science?" The answer is: "Yes. It is therapy-based theory that pretends to be consistent with science but disregards it entirely."

It is critical to be cautious about the fallible nature of memory in response to clients who may have forgotten various events from their pasts. Clients also may claim to be certain that an event took place when in fact it did not. Memories are malleable. Clients may recall one thing from an event in the past, then after spending time with a friend who was also at the event may modify their memory based on what the friend claimed to have remembered.

Studies examining how suggestibility can influence memory illustrate that even when clients are firmly convinced of the accuracy of a memory, that recollection may be seriously in doubt. In other words, when clients feel that there is "no doubt" that an event occurred, they may have been so open to other influences that they were convinced that the event had occurred, despite the fact that it had never really happened (Ceci & Bruch, 1993).

By taking a neutral stance to what clients report, you can avoid much of the tremendous potential for suggestibility. Any encouragement or discouragement can influence client memories of events, especially if they never occurred. Your responses can potentially change client memories; even repeated questioning may influence the quality of recall by leading clients to believe that you "know" they have more hidden in their unconscious minds, perhaps suppressed because of the intense feelings associated with a traumatic experience clients never knew occurred. Alternately, if you act disinterested or change the subject, clients would get the message that the extent and details of an actual traumatic experience are unimportant. In this case, therapy shuts down the conditions for recall.

When clients ask you to uncover memories of events that they worry may have occurred, but there is no concrete evidence that they actually happened, advise them to be cautious. After a century of debate and research on the question of whether traumatic memories are accurate, the generally accepted belief is that the central facts of a trauma are not forgotten. Recollection of the peripheral details is often inaccurate and often fabricated in later stories. It is not possible to distinguish a repressed memory from fake memory without some form of corroborating evidence.

The two main types of explicit memory, episodic and semantic, are distinct yet related (Wheeler, Stuss, & Tulving, 1997). Semantic memory involves language and facts that we use as well as symbols to represent what are and what are not truths and falsehoods. Episodic memory involves an autobiographical sense of self over time. It represents the ability to develop a sense of time and sequencing events that helps children see themselves with a cohesive sense of continuity and an independent person. Therapy is highly dependent on both of these types of explicit memory, and we use them to try to integrate them with implicit memory.

As the name suggests, long-term explicit memory is available for conscious recall for extended periods of time, depending on how strongly the memories have been consolidated. These memories can be available for recall for years if they have been recalled many times and if other associations are made to further strengthen and change them, such as information from family members about the events.

NEUROSCIENCE

While working memory is regarded as generally independent of gene-activated protein synthesis, LTM is mediated by genetically activated structural alterations in the synaptic connections within the neuron network coding the memory (Bailey & Kandel, 1993). Working memory is temporary and involves functional, not structural, alterations in sympathetic strength. LTM is available for extended periods of time but is malleable and never fixed.

LTM differs from STM because the duration is potentially permanent with actual structural changes in the brain. Structural changes involve neuroplasticity, also referred to as long-term potentiation (LTP). To facilitate LTP in the brain, clients must practice the skills being taught in therapy between sessions. Repetition is essentially overlearning, which eventually results in skill building.

LTM goes through a process of cortical consolidation, which involves the reorganization of associated memory traces (Schacter, 1996). For example, a client's memory of a previous day's conversation with his mother is modified by his most recent conversation with her. Perhaps the first conversation was warm, but the one today was heated. Additional information and reconsolidation of those memories occurs each time he remembers or tells a friend about the conversation or dreams that night about talking to his mother.

CLIENT EDUCATION

Every time you recall a memory, it is modified by the context, mood, and vantage point of the present moment.

Much of what becomes reconsolidated is nonconscious, implicit memory. Most clients are amazed to hear that their brains are constantly processing information of which they are not consciously aware. The capacity to consciously attend to challenges that they chose to address while processing other information nonconsciously allows them to drive down the road, brake for a red light while applying the correct pressure on the brake pedal so as to avoid skidding to a stop, while simultaneously talking to someone in the passenger seat.

The reason that people can operate on a conscious level to talk to a friend while on autopilot driving a car is that the brain possesses multiple memory systems. Procedural memory allows us to acquire movement skills and perform them without consciously monitoring movements while engaging in an animated conversation with friends.

The implicit memory systems include both procedural and emotional subsystems. Procedural memory involves motor skills. This is motor or "muscle" memory. When we ride a bicycle, type, or drive a car, we do so without needing to think about it. These motor habits are encoded in our basal ganglia and allow us to operate on autopilot.

CLIENT INFORMATION

You possess the ability to form many good or bad habits that you engage in on autopilot. Our job together is to change the bad ones to good ones.

Implicit emotional memory is activated without conscious attention. An illustration of this type of implicit memory is referred to as the grocery store effect, which represents how, when engaged in an autopilot behavior such as driving, we can forget what we had intended to do. For example, while driving home from work, you forget to stop at the store. This minor error in memory is evidence of two competing parts of the brain, one that creates and maintains habits and the other that is involved in novel learning. Driving home from work is a habit often done on autopilot and involving the striatum, which is part of the basal ganglia, an area of the subcortex involved in movement functions and implicit (procedural) memory. Stopping at the store is a comparatively novel task, involving the hippocampus, the DLPFC, and the explicit memory system.

Procedural and emotional implicit memory combine to make what we are doing and feeling bubble up periodically into conscious awareness, but these feelings are not easily explained experiences. For example, a client, Matt, told me that while driving he felt anxious after he reacted to something his friend said to him with an angry voice. Through our discussion in therapy he became consciously aware that, he felt the same way as a child when his father spoke to him in an angry voice. His amygdala signaled alarm, not only to what his friend said, and also on a nonconscious level he felt danger which spilled over into the feeling that there was something on the road to fear.

CLIENT EDUCATION

Sometimes you may react emotionally to something a friend says or does that feels threatening even though you know realistically that there is no threat. This experience represents your emotional memory that occurs automatically. You can rewire your emotional memory so that you don't feel threatened when there is no threat.

Even strongly motivated clients can engage in negative habitual behaviors and only afterward realize that they have done the very thing they had intended not to do. Clients who suffer from obsessive-compulsive disorder (OCD) often complain, for example, that they have engaged in the behavior they had been trying to extinguish, such as washing hands, only after washing their hands for the 16th time, and despite it being only 10 AM.

Implicit memory can be encoded through classical conditioning, including fear conditioning, resulting in various anxiety disorders. Given that emotion-based implicit memory is driven by amygdala activity, clients may experience a strong generalized emotional valance so that they may fear and avoid situations that even remotely resemble the initial feared situation.

The implicit memory system goes online well before the explicit memory system, so that the former influences the conditions for the latter. In other words, since implicit memories are composed of emotions, habits, and visceral experiences, they set the tone and emotional state through which explicit memories are encoded. In this way, implicit memories set the parameters within which clients encode and retrieve explicit memories. This is what is meant by state-based memories, memories that are coded in a particular mood state.

When clients are in a particular emotional state, they are more likely to trigger explicit memories associated with those emotions. This phenomenon is associated with the concept of transference. Without knowing about how the memory systems can influence one another or for that matter whether there is more than one memory system, psychodynamic theorists have maintained that clients transfer feeling states they had with parents to the therapist. The therapeutic response to those feeling states constitutes the "working through," meaning developing more adaptive (i.e., corrected) feeling states in response to important relationships. More recently, attachment theorists (discussed later in this chapter) have worked on helping clients "earn security" through the therapeutic relationship.

Highlighting the activity of the amygdala as a major player in implicit memory and how it plays a role in the development of anxiety can provide the basis for explaining your interventions. To begin with, clients may be interested to know they actually have two amygdalae deep within their right and left temporal lobes. More activity in the right amygdala is associated with more anxiety and more anxious memories; the left amygdala is associated with less anxiety and positive memories. Both sides of the amygdala add persistence and the subjective characteristics of memory for emotional events and can be traced to a cascade of cognitive, neural, and physiological responses. By drawing attention to the emotional arousal triggers, the memory processes orchestrated by the amygdala can be reconsolidated within the context of the safe emergency.

NEUROSCIENCE

The convergence of the conditioned stimulus (CS) and the unconditioned stimulus (US) leads to neuroplasticity in the lateral amygdala. Then when the CS occurs alone, the potentiated synapses to trigger other amygdala targets in the medial part of the central nucleus which controls conditioned fear responses (LeDoux & Schiller, 2009).

Fear conditioning involves the release of glutamate from sensing fibers in the lateral amygdala, which binds to the excitatory amino acid receptors (alpha amino-3-hydroxy-5-methyl-4-isoxazoleproionic [AMPA]) and N receptors. When the magnesium block is removed and sufficient calcium enters the cell, it activates protein kinesis, which translocates to the cell nucleus and triggers gene expression and protein synthesis.

The amygdala is a relevance detector that aids in the facilitation of attention toward emotionally significant stimuli and in the retention of the motivational value of events (Vuilleumier, 2009). When those events are relevant as potential threats, the amygdala orchestrates a wide range of physiological reactions, including the release of epinephrine and norepinephrine (NE) through the well-known fight, flight, or freeze response. The second phase of the hypothalamic-pituitary-adrenal (HPA) axis response involves the release of cortisol. These networks are described in detail in Chapter 4. The salient point here is that the amygdala-based implicit memory system is key to understanding anxiety disorders and some types of depression.

NEUROSCIENCE

The amygdaloid complex was first identified around 1820. The name "amygdala" is derived from Greek to describe its almond shape. The actual almond-shape part is now recognized as only part of the amygdala rather than the whole region. Nevertheless, most neuroscientists now use the term "amygdala" to denote the entire region of approximately a dozen nuclei.

Because of its role as a relevance detector, the amygdala can also be understood as a sort of smoke alarm, letting clients know that danger is ahead. If clients suffer from anxiety, their amygdala tends to signal danger when there is none. The danger detector function of the amygdala can turn off through it connections with the orbitofrontal cortex (OFC). Clients can be motivated by learning that the OFC can tell the amygdala that everything is okay and there is no reason to fear the situation. In this way, the OFC and amygdala work together to ramp down anxiety, depending on how much affect regulatory control the OFC has learned.

CLIENT EDUCATION

Although the part of your brain that serves as a danger alarm seems to be going off all the time, you can teach it to go off only when there is truly is danger to be alarmed about.

Like the amygdala, the hippocampus is positioned deep within both temporal lobes. Traditionally it had been considered part of the so-called limbic system. However, it plays a smaller role in emotion than does the OFC, which is not part of the limbic system. Hence the concept of a limbic system is outdated. The hippocampus is intricately involved in explicit memory. It is needed temporarily to bind together distributed sites in the neocortex that represent a whole explicit memory. It serves as the librarian, an index to the database of explicit memory. Accordingly, it is a novelty detector, comparing incoming information to already stored knowledge. If there is a difference, the hippocampus triggers a dopamine (DA) increase to facilitate interest in binding new to old information. The hippocampus ceases to play a role in the retention of a specific memory after about 2 years.

NEUROSCIENCE

The hippocampus also plays a role in the modulation of fear expression by the cortex (Fanselow, 2000; Ji & Maren, 2007). It mediates the return of a previously extinguished fear by the memory of the context in which the dangerous situation occurred (Corcoran & Maren, 2001). The neural connections between the hippocampus and the prefrontal cortex (PFC) are involved in inhibiting amygdala activity during incremental exposure to a previously anxiety provoking situation so that it is expressed only in the appropriate context (Phelps, 2009).

Clients often need to understand why it is important to be emotionally engaged outside of their comfort zones to learn new adaptive behaviors. Although the amygdala and hippocampus contribute implicit and explicit memory, respectively, there is an important functional connectivity between them. When the amygdala and hippocampus are working well together, memories are more robust and durable. The amygdala contributes to emotional amplification of explicit memories.

CLIENT EDUCATION

If you make what you want to remember emotionally relevant so that memory is long lasting, you will feel more comfortable in situations that previously you found uncomfortable. For example, if you previously feared being around strangers, consistently putting yourself in contact with strangers will eventually help you enlarge your comfort zone.

NEUROSCIENCE

Emotional arousal increases amygdala activity, which enhances and modulates activity in the medial temporal lobe memory system through the up-regulation of activity in the entorhinal cortex and hippocampus (McGaugh, 2004). In addition, the neurochemical enhancement, including adrenaline, NE, and cortisol through the HPA axis, increases electro-physiological synchrony between neuronal firing in the amygdala and the hippocampus at the theta frequency, which enhances memory-related neuroplasticity (Peres et al., 2007). The same functional connectivity is recapitulated during retrieval of the emotional memories. In other words, explicit memories can be state based (such as when we are depressed, we remember depressing events).

Clients typically want to know why they can feel anxious before having anxious thoughts. One reason for this disparity is that there are two tracks to activate the amygdala, the fast track and the slow track. The fast track sends information directly to the amygdala while the slow track sends information to the cortex before the amygdala. In short, the fast track makes us feel before thinking while the slow track involves thought before feeling. By describing the difference between these tracks, you can provide clarity to how clients can feel a surge of panic and fear without any preceding thoughts triggering the fight-or-flight HPA activation. In other words, clients can feel anxious without knowing why. This fast track facilitates emotional learning at best and fear conditioning at worst. As such, the fast track to the amygdala can trigger flashbacks for clients with PTSD in a sort of bottom-up manner. For example, combat war veterans may hear firecrackers or car backfires through their auditory circuits, and that information is quickly routed through the thalamus directly to the amygdala. In other words, the veterans feel gunfire before they consciously wonder if it is gunfire. For clients with PTSD, the fast-track circuit needs to be integrated with the slow-track circuits, as I will describe in Chapter 7.

For its part, the slow track to the amygdala routes the auditory information to the thalamus and then to the cortex before the amygdala. Consider the situation just described. Combat veterans may respond to a noise by asking themselves "Is that gunfire I hear, or is that a firecracker?" Here, in effect, veterans tell themselves how to respond based on a reality check of what the situation actually calls for. If the booming sound is simply a firecracker, they may then wonder why someone let off a firecracker. They may reflect a moment and say, "Oh, yeah, it's the Fourth of July!"

CLIENT EDUCATION

When you find yourself responding to a situation with immediate and intense fear only to find out that there is no danger, give your slow track time to catch up with your fast track. You can teach your slow track to speed up.

The slow track activates thinking before feeling by sending sensory information to the thalamus, then through the cortex and hippocampus, and finally to the amygdala. When it is too slow or not working at all, fears and phobias can occur because the amygdala "hijacks" the slow track. In other words, the amygdala can dominate the PFC, stirring up unrealistic fears. The work to bolster the slow track to tame the amygdala involves exposure to implicit memories combined with new thinking through which the cortex tones down fear through top-down inhibition.

CLIENT EDUCATION

Because there are two tracks to your amygdala, if you suffer from anxiety, especially posttraumatic stress disorder, your fast track is on too often while your slow track needs to speed up. We will work together to integrate your emotional memory system with your thinking memory system so that feeling and thinking can be in sync. This will slow down your fast track and speed up your slow track.

Your advice to clients to be patient and be persistent can make sense when explaining the two different roles for the amygdala and the hippocampus. The amygdala-based memories are hard to forget; it is as if the memories are engraved in stone. In contrast, the hippocampal circuits, which tell us what to fear and in what context, are easy to forget, like drawings on an Etch-a-Sketch. This means that once a person is traumatized, the residual effects last a lifetime. The explicit memories, however, may be not only forgotten but continually changing based on the current contextual situation. Much of your work in therapy with clients involves integrating the long-lingering amygdala-based memories with newly constructed hippocampal coded explicit memories. By doing so, you help clients put into context what happened in the past within a sense of self-efficacy and confidence felt in the present day.

Consolidating Memories

Memories of events are not snapshots in time, frozen and sealed off from contamination from all the experiences that follow. Nor are memories contained in any particular neuron that somehow goes offline until reactivated when you help clients recall a memory. Memories are encoded in neural nets, clusters of synaptic connections that are modified based on new experiences, including the conditions that you orchestrate in therapy to result in positive rewiring of client brains.

NEUROSCIENCE

Memories of the representations of experiences are stored in the posterior association areas. The PFC directs the process of retrieving memories by matching the retrieval cue with the memory (Wheeler, Stuss, & Tulving, 1997).

Memories of our past, whether they are traumatic or positive, are constantly transformed by the dynamic interaction of our memory systems as we adapt to the present moment and reach for the future. Development through the life cycle essentially involves the establishment and modification of our memory systems. Helping clients understand the memory systems can shed light on why they have difficulty now and how we can help them integrate memory so that they can thrive in the future.

CLIENT EDUCATION

Your brain is not like a computer, remembering every program used or Web site visited. Your memories change based on your experience. That is why we are reworking your memory systems: so that you will feel better.

Therapy necessarily involves constructing new adaptive memory systems. The activation of old memories in the therapeutic context that you help orchestrate can transform those old maladaptive memories based on conditions of the present moment. Technically, the process referred to as "consolidation" involves the conversion of new episodic memories into a more permanent form that is more resistant to forgetting and/or interference. Memory consolidation takes place gradually over a period of time, from hours to years (McGaugh, 2004). Since the consolidation takes place only gradually, its emotion-related effects generally are not detectable immediately after the event but rather evolve over time. Adrenergic and cortisol effects, which begin during the encoding of an emotional event, continue to modulate the consolidation of memory traces afterward due to the stress hormones released during and after the event (Hamann, 2009). This extended consolidation processes takes place in waking consciousness as well as during sleep. There is growing evidence that consolidation of emotional memories occurs during rapid-eye-movement (REM) sleep (Holland & Lewis, 2007). During waking consciousness, cognitive processes, including increased rehearsal of and rumination over an emotional event, reinforce and strengthen emotional memories (LaBar & Cabeza, 2006).

NEUROSCIENCE

Memories are modified through the establishment of synaptic connections, pruned down to even the minutest level with changes to the behavior of a single ion channel or the expression or suppression of specific genes. There are also changes to the shape and number of sprouting new axons modifying their dendritic surfaces and dendritic outgrowth (Kolb & Whishaw, 2009).

(continued)

(*continued*)

> Forming memories is a process that is both intra- and interneuron.
> In the latter case, multiple neural networks fire and wire together
> to form memory. Memory consolidation also involves changes to
> neurons themselves that facilitate connections with one another. The
> synaptic modifications result in, and are facilitated by, many layers of
> biochemical processes, including second messengers. Many of these
> processes were discovered by Nobel laureate Eric Kandel. LTP involves
> the neurotransmitter serotonin and a sequence of neurochemical
> reactions: cyclic adenosine monophosphate (cAMP), then protein kinase
> A (PKA), then cAMP response element-binding protein CREB. CREB
> is a transcriptional control protein that increases the number of synaptic
> connections. CREB1 activates genes; CREB2 represses genes.

A basic principle to convey is that part of your work with clients involves modifying maladaptive memories into adaptive ones. These new memories will form part of the infrastructure of stability and greater mental health. You will modify memories together by bringing up feelings, sensations, and recollections of past events or states of mind and putting them into realistic perspectives. By framing the past through the lens of the present moment within the therapeutic context of the safe emergency, clients gain an improved sense of self-efficacy. They gain hope that the bad "habits" of anxiety and depression can be rewired into good habits, such as feeling calm and positive in varied circumstances.

CLIENT EDUCATION

> We are going to work together to rewire your memory systems so that they
> can serve you more effectively and help you feel better. Doing this will
> require some initial discomfort, but those feelings will pass as we build in
> circuits that will provide you with durable and positive emotions.

Developing Implicit Memory

Infants are born "premature." We spend longer in the care of our parents than any other species. The adaptation to the early caretaking environment plays a major role in the development of the implicit memory system. Most people develop as a result of nurtured nature. However, others, most of whom are our clients, are malnourished, and develop anxiety, depression, and other disorders. Whether nourished or malnourished, the brain and its memory systems that encode our experience form the infrastructure from which we adapt to the world.

Clients typically want to know how they developed their respective psychological problems. The psychodynamic spectrum of psychotherapy emphasized
helping clients gain insight into their development and attachment relationships. Psychological disorders are intertwined in the memory systems. Insight
into how they developed psychologically is, however, but a first step. These
memory systems must be reregulated, and doing that takes more than insight
alone.

Explaining child development helps them make sense of their experiences and
can provide the conceptual framework for brain-changing therapy. Development
illustrates the fundamentals of the "use it or lose it" dynamics inherent to the
brain. By discovering how their brains were wired to meet the challenges of perhaps a chaotic childhood, clients can focus on rewiring those areas that no longer
need to be hypervigilant, such as the amygdala. If clients endured an abusive,
neglectful, or deprived early environment, their implicit memory systems may
have been wired around fear. Repeated abuse experiences wired the brain with
implicit memory circuits representing fear and even terror, and these circuits can
be readily activated later in life, should danger occur.

Child abuse creates havoc in the brain; it ramps up the sympathetic nervous system, including making the amygdala hyperalert to the potential of
more danger with chronically elevated cortisol levels. The residual effects
of child abuse also contribute to structural changes to the brain, including
diminished left-hemisphere and left-hippocampal volume (Bremner et al.,
1997). The impairment of the left hemisphere, which processes positive emotion, results in a vulnerability to depression and anxiety, both associated with
right-hemisphere hyperactivity. There also tends to be less integration of left
and right hemispheres (Teicher et al., 2003). Child abuse is associated with a
wide spectrum of other developmentally inappropriate milestones, such as an
accelerated loss of neurons (Simantov, Blinder, Ratovitski, Tauber, Gabbay,
& Porat, 1996), delayed myelination (Dunlop, Archer, Quinlivan, Beazley,
& Newnham, 1997), abnormalities in developmentally appropriate pruning
(Todd, 1992), and inhibition of neurogenesis in the hippocampus (Gould,
McEwen, Tanapat, Galea, & Fuchs, 1997). These deficits appear to be long
lasting. Adults who were physically or sexually abused as children have been
found to have diminished left hippocampi.

For example, Sarah came to see me with complaints of free-floating anxiety
and hypervigilance in intimate relationships. At age 32, she had never experienced a relationship that lasted beyond a few months. Sarah had survived childhood abuse by her father during the first 6 years of her life, until her mother
finally left him, and she did not want to follow her mother's tendency to put up
with abusive men. Sarah had managed to avoid abusive relationships thanks to
work with a few therapists during her late 20s. However, she was unable to trust
men who were not abusive. Using the BASE perspective, there probably was a
set point, the ratio of activity in the right PFC and the left PFC, favoring the
former, also with overactivity of her amygdala. Our alliance began tentatively.

All her previous therapists had been women. The fact that I am a man pushed her out of her comfort zone. But most important, it offered an opportunity to help her form an alliance with a man in the safety of the therapeutic relationship and with definable boundaries while I orchestrated a safe emergency to help her expand her comfort zone. With my gentle encouragement, she tested out long-term relationships with safe men who did not feel safe initially. With consistent challenges, over time she became better able to maintain healthy relationships.

Deprived environments have also been found to produce more psychopathology, suicides, and medical problems in adults (Felitti et al., 1998). Less severe but also toxic for the brain are deprived environments during the first few years of development. Deprived environments result in the deactivation of the social brain circuits described in Chapter 1. The international example of deprived environments was highlighted by the sad case of 150,000 children who were found languishing in Romanian orphanages at the end of the reign of the dictator Nicolae Ceausescu. Although the orphans were kept clean and fed, they were neglected socially, missing nurturing human contact during critical periods (Kuhn & Schanberg, 1998). This deprivation resulted in sustained impairment if they resided in an orphanage for over 1 year. In such cases, children had a wide variety of impairments, including increased levels of cortisol, impaired OFC resulting in poor affect regulation, and poor social skills. They also had a variety of cognitive impairments, including Attention Deficit Disorder, and various learning disorders.

On a far less extreme level of deprivation, simple failure to activate the social brain networks through nurturing interaction with principal caregivers can cause children to implode. One series of studies called the Still Face paradigm exemplifies the psychological cost of impoverished reflected emotion from a child's principal caregivers (Tronick, 2007). The paradigm places a mother and a 9-month-old child together in a room. Then the mother is asked to show no expression on her face. In response, the baby tries to entice her into playfully interacting, but eventually the baby becomes agitated and distressed and gives up, looking despondent. Babies subjected to prolonged Still Face situations no longer approach novel toys, and their imagination shuts down.

Why would children exposed to the Still Face paradigm react so negatively? Adults generally would have an innocuous reaction to the test, after all. Children and adults differ in how they respond to facial expressions due to the degree to which they recruit the amygdala. Fearful faces provoke more amygdala activity in adults than in children and adolescents. In contrast, neutral faces provoke more amygdala activity and are interpreted as more emotionally negative by children and adolescents than by adults (Tottenham et al., 2009; Tronick, 2007).

The Still Face paradigm demonstrates that ambiguity is the salient factor differentiating children from adults. In response to ambiguous faces, children become anxious, agitated, then withdraw and become depressed. Amygdala activity for neutral faces decreases with age as developing children see more faces in emotionally neutral contexts and their OFCs gain the ability to appreciate ambiguity. This transition illustrates that a shift from subcortical to cortical processing occurs during adolescence and adulthood (Casey, Tottenham, Liston, & Durston, 2005).

Activation of the amygdala during adulthood differs dramatically from young children who do not yet maintain a fully operational OFC. For adults, the OFC and the anterior cingulate cortex (ACC) help navigate through an often-ambiguous world as well as inhibit amygdala overactivity. In contrast to the OFC and ACC, the amygdala is involved in disambiguation of social situations, as it helps people disregard irrelevant information. Combined with the capability of the cortex to add meaning in social situations, fearful faces provoke more amygdala activity in adults than children later in life.

NEUROSCIENCE

The unpredictable nature of human interaction influences amygdala function (Buchanan, Tranel, & Adolphs, 2009). The social environment constitutes an especially ambiguous set of stimuli, and the amygdala is critically involved in their disambiguation. The amygdala helps people disregard irrelevant manifestations to seek out personal information relevant to them.

There are dire implications for the mental health of children if the Still Face paradigm is extended for many months or days, as occurs when mothers suffer postpartum depression. In such cases, developing children are deprived of the emotional nourishment provided by animated facial expressions and engaging emotional relationships.

Infants of depressed mothers display more aversion and helplessness and vocalize less than infants of mothers who do not behave as if they are depressed. The infants have higher heart rates, decreased vagal tone, and more developmental delays at 12 months of age (Field & Diego, 2008). They tend to have overactive right frontal lobes, underactive left frontal lobes, lower levels of DA and serotonin, and higher levels of stress hormones. In fact, there are long-term residual effects of maternal depression. Maternal depression during children's first 2 years of life predicts elevated cortisol production in children at age 7 (Ashman, Dawson, Panagiotides, Yamada, & Wilkinson, 2002).

Treating maternal depression is critically important in preventing childhood depression. Such treatment can contribute to children's improvement if they are already becoming depressed. Mothers can be taught to massage their infants beginning in infancy to reestablish bonding (Field, 1995). Despite being depressed, parents can learn to show positive emotions and care for children (Cumberland-Li, Eisenberg, Champion, Gershoff, & Fabes, 2003).

Explaining the consequences of the Still Face paradigm and depressed behavior to depressed mothers can motivate them to make the behavioral changes necessary to rise out of depression. Most parents will do things for their children that they put off if it would benefit only themselves. Describing the effects of the Still Face experiment on their children can therefore be an important part of therapy.

Whenever I meet a woman with postpartum depression, I am more concerned about her baby than I am about her. This was the case with Deidre. Like all parents, she would do more for her child than she would do for herself. When I told her what could happen to her child's brain if she did not do things to help herself rise out of depression, her first reaction was an expression of guilt. I noted, "If you do things that intentionally hurt your child, then I can understand the guilt. But until now, you haven't. Now you know what you can do to help yourself and help your child."

She complied with my suggestion to bring her baby to the next session. I began by playing peek-a-boo with her child, then asked her to do the same.

"I don't feel like it," she said.

"It's not for you, it's for her."

She nodded with quick recognition. When she began to play peek-a-boo and her baby laughed, she could not help but laugh herself. Then her baby laughed more heartily, and she laughed with pleasure that I had not seen before. You have to be a stone to resist a baby's smile or laugh.

When the principal caregivers provide nurturing interaction to the hungry social brain networks of developing children, the children form an infrastructure of implicit memory that represents a positive adaptation pattern. How and what type of nurturing are offered to children shape their implicit memory system and sets the stage for the degree to which they can control affect, maintain positive relationships, and face challenges throughout life.

Attachment represents the pattern of organizing emotions and behaviors that optimally can serve to support self-esteem, the feelings of lovability and stress tolerance. The more secure the attachment schema, the better the affect regulation. An ineffective attachment schema leads to fear modulation/avoidance behavior, which is associated with overactivating the right PFC and depression as well as anxiety.

Implicit memory begins to develop as children acquire a model of the world based on how they are being cared for and learn to emotionally anticipate future experiences based on these models. The basic developmental components of implicit memory are created through a multimodal model of the interpersonal world from which children can base familiar generalizations about what to anticipate and how to negotiate with those around them. These implicit memories are composed of perceptual biases that continue to be formed throughout our lives.

Repeated positive attachment experiences contribute to a resilient implicit memory system based on being warmly attuned and consistently nurtured. These experiences result in implicit memories of comfort around intimate partners. In contrast, unpredictable, poorly attuned, and inconsistently nurtured attachment experiences all contribute to the formation of implicit memories of discomfort and distrust.

Although they knew little about the amygdala and the implicit memory system, two psychodynamic theorists, Donald Winnicott and John Bowlby, understood the dynamics of bonding and difficulties in attachment. They offered some very useful concepts. Winnicott was one of the contributors to the object relations school of psychoanalysis. His most useful concepts are good-enough mothering and the holding environment, which envisions attachments being formed within the imperfect, flexible, and supportive relationship of the parents. When conflict — what Winnicott called an "impingement" — is encountered in a relationship, the relationship can be enhanced by "repairing" those impingements through using what he called adequate "mirroring." Even though Winnicott did not know about mirror neurons and other social brain networks, he hypothesized that parents reflect back emotional states to strengthen not only the relationship but the developing child's self-efficacy and affect regulation.

Good-enough parents are imperfect, just like human experience. They help prepare children for the often-ambiguous, sometimes stressful life experiences that they will encounter throughout life. Perfect is not "good enough" because people will not encounter perfect situations later in life. In fact, the concept of perfect suggests that when children implicitly feel the need to be gratified without delay and do receive gratification immediately, they will not develop adequate coping skills. High levels of affective matching correlate with insecure attachment, just as low levels of affective matching correlate with insecurity. Good-enough parenting is essentially moderate matching and is associated with implicit feelings of security.

Perfect parenting matches babies' needs immediately and does not allow for the development of frustration tolerance; good-enough parenting, in contrast, matches infants' needs most of the time and especially when those needs are critical. As babies become hungry, cold, warm, or wet, their needs are met warmly by rocking, cuddling, caring, or feeding. These caregiving behaviors help children feel loved and cared for as the attachment is enhanced.

Hyperattunement (i.e. perfect parenting) undermines growing children's capacity to adapt. If every time the baby expresses a need or discomfort, they are tended to with immediate absolute attention. Then they have no time to learn to deal with minor frustrations and to produce the flexible neurocircuitry of arousal. Instead, they respond to frustration with excessive sympathetic arousal and not enough parasympathetic activation. When needs are met immediately, children form very little frustration tolerance and become spoiled, bratty, inflexible, and generally not able to deal with the challenges in life.

Good-enough parenting bolsters the resiliency of the autonomic nervous system so that developing children can rise to the challenge of stressful situations and then calm down afterward to recoup. Good-enough parenting factors in time before babies are soothed so that they can anticipate being soothed and activate their parasympathetic nervous systems when they need to calm down. If, however, babies are matched by instantaneous soothing, they will not develop brakes to the hypothalamic, pituitary, adrenal arousal and not be able to calm down after stress.

John Bowlby, another major figure from the psychodynamic perspective, added to this perspective of how the implicit memory system develops into an effective or ineffective infrastructure for affect regulation. The concept of the "safe haven" represented an optimum psychological situation through which developing children could establish an implicit sense of security with their principal attachment figures and as a result establish a safe haven within themselves.

Bowlby noted that there is a natural tendency of all developing children toward proximity seeking to the attachment figure for safety. Children seek out and are hungry to interact with attachment figures. How parents respond optimally helps children develop the implicit thermostat for resiliency. Bowlby foresaw what occurs with the Still Face paradigm or deprivation of the Romanian orphans from his work on war babies of World War II. Without developing the implicit thermostat acquired through the safe haven in bonding, the individual's ability to adapt to a complex social world is undermined.

Bowlby set the stage for a wide variety of different types of research exploring early bonding. His student, Mary Ainsworth, was the architect of the principal research paradigm to identify the types of attachment. This research paradigm, called the infant strange situation, measures the infant's reaction to four different situations: (1) mother and infant alone, (2) when a stranger is introduced into the setting with the mother and infant, (3) when the mother leaves the room for 3 minutes and the stranger stays with the baby, and (4) when both mother and stranger are absent and the baby is alone.

The key observations occur when the mother comes back. Specifically, how well can the pair calm the baby down and how quickly does the baby return to play? Ainsworth and her colleagues identified three different attachment styles and their associated maternal behaviors. The secure style of attachment is associated with maternal behavior that is emotionally available, perceptive, and effective. The avoidant style is associated with distant and rejecting maternal behavior, and the anxious/ambivalent style is associated with conflictual maternal behavior marked by inconsistent availability. Ainsworth's student Mary Main identified a fourth style, the disorganized, which is associated with erratic maternal behavior.

With secure attachment, there is bidirectional affect regulation between parent and child. Secure attachment results in the development of an implicit infrastructure that enables the person to engage in the world with a positive attitude and respond resiliently to high stress. The parent perceives and responds to the inner state of the child (Fonagy & Target, 1997). If there are conflicts, they are resolved with a correction of the mismatched attunement. The different types of insecure attachment involve either hypersynchronous or asynchronous interactions.

NEUROSCIENCE

Secure attachment results in a durable and flexible autonomic nervous system so that the individual can turn on the sympathetic system when needed and can turn on the parasympathetic system after the challenge has been met. The regulation of the various calming neurotransmitters, such as the endorphin and benzodiazepine receptors which respond to GABA, allows the person to self-soothe and recoup when needed. These neurochemicals, are in short supply in people who have experienced insecure attachment, but they are widely available to securely attached people. Flexible cortisol regulation permits people to ramp up the neurochemistry to deal with a challenge during the daytime; then, during the evening, people can turn down cortisol so that they are better able to restore resources and sleep. In contrast, in the stranger and separation situations, insecurely attached toddlers showed elevated cortisol levels (Nachmias, Gunnar, Mangelsdorf, Parritz & Buss, 1996). Accordingly, there is positive immunological functioning so that a securely attached person is generally healthier. With regard to cognitive development, securely attached children are endowed with better neural growth and plasticity. The thermostat of secure attachment limits cortisol elevation in stressful situations. Early positive maternal care protects the hippocampus from the destructive physiological effects of cortisol (Meaney, Aitken, Viau, Sharma, & Sarrieau, 1989).

Secure attachment is correlated with lower incidence of psychiatric disorders than in the general population (Van Ijzendoorn & Bakermans-Kranenburg, 1996); disorganized attachment is associated with dissociative problems. When mood is assessed corresponding to insecure attachment longitudinally, anxious/ ambivalent and avoidant attachment styles are associated with the development of depression. The avoidant style leads to depression based on a sense of alienation; the anxious/ambivalent style leads to depression based on an internalized sense of helplessness and doubt.

During the last 20 years, some researchers have attempted to assess adult attachment styles. Mary Main and her colleagues have developed the Adult Attachment Interview (AAI), an 18-question interview about attachment history that primes the implicit attachment system in adults with inquiry of their explicit memories. Adult attachment as assessed by the AAI can predict with 80% accuracy the parents' attachment style and can help predict the attachment style of unborn children. A meta-analysis of the AAI studies indicates that insecure attachment is correlated with anxiety and mood disorders.

There appears to be a strong correspondence between the attachment styles identified by the infant strange situation (ISS) and the AAI. For example, the AAI-identified preoccupied style shows strong relational similarities to the ambivalent style of the ISS. Ambivalent babies typically have preoccupied parents, and they often become preoccupied adults themselves. They tend to be obsessed with love and loss and are emotionally underregulated.

The AAI-identified dismissive style shows strong correspondence to the ISS-identified avoidant style of attachment. Avoidant babies learn to deal with parental insensitivity by shifting attention away from emotions. When they grow up to be dismissive adults, they know little about their own feelings or those of others. These people often state that they tend to have few explicit memories of their childhood, not because they are repressing difficult memories but rather because of little amygdala activity to amplify the hippocampus-based explicit memories during development. Dismissing adults tend to be overregulated and rigid. But separations still provoke spikes in their levels of cortisol.

The fourth category identified by the ISS, referred to as the disorganized style, is associated with the unresolved type identified by the AAI. For the disorganized style, attachment figures inspired fear. The developing child both approached and avoided contact with that attachment figure, as trauma is common. There appears to be strong transgenerational effects of the attachment styles, especially the disorganized/unresolved types. For example, if the parent is unresolved, there is an 80% chance the baby will be disorganized.

The intent of brain-based therapy is to discover and highlight common denominators among theoretical perspectives. The psychodynamic school always attempted to focus on interpersonal dynamics and to bring the unconscious to consciousness. By discarding the theory-laden term "unconscious" and replacing it with the parsimonious term "nonconscious," we can envision psychotherapy as providing the means through which implicit memory is integrated into explicit memory.

When attachment is considered from a transtheoretical perspective, the concept of the common factors of security appears to overlap among various theoretical perspectives. Security in adulthood is based on the capacity to develop the ability to hypothesize what may be occurring in the other person's mind. Developmental psychologists have called this the theory of mind (TOM). People with autism spectrum disorders possess an underdeveloped TOM ability. Mentalization can be thought of as a psychodynamic view of TOM. From a psychodynamic perspective, the capacity for intersubjectivity relates to the ability to share a frame of mind. Intersubjectivity from a developmental perspective describes the sharing of subjective states by the nonverbal communication of infants, young children and their parents (Stern, 1985). The psychoanalytic concept of mentalization attempts to explain the ability to understand the mental state of oneself and others just like the TOM, which describes the ability to attribute mental states, beliefs, desires, and intentions that are different from one's own. From a psychoanalytic perspective, individuals without secure attachment have difficulties in the development of mentalization abilities (Fonagy & Target, 1997). In contrast, securely attached individuals tend to have had mentalizing primary caregivers and so have more robust capacities to represent the states of their own and other people's minds. Metacognition, defined as "cognition about cognition" or "knowing about knowing," includes knowledge about when and how to use particular strategies for learning or for problem solving.

Therapy can be explained to clients as a method through which the therapeutic relationship can help in rewiring attachment so that an insecurely attached client can earn security through the corrective experience of a secure alliance in therapy. Change can occur through the transformation of the insecure style to the secure style through the promotion of positive relationships and moderate levels of stress. Unfortunately, the transformation can also go from secure to insecure when people encounter sustained environmental and familial stressors. This is often seen in negative changes in caretaking and marriage, including domestic violence situations, as well as loss and complicated bereavement. Relationships can become severely compromised in societal chaos with severely decreased resources.

When thinking about the issues raised by memory and attachment research, the therapeutic extrapolations to consider include examining how clients implicitly respond to good-enough interventions. Negative effects and reactions can be a plus because you can utilize them for repairing ruptures and to build stronger alliances. Effective therapy can be understood as good-enough therapy. Attempts to offer "perfect" therapy are not only impossible but fail to provide the interpersonal conditioning from which to develop resiliency. You should be alert to avoid premature terminations and idealized transferences, it is best to be aware of nonverbal communications as well as use outcome management protocols to ensure that clients are revealing their thoughts and feelings about the alliance.

Developing New Memory

The process of developing new adaptive and integrated memory systems lies at the heart of psychotherapy. By helping the client establish an infrastructure of frustration tolerance and viable affect regulation, even if the developmental background of the client may have undermined those skills, they can be rewired to form a firm foundation of resiliency.

Attention is the initial critical factor to maximizing memory in therapy. If the PFC, especially the DLPFC of clients is not activated, then their working memory does not transfer information to their hippocampus. If their amygdala is activated by emotional arousal simultaneously with the hippocampus, memories can be encoded with greater likelihood of recall. Given that the amygdala is a relevancy detector, emotional engagement in therapy provides the most durable effects. By breaking new ground and getting clients out of their comfort zones, they not only increase competency but make what is covered in therapy new and fresh. Along with the relevancy detector function of the amygdala, the hippocampus serves as a novelty detector. They can work together in therapy by maximizing emotional engagement and novelty. Accordingly, the associations that you co-construct in therapy should be time rich, enduring, and consistent with building a secure attachment infrastructure.

Many clients state that they do not yet "feel ready" to take on the challenge of trying anything new. Perhaps because of early trauma or abuse, clients may argue that they will never feel secure or safe enough for the challenge. By explaining the safe emergency of moderate activation, which you can illustrate by the inverse U discussed in Chapter 1, you can encourage clients to take the first step of getting out of their comfort zones. Since much of memory consolidation, especially implicit memory, involves classical conditioning, applying titrated exposure can defuse clients' fear-based memory. Their previously hypersensitized amygdala can be toned down through the enhanced affect regulation provided by the PFC systems.

Integrating explicit with implicit memory involves forming adaptive associations that are context specific and provide memory landmarks. Teaching clients to use memory landmarks can provide them with memory cues for skills learned in therapy so that they can incorporate the skills in everyday life. For example, Nancy came to see me for help overcoming the anxiety she felt when talking in staff meetings and occasionally giving presentations. She had previously worked with a therapist who helped her develop the insight that she was humiliated by her father during dinnertime discussions and so felt the same way in meetings. Then the therapist moved on to relaxation exercises. While both methods were acceptable beginning points, they failed to integrate Nancy's memory systems, and she experienced no improvement despite working with the therapist for over a year.

I explained that her implicit memory system needed to adapt to her current life conditions and that her amygdala cannot switch off by insight alone, even when followed by relaxation exercises. Rather, our work together challenged her to activate her implicit reactions that did not "feel right." In time, through integration with her explicit memory system and conscious awareness, the reactions would feel right in the future. The initial change was to shift her behavior in the staff meetings from an avoidance orientation to an approach one. While making that shift, I asked her to discover some issues raised during the meeting that she felt either enthusiastic about or disturbed by and express that feeling in the meeting. Doing this involved getting her amygdala and hippocampus to work together with a little more left-PFC activity than right-PFC activity. I explained that this would serve to activate tolerable emotion and develop her resiliency. Given that neuroplasticity requires repetition, increased challenge, and consistent practice, I suggested that we monitor her progress over the next few months.

CLIENT EDUCATION

You may wonder if what you learn about in therapy is transferable to everyday life. The context and similarity of what we discuss to what you previously experienced are points to keep in mind as you practice new behaviors. For example, where you learn, including the situation and your surroundings, has a significant impact on your recall and ability to apply new skills. Practice in the same place where you will perform or need to apply the new skills.

One of the many problems with the memories from a trauma is that thoughts (explicit memories) and emotions (implicit memories) become fragmented and dysregulated in the brain. These dysregulated memories need to be integrated and re-regulated. Placing past events in the context of clients' ongoing autobiographical memory allows them to integrate past experiences into a cohesive sense of self in their world, which, although unfair, can be understood and accepted (Fivush, 1998).

Memory just after an event is unstable, fragile, and labile until a sufficient period of time has passed during which it gradually becomes stable and consolidated. But memories can give way to dynamic and malleable change every time a memory is retrieved. During this time, the underlying memory traces once again become fragile and labile and go through another period of consolidation referred to as reconsolidation. Successful therapy, therefore, involves adaptive reconsolidation. Given that much of anxiety involves maladaptive fear-based memories, therapy involves the reconsolidation of those memories so that they serve as realistic responses to stress.

The state of mind and mood of clients at the time of reconsolidation plays a major role in how they will recall those memories, known as state-based memories. Clients will recall them easily when they are in the same state again. This is why your orchestration of the safe part of the safe emergency is critical. Therapeutic approaches that attempt to integrate implicit and explicit memory of traumatic experience do so by constructing an adaptive narrative while simultaneously evoking implicit memories through exposure, either in vivo or through imagery.

NEUROSCIENCE

Given that protein synthesis is required for the consolidation or reconsolidation of memory, blocking protein synthesis has been shown to block the consolidation of fear memories. When anisomcyin, a protein synthesis inhibitor, is injected into the rat amygdala, it aids in blocking

(continued)

(continued)

> the reconsolidation of the fear-based memory (Nader, Schafe, & LeDoux, 2000). The administration of propranolol, a beta-adrenergic antagonist, blocks reconsolidation by indirectly influencing protein synthesis in the amygdala (Debiec & LeDoux, 2004).

The context in which explicit memory is encoded represents an efficient manner of therapeutic retrieval of that memory. This best occurs when there is a match between the retrieval cue and the memory representation. In other words, when you ask clients about an event earlier in their lives, the context of the therapy session may not provide retrieval cues to match the episodic memory. If, however, clients present a memory cue, such as a gun or knife, and tell you about events leading up to the memory, there is a closer match for the context-dependent explicit memory.

NEUROSCIENCE

Some researchers have identified the left frontal lobe as playing a dominant role in encoding episodic memory and the right frontal lobe as being dominant in retrieving episodic memories (Tulving, Kapur, Creik, Moscovitch, & Houle, 1994). Since eye movements to the left are associated with activation of the right hemisphere and vice versa, during recall of episodic memories people gaze to the left.

Therapy combines reconsolidation and storytelling. Throughout human history, the telling of stories has served multiple functions, including enculturation, so that members of a society can agree to common origins and give meaning to their existence as well as morals, ethics, and general customs to provide cultural cohesion. Stories have also served a fundamental role in the interaction between parent and child. Following the development of the explicit memory system, which is dependent on the hippocampus going online around age 2½ to 3, children and their caregivers co-construct narratives that describe and make sense of the children's existence. So too does co-constructing a client's autobiographical memory serve to reconsolidate a more durable and resilient sense of self.

Narratives that you co-construct with clients are multilayered because people experience innumerable events in their lives. The contexts for those experiences are forever changing, with no single narrative underlying the experiences. Since clients may continually interact with multiple people, the context of an interaction and client expectations play a significant role in narratives that you can effectively use with them. The fluid and changeable nature of social experiences means that how clients remember themselves through narratives is constantly changing with every new social context. Through the process of co-constructing narratives, they learn how to narrate to themselves. These narratives contribute to the formation of the explicit memory system within which autobiographical and episodic memories form part of clients' psychological infrastructure.

Chapter 4

AUTOSTRESS DISORDERS

E veryone experiences stress periodically because life typically presents challenges. And some people engage in extreme challenge for fun, such as skydiving and mountain climbing. Yet many clients believe that stress itself is something to avoid at all costs. In fact, stress by itself is not harmful, but some people are more durable than others. What is important is how much and for how long people experience stress, whether the stress is extreme and/or persisting. The implicit memory system in people with very little social support or insecure attachment sets their frustration tolerance extremely low.

In some people, the stress reaction to perceived intolerable conditions remains activated well after stressful or dangerous conditions subside. In such cases, prolonged stress reactions can become ongoing anxiety. In other words, the stress reaction system gets turned on inappropriately and becomes an anxiety disorder. From this perspective, an anxiety disorder feeds on the stress response system and so can be understood as an autostress disorder. Like autoimmune disorders that hijack the immune system, attacking the body instead of protecting it, autostress disorders transform the stress response system into something that attacks the self rather than protecting it. A consistent pattern of false alarms transforms to an autostress disorder, which we refer to as an anxiety disorder. Stress becomes anxiety when the stress system is turned on too often and signals danger when there is none.

You can convey to your clients that a little stress need not transform into anxiety. Without some stress, people would not get out the door to go to work on time, stay in the right lane while driving, or move out of the way if when crossing the street a semi-truck speeds toward them. People need the feeling of sharpened alertness facilitated by the sympathetic branch of the autonomic nervous system to keep them safe. The sympathetic branch comes in handy dealing with the challenges of life.

TOP DOWN AND BOTTOM UP

It is often helpful to introduce information about stress by describing how all species have similar self-protective mechanisms. All animals, down to the most primitive, possess an alert system that keeps them safe while allowing them to stay engaged in the world to thrive. Humans are no exception. Our alarm system just happens to be more elaborate thanks to an enlarged cortex, especially the prefrontal cortex (PFC).

Of course, it is easy to tell clients that they have the capacity to shut off anxiety; actually shutting off that anxiety is more difficult. In fact, mental health professionals have described different, seemingly contradictory, aspects of the alarm system for over a century. One of the first to weigh in was the founder of American psychology, William James, who argued that stress is bottom up. In a paraphrase of the theory he said, "My hands are shaking; I must be nervous." This perspective became known as the James-Lange theory of emotion. Objecting to that perspective, James's student Walter Cannon stated that stress and anxiety are determined "top down," as decided by the mind. Cannon went on to propose that all living organisms maintain health by a process of homeostasis, essentially balancing high and low arousal. When extremely stressed, organisms can react with a fight-or-flight response to danger.

Since many clients have heard about the fight-or-flight response, you can use the concept to help them put in perspective what is actually worthy of fight or flight and what is really dangerous. Trauma researchers examining extreme stress have identified two other responses: freeze and paralysis. Freezing ranges from the deer-in-the-headlights reaction all the way to catatonia. When stress is severe, people's muscles stiffen, as if they are preparing for a mortal blow. This has been described as being "scared stiff," involving tonic immobility.

When people feel that death is imminent, they may collapse, frozen in fear. Collapsing, going numb, and being immobilized euphemistically has been called "playing possum." Since most predators, such as mountain lions, abandon motionless, seemingly dead animals, especially if they emit a putrid odor, this tactic is a hardwired last-ditch defensive instinct. During the period of immobility, the captured animal is amnestied briefly in a coma-like state by endogenous opiates in preparation for pain relief if it were to be torn apart by the predator. The lion may even drag the limp and paralyzed prey back to the den, then go fetch cubs to share in the feast. During that unguarded moment, the captured animal awakens from the stupor, shakes or twitches, then bolts in a hasty escape. Similarly, people who were deeply traumatized and had used paralysis as a last-ditch defensive system may twitch and shake in a state of frantic agitation during the early therapeutic recovery phase (Levine, 2010). Thus, they emerge from the immobility stage of defense, which may include dissociation, into the fight-or-flight phase.

CLIENT EDUCATION

Like all other species, you have an emergency response system that is available when you encounter true danger. Since most situations do not require that you fight or take flight, your job is to keep your emergency response system handy for only those times you really need it for real danger.

How the stress system can be hijacked by top-down processes and transformed into anxiety was illustrated by social psychologists who demonstrated that the social context frames and defines what is stressful. The researchers showed that people search the environment for cues to label and interpret unexplained physiological arousal (Schacter & Singer, 1962). In Schacter and Singer's now-classic experiment, subjects were first given an injection of epinephrine (adrenaline) to promote arousal. Then they were put into a social situation with a happy or sad "accomplice" who influenced the subjective appraisal of the situation, with a happy response or anxious behavior, which influenced the subject's top-down response. Using a large body of facial expression research, Paul Ekman provided support for William James and his bottom-up perspective. By asking subjects to move their facial muscles, he demonstrated that changes in emotions occur in a bidirectional flow of information among the mind, brain, and face. For example, subjects felt happy when they smiled and felt sad when they frowned.

In a similar study, subjects were asked to hold a pencil in their teeth, which simulated a smile, or to hold a pencil by their lips, simulating a frown. After 1 hour, the first group reported happy memories while the second group reported sad memories.

Accordingly, when a client asks, "What do you want me to do, go to that party and put on a happy face?" I respond by saying "That's a great idea. Yes!" Even without knowledge of neuroscience, people in 12-step programs recommend that members fake it until they make it.

CLIENT EDUCATION

Behaving as if you are happy or sad will make you feel that you are happy or sad.

The psychodynamic and emotionally focused therapies adopted the bottom-up version of stress theories. Cognitive-behavioral therapy (CBT) and, recently in the United Kingdom, cognitive bias modification, have offered the top-down approach. Taken altogether, these research and theoretical paradigms illustrate that neither the top-down nor the bottom-up perspective offers an exclusive and complete explanation for the development of anxiety or how to shut it off. A brain-based therapy approach to neutralize stress should orchestrate both bottom-up and top-down neural networks.

To put the bottom-up network into perspective, it is useful to introduce the amygdala. It plays a key role in generating the emotion required to transform stress into anxiety. Clients may be interested to know they actually have two amygdalae deep within their right and left temporal lobes. The cluster of neurons was named the amygdala in 1820, because the neuroanatomist who first identified it thought it looked like an almond. Derived from the Greek word *amydale* for "almond," it was later Latinized to the "amygdala."

The amygdala serves many functions. Primary among them is the generation of emotion. Although the amygdala it is not the only part of the brain associated with emotion, it is key to understand how, under certain circumstances, stress can transform into anxiety. The amygdala in general is a relevance detector, letting clients know if anything in the environment is relevant to them. As a sort of smoke detector, it alerts clients when there is danger ahead. If clients suffer from anxiety, their amygdala has been conditioned to signal danger when there is none.

CLIENT EDUCATION

The smoke detector function of your amygdala need not be stuck in the on position. You can turn it off through its connections with the orbitofrontal cortex, which you can train to tell your amygdala there is no danger when there is none.

Because the amygdala governs the emotion-based implicit memory system, clients should know that they can feel fear without knowing why. The amygdala can be trained to dampen down its implicit fear response.

NEUROSCIENCE

Individual differences in amygdala activation have been investigated, including the underlying cellular and molecular mechanisms. In particular, genetic systems have been noted to have variance at the molecular level that relates to variance in amygdala function. Specifically, variation in the serotonin transporter gene (5-HTT) and in the tryptophan hydroxylase gene have been noted to influence variation in amygdala activity. 5-HTT influences the transport of serotonin from the synaptic cleft. 5-HTT has a common variation in the central transcription region that results in either the short (S) or the long (L) variant (or allele). Since each person carries two alleles of any gene (inherited from each parent), there are three 5-HTT categories of individuals: those with two long alleles (L/L), those with two short alleles (S/S), and those with one of each (S/L) (Canli, 2009). Individuals carrying either one or two copies of the short allele group (S/L or S/S, referred to as the S group) scored higher in self-reported neuroticism than individuals in the L/L or L group (Lesch et al., 1996). These variations have been associated with variations in amygdala activation. Whereas activation in the S group is significantly greater than for the L group, the S group is characterized by elevated amygdala resting activation and amplified by life stress experiences (Canli, 2009).

Variation in the tryptophan hydroxylase-2 (TPH2) gene was also found to modulate amygdala processing of emotional stimuli, regardless of valence. Carriers of the TPH2 allele tend to have more amygdala activity in response to happy, fearful, and sad faces when compared to neutral faces (Canli, 2009).

Learning that the OFC and amygdala work together to ramp up or tone down stress can motivate clients to work with you to train their OFCs to calm the amygdala when there is no realistic danger. Knowing that the feelings of anxiety represent a hijacking of the stress system offers clients a tangible explanation for what is occurring and a reason to be motivated to work on mastering the ability to turn it off.

One way to explain how bottom-up and top-down stress reactions can transform into anxiety is by describing the two tracks to the amygdala, the fast track and the slow track. I often tell people who overreact to stress and have developed an autostress disorder that their fast track is on too often while their slow track hardly works. Here is what happens: Let's say I'm hiking down a trail in the Grand Canyon, and I detect in my peripheral vision a long, slender object. My retina signals my thalamus, which is positioned in the middle of my brain and functions as sort of a central switchboard, to signal my amygdala directly. In this scenario I "feel" *snake* before I "think" *snake*. In other words, I "feel" very anxious but I don't know why.

In the slow-track scenario, my retina detects a long slender object, then signals my thalamus, which sends that information to my cortex (the center of thinking), and I think, "Oh, there's a long stick that looks very much like a snake, but it's not." In this slow-track case, the reality testing works well to calm me down when I do not need to get into a fight-or-flight mode. If the object actually were a snake, my cortex can tell me there is no danger because the snake is a safe distance away. Of course, even the slow track can be faulty, as would be the case if the snake was very close and coiled, ready to strike. To take this scenario one more ridiculous step, my cortex decides that it is a friendly rattlesnake and that I can sit down next to it so that I can pet its head. In this case, not only is my cortex not doing its job, but my amygdala is not signaling enough danger.

CLIENT EDUCATION

If you experience surges of anxiety, the fast track to your amygdala is on too often and your slow track needs to speed up. We can work together to slow down your fast track and speed up your slow track.

The tracks going up from the amygdala to the orbitofrontal cortex (OFC) are stronger than those going down from the OFC to the amygdala. There are plenty of good reasons for this disparity; first among them is that it is better to be safe than sorry. Because the nerve fibers going up are stronger than those going down, true danger has precedence over any other situation. Clients can benefit by learning that if the track going down from the OFC to the amygdala is abnormally weak and not well exercised, their ability to distinguish what is really dangerous from what just feels like danger can cause a needless stress reaction and promote an anxiety disorder. This scenario amounts to feeling danger without verifying it, which is not based on sufficient reality testing and is essentially mindless. This lack of realistic thought provided by an abnormally weakened slow track underlies much of the problem for those suffering from anxiety disorders.

Also important to point out is that the amygdala can hijack not only the OFC but the rest of the PFC. In this case, the entire PFC will conjure up all sorts of semiplausible reasons why clients feel fear. They may even tell themselves that feelings are wiser than thoughts or "since I feel anxious, there must be a good reason for the anxious feelings." Perhaps they may think of themselves as especially intuitive and regard the anxious feelings as premonitions that something bad is about to happen. I am not arguing that we should tell clients that intuition is impossible. But if clients suffer from excessive stress and even anxiety without identifiable stressors, those feelings probably are not intuition but signs of an autostress disorder.

You can explain that the problem with most anxiety disorders is that when the amygdala is overactive and not monitored and calmed by the PFC, the anxious feelings can fuel anxious thoughts. Heightened and unchecked amygdala activity tends to increase anxiety symptom severity.

CLIENT EDUCATION

When you feel anxiety without any apparent danger, your amygdala needs to be put in check by the more advanced part of your brain called the prefrontal cortex.

NEUROSCIENCE

Consistent with the concept of affect asymmetry, the more activity there is in the right amygdala, the more anxiety and more anxious memories there are. In contrast, more activity in the left amygdala is associated with less anxiety and more positive memories.

Teaching clients about the stress systems and how anxiety can develop should also involve a description of both branches of the autonomic nervous system, the sympathetic and parasympathetic. When the sympathetic branch activates, the parasympathetic branch relaxes. So far in this chapter we have focused on various aspects of the sympathetic branch of the autonomic nervous system. The parasympathetic branch provides the counterbalance to the sympathetic branch, offering an opportunity to recoup energy to deal effectively with stress later by saving the body and brain from wear and tear. In clients who self-generate stress into anxiety disorders, the parasympathetic branch of the autonomic nervous system needs bolstering.

Clients are often fascinated to learn that the ability to calm down during or after a stressful situation is connected with both the social brain networks and the parasympathetic system. Helping clients access their parasympathetic nervous systems not only helps them lower anxiety but also helps them increase social skills. Most clients understand that feeling calm in social situations is important, but few understand that the parasympathetic nervous system is connected to the social brain.

NEUROSCIENCE

The vagal nerve system provides much of the neurological basis for the parasympathetic nervous system (Porges, 2011). The vagus complex is not a single nerve but a system with many branches. Two general routes of the vagus include the dorsal vagal complex and the ventral vagal complex. The dorsal vagal complex begins in the brain stem and sends axons down into the abdominal organs, including the heart. The ventral vagal complex extends from the nucleus ambiguos. The ventral system is faster than the dorsal system, in part because its nerve fibers are covered with myelin to increase conductivity. The vagus comes down from the 10th cranial nerve area, extending to many of the organs in the thoracic cavity, including the heart. Humans possess a much more elaborate vagal nerve system than other species. The so-called smart vagus nerve is myelinated and found only in humans (Porges, 2011). This expanded and highly efficient vagus nerve allows humans to use the parasympathetic nervous system to calm down.

When describing the parasympathetic nerve system to clients, you may note that variations in vagal tone correspond to how well clients can calm themselves down during or after a period of high stress. Higher vagal tone provides better self-soothing capacity, more reliable autonomic responses, and a greater range and control of emotional states than low vagal tone. Secure attachment is correlated with higher vagal tone. As explained in Chapter 3, the better the early relationships, the greater the chance of enhanced affect regulation. Lower vagal tone correlates with anxiety and impulse control problems, hyperactivity, attention deficit and distractibility, and irritability as well as insecure attachment styles. The vagal brake serves as a mechanism to slow heartbeat. When clients' vagal brake is off, there is an increase in heart rate and they feel like they are in a constant state of emergency.

The myelinated vagus nerve has been called the social engagement system because nerves enervate the lower facial muscles so that changes in the activity of the organs in the thoracic cavity are reflected in the face. For example, if clients' hearts race, their faces will reflect the discomfort. The bidirectional relationship between the face and the brain is echoed in the brain and the organs. If clients smile, they will feel more relaxed. In a social context, if another person smiles or glares at clients, their vagal system will respond by engaging or disengaging the parasympathetic system.

The neurochemistry involved in the feeling of comfort includes the neurohormone oxytocin, which has receptor sites on the vagus. Until recently, it was assumed that oxytocin was relevant only to women during childbirth. It turns out that both women and men utilize oxytocin as a means to increase comfort and enhance bonding by activating the parasympathetic nervous system.

The oxytocin effect occurs not only through physical touch but also through proximity. The release of oxytocin can occur even when people talk on the phone with someone they love. For example, oxytocin levels were taken of college freshman girls before and after they called their mothers. After the call their oxytocin levels shot up, and they reported that their stress levels were down.

If vagal brakes of clients are weak, their alarm response can be sustained well after encountering stress, resulting in elevated epinephrine and cortisol over many days. In such situations, they experience stress overload when the stress demands exceed the gains from rest and recuperation (McEwen & Chattarji, 2007). In other words, chronic stress occurs when clients go beyond their limits.

To discuss how to manage stress so that it does not transform into an autostress disorder, we must address the term "stress" itself, because it fails to describe the dynamic nature of challenges to client experiences. The mid-20th-century researcher Hans Selye initially popularized the term "stress," adopting it from engineering, where it was used to describe such things as how much weight (i.e., stress) a bridge can bear before collapsing. It has become popularized to mean that everyone should strive for a "stress-free" life, which is impossible, and for that matter boring.

The old fight-or-flight model and the term "stress" have been updated. The new model, referred to as allostasis, describes the ebbs and flows of stress and challenges of daily life and achieving stability through change (McEwen & Chattarji, 2007). Many systems promote allostatic adjustments. The brain structure that plays a major role in maintaining allostatic adjustments is the hypothalamus, a word that means "below the thalamus." Although the hypo-thalamus is a relatively small structure, it is very much like "Alice's Restaurant" from the Arlo Guthrie song: You can "get everything you want" there. For this reason, many brain systems try to influence the hypothalamus. It turns on the parasympathetic (relaxation) circuits and the sympathetic (stress) circuits. Many popular lectures on the brain note that the hypothalamus can trigger the 3 Fs: fight, flight, and f___ (sex).

NEUROSCIENCE

Allostatic adjustments are made by the brain and the rest of the body to deal with daily challenges. These adjustments occur through regulation of neurochemicals, such as cortisol, to help orchestrate adjustments by enhancing or inhibiting gene transcription, regulating brain-derived neurotrophic factor (BDNF), up-regulating amygdala activity, and targeting prefrontal systems involved in stress and the emotions (Sullivan & Gratton, 2002).

Allostasis is the process of adaptation that regulates levels of epinephrine (adrenaline) and cortisol to promote adaptation to short-term stressors. However, if the alarm response is sustained and results in elevated epinephrine and cortisol over many days, the allostatic state breaks down and leads to allostatic load. Allostatic load conceptually replaces Selye's exhaustion phase. With allostatic load, there is significant wear and tear on the body. It potentially leads to the acceleration of atherosclerosis, abdominal obesity, loss of minerals from the bones, immunosuppression, elevated blood sugar levels, as well as atrophy and damage to the brain, especially the hippocampus.

CLIENT EDUCATION

Just as your car has shock absorbers that enable you to drive on a bumpy road, so too can you develop the ability to adapt to the challenges that you encounter daily.

Mental health is not a static state. Rather, it involves adjustments, adapta-tions, mood wings—life changes, and so do we. The capacity for resiliency, there-fore, can be understood as dynamic equilibrium between the activation of the sympathetic and parasympathetic branches. We can be aroused one moment, stressed at another moment, and recoup later. Optimally the systems of allostasis balance each other in dynamic equilibrium. Resilience is dependent on the person's dynamic equilibrium, his or her ability to shift state as the situation demands.

Although ramped-up and extended stress contributes to allostatic load and to autostress disorders, making it difficult to concentrate, mild to moderate stress actually can help people stay alert and focused. Moderate and fluctuating levels of cortisol energize people to engage in the challenge at hand. Sustained and escalating stress ramps up levels of norepinephrine (NE). The combination of high levels of cortisol, corticotropin-releasing hormone (CRH), and NE further overactivates the amygdala, which can interfere with prefrontal brain areas, making attention and working memory falter (Chajut & Algom, 2003).

Enjoying a safe and stimulating life requires that clients know the difference among healthy, mild, and intermittent stress, which alerts them to challenges and unhealthy anxiety that plagues them for no practical reason. Realistically, it makes no sense to help clients try to achieve stress-free lives. The stress system, like the immune system, is a necessity, as it keeps us safe and healthy. If, however, clients suffer from chronic stress when there is no practical reason for it, you can suggest that the goal is for them to transform the stress system back into a realistic alarm system that keeps them truly safe while allowing them to durably engage in the world.

NEUROSCIENCE

Research that involves inducing mild doses of stress appear to result in subsequent stress resilience. For example, rat pups and young squirrel monkeys were separated from their mothers periodically. Upon their return, they were able to deal with stress better whether they received increased maternal attention or not (Parker et al., 2006).

A graphic way to explain how a healthy allostatic system kicks into gear would be to describe how a person may respond in a life-threatening situation. Consider the case of a woman who was in a relaxed mood in a shopping mall, looking over books on display. Then a crazed man with an automatic assault weapon rushes in, yelling obscenities. The woman's amygdala and the rest of her emergency response system jumps into action, resulting in the release of a wide range of neurochemicals. Through the amygdala's direct connections with the locus coeruleus (LC) the release of NE triggers brain systems to maximum alert. Activity in the right PFC (R-PFC) increases, promoting avoidance and withdrawal behaviors.

The amygdala's rich connections with the hypothalamus promotes the release of CRH to activate a range of alarms, including signaling the pituitary gland to release adrenocorticotropic hormone (ACTH). ACTH bursts into the bloodstream and reaches the adrenal glands, where it triggers the release of adrenaline (epinephrine). Adrenaline acts to ensure that available glucose is used for fuel to take flight or to fight. Meanwhile, the woman's cortex assesses the situation and determines that fighting would be suicide, so she looks for someplace to hide. Her adrenals also release cortisol to further ramp up her stress system. If the horrific situation continues, the woman's adrenal glands continue to release cortisol by making use of any available stores of glucose, even from fat cells, to ensure that her body gets all the energy it needs. Cortisol also ensures that other activating neurotransmitters are released to deal with the challenge of protecting herself. This part of the stress system represents his HPA axis in action.

If the guy with the assault rifle is still rampaging around, CRH triggers the amygdala to ramp up activity while also triggering the locus coeruleus to release even more norepinephrine. CRH also acts as a hyperactivating neurotransmitter. In fact, there has been a considerable amount of recent research on CRH due to its involvement in agitated depression as well as anxiety disorders.

NEUROSCIENCE

The role of CRF in depression has gained considerable attention because elevated levels of CRF have long been found in depressed patients; the cerebrospinal fluid of depressed suicide victims also shows elevated CRF concentrations (Arato et al., 1989). It is therefore no wonder that big pharma is actively developing drugs that target CRF.

There are two CRF receptor subtypes, CRF1 and CRF2, which have distinct neuroatomic characteristics and receptor pharmacology. The CRF1 subtype reportedly plays a central role in mediating depressive and anxious behaviors. Pharmacological research has shown that compounds that block this receptor may possess antidepressant and anxiolytic effects (Zobel et al., 2000).

Hypersecretion of CRF early in life, due to maternal deprivation or severe stress, may result in an altered set point for activity of the CRF neurons and the HPA axis. These changes contribute to an overreaction to stress during adulthood as well as subsequent depression (Newport, Stowe, & Nemeroff, 2002).

Throughout the horrific shopping mall ordeal, the woman's PFC had been trying to decide how to make sure that she can remain safe. Depending on how well it does its job, it will make decisions about what to do about the situation. Some decisions are smart while others are not so smart. The smart decisions involve the activity of both the left PFC (L-PFC) and the R-PFC. The not-so-smart decisions involve just the R-PFC. As a result of total avoidance, the woman's amygdala is overactivated. In this case, she may decide to avoid taking any kind of action, despite the fact that it may be smart to take action. But what if people are rushing to safety during a window of time when the gunman is in another area? The L-PFC–generated smart thing to do would be to flee to safety.

Allostatic Load

Chronic stress cranks up the same stress circuits that are activated during a trau-matic situation, but over an extended period. Highly stressed clients often have a difficult time understanding why they suffer a wide variety of physical problems. Cortisol acts to shut down many body functions, such as digestion, immune func-tions, sexual systems, and metabolism, that are not related to putting the entire body onto maximum alert. During allostatic load, cortisol acts to raise levels of adrenaline, NE, and cholesterol and to increase blood pressure and heart rate (McEwen & Stellar, 1993). When prolonged, the increased cortisol, epineph-rine, and NE can contribute to cardiovascular problems, including increased heart rate and blood pressure and damage to the inner surface of the heart. Blood vessels tend to constrict, and the heart's rhythm can decrease in variability, increasing the risk of sudden heart attack and possibly death. All of these corro-sive effects on the heart vindicate J. M. DeCosta's description of health-related effects of trauma incurred during the Civil War, which he dubbed "soldier's heart." He argued that the actual physical ill effects on the heart were not just a metaphor (DeCosta, 1871).

Excessive cortisol has a corrosive effect on many areas of the body. For example, women who have been chronically depressed also have been found to have high levels of cortisol and decreased bone mineral density (Michelsen et al., 1996). Cortisol can shut down the reproductive system, affecting both sexual perfor-mance and reproduction. These detrimental effects are all too common to young couples struggling to begin careers while simultaneously attempting to start a family.

During stress, cortisol acts to:

- Increase heart rate.
- Increase blood pressure.
- Constrict blood vessels.
- Decrease heart rate variability (upping the risk of sudden death)
- Increase cholesterol.
- Increase epinephrine.
- Increase NE.

Chronic stress, including chronic depression, leads to a wide range of changes to neurotransmitters and neurohormones involved in the stress response that work with each other synergistically. Chronically high cortisol in the PFC augments catecholamines by blockading their reuptake, so that clients stay on alert for more negative experiences. Also, because high levels of cortisol further activate the amygdala, clients tend to be more alert to any sign of new threats. With less PFC activity, clients are even less able to inhibit amygdala overactivity, so their working memories are inhibited (Rovzendaal et al., 2004).

The combination of many factors can impair the PFC and its ability to inhibit anxiety; these include: low serotonin, which leads to a reduction of the ability of the OFC to inhibit amygdala overactivation; elevation of NE through activation of the adrenoreceptors receptors; and increases in cortisol and its interactions with catecholamines. These factors ramp up anxiety by unleashing the amygdala and further releasing NE through the LC and dopamine (DA) via the ventral tegmental area, as well as acetylcholine via the dorsolateral tegmental nucleus to further dampen the PFC's capacity for problem solving and rational behavior. Consequently, clients are prone to heightened startle responses, vigilance, insomnia, flashbacks, intrusive memories, and an increase of further fear conditioning.

Whereas high stress and associated anxiety make it difficult to concentrate, mild to moderate stress actually can help clients stay alert and focused. Healthy levels of cortisol energize people to engage in the challenge at hand. Sustained and escalating stress, however, kicks in another neural system that secretes high levels of NE. The combination of high levels of cortisol and NE activates the amygdala and interferes with the prefrontal areas, especially the L-PFC, making affect regulation, attention, and working memory falter (Chajut & Algom, 2003).

CLIENT EDUCATION

Chronic stress has temporarily changed your brain chemistry so that your negative experiences are amplified. Also, a hyperactive amygdala can hijack your prefrontal cortex to narrow your attention to potential danger. This makes positive experiences that are unrelated to threat fade out of focus. These are all the symptoms of chronic stress, not signs of danger ahead. Let's work together so that you can regain control.

Since the early 1990s, considerable attention has been devoted to the neurophysiological consequences of chronic stress, trauma, and PTSD. The initial research was done with rats and baboons. With the new brain imaging tools available, the studies moved to humans. The long-term effects of stress can contribute to multiple destructive effects to the brain. Essential fatty acids form a significant part of the brain, and stress can have a destructive effect on them, including inadequate replacement of lost fatty acids and destruction (rancidity) of long-chain fatty acids. Depletion of long-chain fatty acids in the brain contributes to depression (Hibbeln & Salem, 1995).

NEUROSCIENCE

High levels of cortisol can also increase the toxic effects of glutamate, the principal activating neurotransmitter. While moderately elevated glutamate is optimum for neuroplasticity, there is a corresponding decrease in the amount of glutamate necessary to make the next transmission, which lowers the threshold and strengthens the connection (long-term potentiation LTP) via a glutamate receptor called N-methyl-D-aspartate (NMDA). Chronic stress raises glutamate levels too high, which overactivates the NMDA receptors, letting in too much calcium, which generates free radicals. A syndrome called excitotoxicity results, which results in cell damage.

It is well established that traumatic as well as chronic stress ramps up the neurochemistry necessary to keep people hypervigilant to prepare for a repeat of the threat. The continued heightened level of stress-related neurochemistry leads to a syndrome referred to as the stress cortisol cascade, in which excessive cortisol and other neurotransmitters, such as NE, are produced. Excessive cortisol causes dendrites in the hippocampus to shrivel up (Sapolsky, 2003).

Meanwhile, the excessive and prolonged rise in the level of cortisol leads to heightened hyperreactivity of the amygdala. Normally, with periodic and moderate levels of cortisol, the hippocampus plays a role in turning off the HPA axis, much like a thermostat acts as a negative feedback mechanism to turn off the heat. Excessive and prolonged levels of cortisol lead to even more cortisol release, damaging the hippocampus. Because of the elevated levels of cortisol, clients who have experienced chronic stress or depression may have smaller hippocampi than other clients (Bremner et al., 1999). With the thermostat function broken, clients will be less able to turn off the stress response. And with the corresponding feed-forward amygdala activity, clients tend to be hypervigilant. This combination of the inability to turn off the stress response coupled with the ramping up of stress reactivity puts clients in unbearable and confusing stressful situations. Additionally, because the hippocampus functions as a key part of the explicit memory system, clients' ability to remember insights derived from sessions may be compromised.

NEUROSCIENCE

A 20-year assessment of the neuropathological consequences of stress indicated that the greater the perceived stress, the smaller the volume of the hippocampus (Gianaros et al., 2007). Whereas hippocampal volume decreases after years of depression, amygdala volume has been reported to increase after the first depressive episode (Frodl et al., 2003; MacQueen et al., 2003).

CLIENT EDUCATION

Although the thermostat function in your brain may be impaired, we will work together to rebuild it so that you will no longer react to normal situations as if they are dangerous and so you can turn off your stress response system when it is not needed.

NEUROSCIENCE

The stress cortisol cascade syndrome is associated with a range of brain deficits, including increased blood flow in the amygdala, reflecting its overactivity. The PFC, which normally can inhibit amygdala overactivity, appears to lose volume; there is evidence of reduced gray matter volume in the medial PFC (mPFC); (Carrion et al., 2001; Pissiota et al., 2000). The decrease in gray matter in the ACC is associated with reduced neurointegration and reduced cortical volume (DeBellis, Keshavan, Spencer, & Hall, 2002).

Hippocampal function becomes impaired due to a combination of high levels of cortisol, excitotoxicity, and/or blocking of neurogenesis. These reductions in hippocampal volume have been reported in clients with combat-related PTSD (Bremner et al., 1995) and in those with PTSD related to childhood physical and sexual abuse (Bremner et al., 1997). These impairments result in inadequate top-down inhibition of the amygdala. With the increased amygdala activation, there is a corresponding increase in a general response for false positives for threats.

Chronic stress has been correlated not only with HPA axis hyperactivation but also with its hypoactivation (Charmandari, Tsigos, & Chrousos, 2005; Chrousos, 1995). These deceptively contradictory findings have been the focus of considerable inquiry. Normally, there are variations in catecholamine, cortisol, and CRH levels. Hypersecretion of CRH and cortisol has been associated with melancholic depression

(continued)

(continued)

> (Gold, Gabry, Yasuda, & Chrousos, 2002). A wide spectrum of conditions, including panic disorder, obsessive-compulsive disorder (OCD), anorexia nervosa, and alcoholism, has been associated with increased and prolonged activation of the HPA axis (Charmandari et al., 2005). Hypoactivation of the stress system, including chronically reduced CRH secretion, may result in fibromyalgia and chronic fatigue syndrome.

Helping clients tone down the stress response system involves orchestrating activity in neural circuits that are underactive in order to modulate fear. Moderating stress should include the hippocampus with its projections to the ventromedial PFC that inhibit amygdala activity, so that emotions are expressed in the appropriate context (Phelps, 2009). The dorsolateral PFC (DLPFC) also needs to be involved in the effortful manipulation, or interpretation, of the anxiety-provoking situations that are encountered.

Given that anxiety disorders are associated with an overactivation of the R-PFC, with hyperactivity in the amygdala and an underactivation of the L-PFC, fears add to a feeling of timelessness, with all thoughts tumbled together in one overwhelming gestalt. The trauma feels like it is happening now, leading to further kindling and the potential for further flashbacks. Failure to inhibit anxiety by action generated by the L-PFC ramps up the stress response system.

CLIENT EDUCATION

> You may be not only frightened but confused by your tendency to overreact to normal experiences with intense anxiety. Although your stress response circuits are set too high, they can be reset to turn on when they are really needed. Rewiring your stress response system will take a little time and effort, but after our work together, through a period of discomfort your needless anxiety will subside.

To motivate clients to work with you to reset their emergency response system, tell them that being in a constant state of alert can be taxing to their entire bodies, including the brain. Prolonged high levels of cortisol can be damaging to the brain, because there are many cortisol receptors on the hippocampus. If the stress is chronic or extreme, the high levels of cortisol may have shrunk some of the dendrites in the hippocampus. As a consequence, clients' explicit memory skills may falter while their implicit memory may be exaggerated, making them feel anxious much of the time. You can work together to tone down clients' alarm systems so that there is a moderate level of cortisol or even brief elevated levels function like a thermostat, turning off cortisol release.

You can encourage clients to do a variety of things to turn off the excess cortisol levels. All of the SEEDS factors described in Chapter 2 will help lower stress. For example, engaging in aerobic exercise in the late afternoon or early evening will help burn off excess cortisol and also raise gamma-aminobutyric acid (GABA) levels so that clients will be more relaxed and sleep will be deeper.

Patterns of dysregulation correspond as to whether the stressor has passed or is still present. The more time that elapses since the stress first emerged, the lower a person's morning cortisol, daily volume of cortisol, ACTH, and post-examethason cortisol. When chronic stressors are still present in the environment, morning, afternoon/evening, and daily cortisol output is significantly higher.

If stress involves being physically threatened, there tends to be a higher and flat cortisol output. Although morning cortisol can be lower, afternoon/evening overall output is higher. If the stress is of a social nature, such as divorce, the overall cortisol output is higher in the morning, afternoon, and evening. Some studies have shown that initial low urinary cortisol concentrations immediately after the trauma predict subsequent PTSD diagnosis in adults (Delahanty et al., 2000; Yehuda, Resnick, Schmeidler, Yang, & Pitman, 1998).

NEUROSCIENCE

Increases in CRH target the LC, the principal part of the brain that releases NE, which plays many roles in stress, including further activating the amygdala. In fact, CRH itself targets the amygdala during extreme allostatic load, especially when the pituitary shuts down due to too much CRH. Pituitary volumes have been reported to be higher in pubertal/postpubertal posttraumatic stress disorder (PTSD) patients (Thomas & DeBellis, 2004). The HPA axis can shut down the release of cortisol; however, the traumatized individual remains hyperalert to the possibility of more danger. For example, after prolonged and extreme stress there can be adaptive down-regulation of CRH receptors in the anterior pituitary so that there is not too much cortisol floating around (Bremner et al., 1997).

Hypersecretion of CRH by the hypothalamus may lead to a down-regulation of CRH receptors in the anterior pituitary (Bremner et al., 1997). The down-regulation of CRH may be adaptive in response to pituitary hypertrophy because during extended and/or severe trauma elevated CRH would result in higher cortisol levels and damage to multiple systems, including the hippocampus. This stress mechanism, therefore, involves a feedback system that is an attempt to put on the brakes. But it is not without adverse consequences. Pituitary volumes have been found to be significantly larger in pubertal/postpubertal children with PTSD than children without PTSD (Thomas & DeBellis, 2004). The duration of the abuse correlates negatively with pituitary volume.

The process known as priming or sensitization occurs when repeated stress increases in magnitude and the compensatory adaptation of the amygdala-HPA axis occurs long after trauma so that ACTH and cortisol are set at lower 24-hour levels. Meanwhile, hormones such as arginine, vasopressin, and the catecholamines act synergistically with CRH to increase the stress response. When people experience a new emotional stressor, the amygdala-HPA axis responds through even higher ACTH levels, making this primed system hyper-respond to stress (see DeBellis, Hooper, & Sapia, 2005, for a review).

The interaction between the noradrenergic system and CRH results in dys-regulation of serotonin and increases the risk of comorbid depression. Therefore, people suffering from PTSD are at risk for developing a major depression. In fact, the onset of major depression is significantly increased for people who have been traumatized compared to those who are not exposed (Breslau et al., 2001).

Psychoneuroimmunological Interface

One of the most exciting areas in healthcare is psychoneuroimmunology, the study of the intersection of the mind, brain, and immune system. From a psycho-neuroimmunological perspective there are a wide variety of ways that allostatic load can wear the body down and lead to a systemic breakdown of the ability to recoup resources. For example, high levels of cortisol in the evening impair sleep. Sleep deprivation ramps up even more cortisol and glucose the next day and evening. This leads to a drop in vagal tone and, correspondingly, less para-sympathetic and more sympathetic nervous system activity. R-PFC overactivity leads to a drop in natural killer cell activity, resulting in an impaired immune system.

Vince Fellitti, a primary care physician in Kaiser Permanente, examined the health and social effects of adverse childhood experiences (ACEs) throughout the life span of 17,421 members of the Kaiser Health Plan in San Diego County (Fellitti et al., 1998). The ACEs included: childhood abuse and neglect; growing up with domestic violence, substance abuse, or mental illness in the home; parental discord; or crime.

Since many people with chronic health problems may have multiple health problems, the study was meant to explore the long-term health consequences of ACEs. Psychologists have long debated why people who experience ACEs may be driven to perpetuate conflict. The traditional explanation emphasizes that people model what they learned from family members who engaged in constant conflict. The brain-based explanation that underlies this tendency describes how people who experienced ACEs respond to stressful situations with excessive cortisol. (Marinelli & Piazza, 2002). In some people who experienced ACEs, social stressors produce the odd mix of elevations in both DA and cortisol (Pruessner, Champagne, Meaney, & Dagher, 2004). These dynamics reflect the seemingly contradictory mix of stress and anticipated enjoyment. This ramping up of cortisol for the cheap thrill of DA only serves to add to allostatic load.

Other measures of the mind–body breakdown in people who experience ACEs include high blood pressure, which leads to a host of cardiovascular problems. Also, people with ACEs have high blood cholesterol, glycosylated hemoglobin, higher cortisol, and higher NE in overnight urine. From this perspective, we can see how allostatic load can potentiate many health problems, including type 2 diabetes. The stress alarm system involves the stimulation of the adrenergic receptors at the blood vessels, which leads to an increased uptake of glucose and a corresponding increased energy metabolism. Stimulation of adrenergic receptors in a type of glial cell called astrocytes triggers the release of glucose that the astrocytes had been storing. Cortisol acts to up-regulate the amount of glucose people have available to deal with challenges, but instead of using the extra fuel to fight or flee, clients implode.

High-stress situations put the alarm on for the entire body, signaling that cells need more glucose for fuel to deal with increased demands. Chronically high levels of cortisol have been associated with dampening the effects of insulin and have been seen as a risk factor for type 2 diabetes (Konen, Keltikaga-Jarinen, Addercreutz, & Hautenen, 1996). Insulin's principal job is to manage glucose levels so that cells can receive optimum levels of fuel. This works fine when the stress is short-lived. But in high-stress situations that are extended or chronic, the endocrinological and stress systems begin to break down.

Even down to the genetic level, high stress activates genes in cells to increase glucose uptake. High levels of adrenaline and cortisol also raise blood glucose by triggering the liver to convert protein to glucose. The resulting excessive level of cortisol contributes to excessive glucose and receptors that become resistant to the effects of insulin. Thus, high levels of cortisol increase the risk of insulin resistance and type 2 diabetes.

The mediators of allostasis operate as a nonlinear network with reciprocal regulation by each mediator (McEwen, 2012). The dysregulation of this network through stress and trauma leads to a systemic breakdown (allostatic load). While sympathetic activity increases proinflammatory cytokine production, parasympathetic activity is anti-inflammatory (Bierhaus et al., 2003; Borovikova et al., 2000). These nonlinear interactions also occur in the renin-angiotensin system, a hormone system that regulates blood pressure and water balance and plays a role in promoting proinflammatory responses and elevated blood pressure (Saavedra, Benicky, & Zhou, 2006).

NEUROSCIENCE

It has long been known that there exists a negative feedback loop between the activation of cortisol and the dose-dependent conditions in which glucocorticoids have proinflammatory effects (Sorrells & Sapolsky, 2007). Glucocorticoid resistance is a condition that occurs in proinflammatory states as well as depression (Raison, Capuron, & Miller, 2006).

Cytokine proteins are involved in communication between immune cells and exert far-reaching effects throughout the body and the brain. They have multiple functions, including a role in inflammatory immune responses. Inflammation is a vital response to infection or injury, but chronic or excessive inflammation contributes to significant impairments throughout the body and certainly the brain. Excessive anti-inflammatory control can lead to increased risk for infection and illness, and chronic inflammation has been associated with serious medical conditions, including type 2 diabetes, cardiovascular disease, arthritis, inflammatory bowel disease, and dementia.

As some cytokines have pro and others have anti-inflammatory characteristics, they are generally classified as either pro or anti-inflammatory. The proinflammatory cytokines include interleukin (IL)-6, IL-1, and tumor necrosis factor. Anti-inflammatory cytokines include IL-10, which acts as a regulator of the immune response, in part by inhibiting the production of proinflammatory cytokines (Parham, 2005).

Proinflammatory cytokines rise in response to acute stressors, including public speaking or even mental arithmetic (Brydon et al., 2004). Circulating IL-6 and IL-1 cytokines have been noted to increase up to 2 hours after completing complex cognitive tasks (Steptoe, Willemsen, Owen, Flower, & Mohamed-Ali, 2001). Chronic stress as seen in older women who were caregivers led to a 6-fold greater increase in IL-6 over a 6-year follow-up (Kiecolt-Glaser et al., 2003). Chronic stress can accelerate aging due to a combination of many factors, including inflammation (Christian, Deichert, Gouin, Graham, & Kiecolt-Glaser, 2012). At the chromosomal level, chronic stress is associated with a shortening of the telomeres (the caps on the ends of the chromosomes), which results in accelerated aging (Epel et al., 2004).

Allostatic load occurs when the feedback loops that maintain homeostasis break down. In healthy individuals, after the HPA axis activates, the levels of cortisol rise, signaling back to the HPA axis that the stress response can be terminated. This negative feedback loop works quite well if all the systems are intact, such as the hippocampus with its many cortisol receptors. Cortisol also functions as an anti-inflammatory agent on the cytokine-producing cells. However, this system breaks down with repeated or chronic stress, which results in prolonged and elevated levels of cortisol. The cortisol receptors in the hippocampus atrophy, and cortisol insensitivity in the HPA axis and cytokine-producing cells provokes greater production of proinflammatory cytokines. In other words, the breakdown results in the detrimental effects of both high cortisol and high cytokines. This combination of elevated cortisol and inflammatory cytokines results not only in increased depression and anxiety but also susceptibility to, severity of, and duration of infectious illness (Christian et al., 2012).

One factor that has multiple ramifications is that extra fat cells leech out inflammatory cytokines, which have destructive effects on the body and the brain. As described in Chapter 9, an increase in inflammatory cytokines is associated with "sickness behavior," which appears very much like depression, as well as cognitive problems and, worse still, dementia. Recently, Rachel Witmer of Kaiser Permanente surveyed thousands of records and found that if middle-age people have a waist-to-hip ratio much greater for their waists, their risk for developing dementia jumps up dramatically. This increase in abdominal fat contributes to dementia and mortality for a number of reasons. In addition to a poor diet, impoverished sleep, and lack of exercise, the increase in abdominal fat results from the high levels of cortisol receptors in the abdomen, the corresponding high levels of cortisol occurring with chronic stress, and the increased levels of inflammatory cytokines.

The emergence of an autostress disorder (anxiety) from excessive stress is augmented by avoidance, which overactivates the R-PFC. With less L-PFC activity in meeting the challenges associated with stress, the amygdala tends to become even more active. Another contributor to the emergence of an autostress disorder is the client's excessive focus on stress symptoms. Hypersensitivity to any sensation associated with those symptoms results in a sort of hijacking of the PFC by the amygdala and the increase in fear-centered thoughts that justify anxious feelings.

Clients seek help from mental health professionals when their stress management skills and allostasis break down. Their usual methods of dealing with intolerable feelings only increase their distress.

Your work on building clients' sense of self-efficacy, confidence, and self-esteem builds allostasis back in negative feedback loops and minimizes allostatic load. Studies have shown that clients with poor self-esteem and low internal loci of control have 12% to 13% smaller hippocampi as well and higher levels of cortisol (Pruessner et al., 2005). Loneliness and low self-esteem have been associated not only with higher levels of cortisol but also with high fibrogen responses to stress (Steptoe et al., 2004). In contrast, positive outlook is associated with lower levels of cortisol as well as higher parasympathetic activity and lower fibrinogen activity (Steptoe et al., 2007).

It has long been understood that chaos at home plays a key role in the etiology of poor self-regulatory behaviors, helplessness, and distress (Evans et al., 2005). Multiple pathophysiological syndromes result from early stress and deprivation, including elevation of proinflammatory processes, as measured by C-reactive protein levels decades later in life (McEwen & Chattarji, 2007). To deal with the adverse effects of inflammation, activation of the parasympathetic nervous system through activities such as yoga, meditation, and tai chi improves mood and boosts the immune system. Beneficial immunological effects include decreased production of interferon gamma (IFNγ) and increased production of IL-4, an anti-inflammatory cytokine, by stimulated T-cells (Carlson, Speca, Patel, & Goodey, 2003).

This chapter has shown how we can help clients understand not only how anxiety disorders develop but also how to alleviate them. The next two chapters address how anxiety can be either generalized or focused on one or more specific fears.

Chapter 5

WHEN ANXIETY IS GENERALIZED

Once the stress system has been ramped up and stays abnormally active despite the fact that the threat has passed, an autostress disorder can be self-generated and different types of anxiety disorders may develop. A variety of types of anxiety disorders have identified between the third edition of the *Diagnostic and Statistical Manual of Mental Disorders* and the fifth (*DSM-5*)(APA, 2013). In this chapter, we address how anxiety becomes generalized and how to help clients understand and deal effectively with it.

The degree to which the stress system stays activated in generalized anxiety disorder (GAD) metaphorically differs from panic disorder, just as chronic pain differs from episodic acute pain. While symptoms of GAD are not acute like panic, there is a constant nagging feeling that things are not right and that something bad may happen at any minute. The underlying physiology of GAD involves less parasympathetic and more sympathetic nervous system activity, so people feel a chronic sense of uneasiness, as if something terrible could happen at any moment.

Consistent with the autostress disorder concept discussed in Chapter 4, GAD is fueled by a breakdown in the dynamic equilibrium between the two branches of the autonomic nervous system. The parasympathetic branch, which provides rest and relaxation, needs to be in balance with the sympathetic branch, which provides arousal and the emergency response system. In GAD, the dynamic balance normally maintained by negative feedback loops becomes dysregulated, and a positive feedback loop is set in motion. The associated emotional dysregulation is partly due to the disinhibition of the vagal brake and hyperstimulation of the heart.

Two major tendencies that contribute to GAD include free-floating anxiety and excessive worry. Symptoms of free-floating anxiety include feelings of constant tension, insomnia, and the tendency to become easily stressed; these can be considered the bottom-up aspects of GAD. The tendency to worry constantly can be considered a breakdown in the capacity of top-down control neural circuits that feeds free-floating anxiety.

Although the feeling of free-floating anxiety and constant worry are not always intense, clients may intensify stress from situations that others find innocuous. For example, in addition to feeling like being on edge throughout the day, driving during rush hour may make clients' anxiety peak, spurring hypervigilance, and perhaps even braking abruptly when the car in front slows down.

A combination of many factors can impair the top-down regulatory capacity that is largely a function of the prefrontal cortex (PFC). The PFC top-down ability to inhibit amygdala overactivity and anxiety can be undermined by the failure to make sensible decisions about self-care such as diet, the bottom-up foundation. For example, because there are many serotonin receptors in the orbitofrontal cortex (OFC), low serotonin leads to a reduction of capacity to inhibit the overactivation of the amygdala. In other words, a poor diet that is deficient in tryptophan can undermine the top-down regulation of anxiety.

CLIENT EDUCATION

A bad diet—especially one low in tryptophan, the amino acid your body uses to make serotonin—will deplete serotonin and therefore the capacity of your orbitofrontal cortex to calm your amygdala when it gets unnecessarily overactive. Even just skipping breakfast will undermine your orbitofrontal cortex and cause needless stress and anxiety.

Sara came to me complaining of constant free-floating anxiety. She had been to see two therapists who both reportedly believed that therapy was simply an art and that science got in the way. Through these therapists, Sara developed the idea that "emotions are wise" and that they "revealed what is truly is in the heart."

Over the last 40 years, I have become all too aware of many well-meaning therapists who had been trained in academic programs that were short on science while being very high on sugar-coated pop psychology. Understandably, many such programs have lost their accreditation, but a few still exist. In many ways, Sara suffered not only anxiety but the ill effects of pop psychology.

One of her therapists had her take the Myers-Briggs test, which was loosely based on the work of the venerable Carl Jung. I have been, and still am, deeply appreciative of Jung's contribution, but not the New Ageisms tacked on like barnacles that need to be scraped off a stately ship. The use of the Myers-Briggs test with a person such as Sara who suffered from free-floating anxiety was irrelevant at best. The results of the test served to reinforce her belief that she was "too sensitive" for a complex "toxic world."

BALANCING THE AUTONOMIC NERVOUS SYSTEM

For at least a few thousand years before the advent of psychotherapy, practitioners of meditation, yoga, and prayer have cultivated a balance between the branches of their autonomic nervous systems. Although they may not have known the physiology, these practitioners all calmed their minds as they focused on breathing.

Within the world of psychotherapy, breathing retraining has been part of the repertoire of therapeutic techniques such as hypnosis, autogenesis, and systematic desensitization (the latter since the days of Joseph Wolpe in the late 1950s). The concept of reciprocal inhibition described how two opposing feelings, such as relaxation and anxiety, could not occur at the same time. Breathing retraining has served as one of the common methods to induce relaxation, and it has long been practiced by therapists from many disciplines.

Yet it is not without critics who argue that teaching clients how to control their breathing to avoid or reduce panic symptoms can be countertherapeutic because it may prevent them from learning that their feared sensations are not dangerous (Meuret, Wilhelm, Ritz, & Roth, 2003; Schmidt et al., 2000).

Although research on the utility of breathing retraining is still being debated in CBT circles, David Barlow and Michelle Craske (2007) suggest that it be offered to "facilitate movement forward" in exposure, not as a panic control strategy. They caution that breathing retraining not be used with clients who may use the skill to "control" their panic symptoms. Breathing retraining is, however, a good way to help clients access their parasympathetic nervous systems, especially for clients with GAD. For this reason, we are addressing breathing retraining in this chapter.

There is a significant difference between relaxed deep breathing and overbreathing. Most people breathe 9 to 16 breaths per minute, but people with GAD at times tend to intensify sympathetic arousal by overbreathing, which can occur at the rate of 27 breaths per minute or more. Also called hyperventilating, overbreathing pulls in too much oxygen, which forces down the carbon dioxide (CO_2) level in the bloodstream. This imbalance creates a problem because CO_2 helps maintain the critical acid base (pH) level in the blood. Lower pH levels cause nerve cells to become more excitable, and people associate these feelings with anxiety.

NEUROSCIENCE

With overbreathing, the excessive dissipation of CO_2 leads to hypocapnic alkalosis, in which blood is more alkaline and less acidic. This leads to the following symptoms:

- Vascular constriction, resulting in less blood reaching the tissues.
- Less oxygen released to the tissues and the extremities.
- Dizziness, light-headedness, and cerebral vasoconstriction, which leads to feelings of unreality.
- Peripheral vasoconstriction, which leads to tingling in the extremities.
- Feelings of suffocation, due to CO_2 receptors in the brain stem. This dyspnea (the feeling of not getting enough air) can spur anxiety, panic, and more hyperventilation.

Jana complained of a "never-ending feeling of being wired." As she talked, she could barely take a breath. Her breathing was so shallow that as the words came out, rapid fire, they were increasingly laced with tension. She seemed to have the nervous energy of a person who just drank a pot of coffee, but she had not. She reported that she had "always had a problem with nerves, as far back as I can remember."

Her mother, too, had the same problems. When they talked together, both would need to "take a break to catch their breath," because they stirred each other up, amping up their breathing speed and rapidity of speech. As Jana told me about the conversations with her mother, she cranked up her breathing and not only the quickness of her words but also their volume.

I asked her to pause for a moment and take a deep breath. She tried to, but soon started breathing quickly again. In response to a gentle nod from me to slow down again, she responded, "Oh, sorry," then took another breath, this time deeper.

I began modeling deep breathing, saying "Make sure that your belly rises with the inhales. Then exhale out more air than you thought you had to let go." I told her that her exhales were engaging her parasympathetic nervous system, which helps her calm down. She had the patterns reversed with sharp, shallow inhales and exhales seemingly long enough only to inhale again with bursts that were more like gasps for air. She did her best to slow down her breathing, appearing to reflect on her thoughts as she did so.

"Notice how your thinking changes as you slow down your breaths," I said.

"They're not as jumbled."

"Pick a melody from a song that you enjoy with a slow tempo," I told her. She reflected for a moment, then chose "Silent Night." "Now, tell me about when you first heard it, trying to carry the same melody." As she told me about the holidays and the melody of "Silent Night," she began to smile and her eyes dilated.

Just as with Jana, establishing a connection between how clients breathe and their mental state can help them gain a better working understanding of the mind–body interplay. It is perhaps the clearest example of biofeedback without the need of instruments.

CLIENT EDUCATION

Your breathing and your heart rate are interconnected. As you learn to breathe more deeply, your heart rate will slow, and you can enjoy a calm and clear frame of mind.

One way to describe the connection between breathing and the two branches of the autonomic nervous system is to say that exhaling accesses the parasympathetic branch while inhaling accesses the sympathetic branch. A good illustration of this difference is that we laugh and sigh when we exhale, which accesses the parasympathetic nervous system. In contrast, a gasp is an abrupt inhale that activates the sympathetic branch of the autonomic nervous system. Ask clients if they tried to laugh when abruptly inhaling. You may even demonstrate an attempt to laugh with an inhale to illustrate the ridiculousness of a gasp as a laugh.

The point is that there should be a dynamic balance between the two branches of the autonomic nervous system and that clients can learn to cultivate easier access to the parasympathetic branch. The ability to access it represents a critical function of allostasis, which generally is diminished for clients with GAD. Given that they tend to feel tense and anxious much of the time, mindfulness, yoga, and self-hypnosis can be excellent relaxation methods to help them cultivate easier access to the parasympathetic nervous system.

CLIENT EDUCATION

There are several methods for you to access your parasympathetic nervous system. The ones listed next are common to prayer, meditation, relaxation exercises, and hypnosis. These common factors can calm your mind:

1. Deep, deliberate, and focused breathing allows you to slow your heart-beat and find you an accessible focal point for attention.
2. By shifting attention to the here-and-now, you can transform each moment into a poignant and tranquil experience in the present. This mindful presence activates your prefrontal cortex to calm the over-reactivity of your amygdala.
3. A relaxed posture can defuse body tension. This can include sitting in a relaxed posture or stretching through traditional yoga or a hybrid yoga, which includes stretching and mindful focusing.
4. A quiet environment will provide you with an opportunity to learn how to relax without distractions. Later you can relax in less quiet environments.
5. Through an accepting and nonjudgmental attitude, you can help shift yourself away from rigid expectations of what needs to be in place to feel calm.
6. Observing bodily sensations and thoughts allows you to detach from anxiety while simultaneously not denying its existence.
7. Labeling what you experience serves to access your prefrontal cortex and detach from anxious feelings.

In general, the approaches to helping clients suffering with GAD include parasympathetic activation that involves somatic exercises, such as hatha yoga, mindfulness, and relaxation training that emphasizes breathing and stretching. Clients should not engage in these methods as a form of avoidance but rather as a way to cultivate easy access to the parasympathetic nervous system.

NEUROSCIENCE

Consistent with the research on affect asymmetry, patients with lesions in the right amygdala recollect more high-intensity pleasant autobiographical memories and fewer high-intensity unpleasant memories. In contrast, patients with left-amygdala lesions recall fewer high-intensity positive memories and more high-intensity negative memories (Buchanan, Tranel, & Adolphs, 2005).

The point is, when the right hemisphere is impaired, the left is dominant, and vice versa. From a practical point of view, since the left hemisphere is associated with approach behaviors and the right is associated with avoidant and withdrawal behaviors, encouraging clients to approach life with a can-do attitude helps balance out the activity in the two hemispheres.

Using antianxiety medications is a form of avoidance. Many clients have been prescribed such medications unnecessarily. I have found that those who attend my anxiety class are interested to learn that those medications target the neurotransmitter gamma-aminobutyric acid (GABA). The role of GABA is highlighted by the effect of benzodiazapines, which include Valium (diazepam), Ativan (lorazepam), Klonopin (clonazepam), and Xanax (alprazolam). These drugs target the GABA receptors in the brain and provide initial effects that include the easing of tension and anxiety as well as some sedation. Because of these immediate effects, benzodiazepines, especially Valium, were prescribed very often some 30 years ago. The major problem with these drugs is that they provide brief relief followed by rapidly diminishing benefits. They lead to tolerance, which means that after regular use, clients must take more of the drug to gain the same effect. Eventually clients find themselves needing more of the drug to feel calm. Clients find it increasingly difficult to get off the drug because withdrawal increases anxiety. Generally the use of benzodiazepines leads to what psychologists call anxiety sensitivity, meaning that the sensations of anxiety increase as the drug wears off. Since tolerance is a factor when used on a regular basis, clients experience increased anxiety over time and each time the medication effects wear off.

Many people who have come to my anxiety class as well as some I have seen individually initially ask if medication is the answer to their anxiety and/or depression, hoping to get their brain to operate in a healthy manner. In most cases, medication is unnecessary; it can even complicate recovery. In particular, the use of benzodiazepines on a regular basis can prolong anxiety.

Overall, it is critical to point out that the long-term use of these drugs is countertherapeutic, meaning they make anxiety worse. When people who are on benzodiazepines come to my anxiety class, I work with them and their prescribing physician to titrate them off the drug. True rewiring of their brains is possible only after they are completely off the drug. A similar effect occurs with alcohol. A person does not have to be an alcoholic to suffer anxiety effects from alcohol. A host of neurotransmitters, especially GABA, are down-regulated for days and even weeks after your last drink.

Cognitive Avoidance

Avoidant behavior has been the subject of psychological inquiry well before there was an understanding of the underlying brain circuits and their associations with anxiety. There is a long history of theoretical development related to tempera-ment which described two general patterns, introversion and extroversion. The levels of arousal across a wide range of performance domains were first hypothe-sized by Carl Jung and then supported by the research of Hans Eysenck (Eysenck & Eysenck, 1985).

Jeffrey Gray went on to frame the introversion and extroversion paradigm within two major neurobiological systems. This model has received impor-tant revisions, which are quite relevant to understanding anxiety (Gray & McNaughton, 2000; McNaughton & Corr, 2004). The two major motivational systems of any viable organism include: (1) the need to avoid noxious stimuli, such as predators; and (2) the need to approach stimuli that are important for survival, such as food and sex.

As noted in Chapter 4, avoidant behavior paradoxically increases anxiety, even though clients feel temporary relief. With GAD, the avoidant behavior is not as obvious as it is with panic and phobias. Avoidant behavior with GAD takes a cognitive route by kindling the worry circuits so that clients worry as a method of avoiding uncertainties.

A large literature base describes worry as one of the main factors of GAD (Ouimette, Moos, & Brown 2003). Underlying worry is a general intolerance to uncertainty combined with poor problem solving and positive beliefs about worry. Worry can be seen as cognitive avoidance that attempts to problem-solve possible future negative events. Excessive worry attempts to reduce or inhibit aversive mental imagery, emotional experience, and physiological sensation. Clients struggling with GAD find themselves in a difficult bind in that they worry about uncertain situations, and most situations in life are uncertain.

There is a bidirectional relationship between excessive worry and simultane-ously feeling tense and anxious much of the time. Clients with GAD tend to be chronic worriers who can torture themselves with what-if thoughts throughout the day. Constant worries contribute to overreacting to stress, which only creates more anxiety.

Clients try to think themselves out of discomfort only to find them-selves more uncomfortable. Worry is both consciously and unconsciously self-reinforcing. Yet the intolerance to uncertainty leads many clients with

GAD to believe that worry is somehow helpful, which only feeds into the self-reinforcing tendency. The beliefs about worry may include "Worrying helps me cope," "If I worry, I can prevent bad things from happening," or "My worries are uncontrollable."

One of the self-reinforcing habits that keep worry cranked up occurs when clients search for ways to verify that things will be okay. It is quite common for clients with GAD to ask other people for reassurance that a particular worry is unjustified. Despite the fact that the reassuring people are trying to be kind, their effort serves only to feed clients' insatiable worry loop.

Because worry is a form of cognitive avoidance, different therapeutic approaches have been used to address it. In recent years, there have been some common themes among the popular approaches, such as acceptance and commitment therapy (ACT), dialectical behavior therapy (DBT), and cognitive-behavioral therapy (CBT), which all promote some form of cognitive, emotional acceptance and physiological exposure. In DBT, distress tolerance is promoted with parasympathetic activation such as breathing. Clients are asked to experience emotions like waves and ride through them. The emerging consensus is that clients are best served by getting comfortable being uncomfortable.

While there is a natural tendency to comfort clients by helping them resolve a worry, that comfort can be a short-lived fix if you address only specific worries instead of the *tendency* to worry. If you help clients reassure themselves that a specific worry is not worthy of concern because "all will be okay" in the end, they will move onto another worry. You can warn clients that you are not doing them any favors by explaining that there is certainty in life. By helping clients to acknowledge and accept that there is no absolute certainty, you could be helpful. The key point to raise with clients is that therapy can help them learn to accept and appreciate that there is no such thing as absolute certainty. And, for that matter, that is what makes life interesting.

CLIENT EDUCATION

The next time a well-meaning person tries to reassure you that there is certainty that everything will be okay, say, "Thanks so much, but I'm learning how to appreciate uncertainty."

In addition to examining the accuracy of dysfunctional thoughts and traditional relaxation skills, therapy should orchestrate and encourage exposure to anxiety-provoking and worry-related mental imagery (Borkovec, 2006). Helping clients improve problem-solving skills directed at solvable problems must be balanced with the recognition that some things people worry about are unsolvable. For problems that are unsolvable, exposure to and acceptance of the uncertainty is critical.

NEUROSCIENCE

Clients with GAD tend to have a significantly larger superior temporal gyrus and also more pronounced right–left symmetry in total white matter, and the volume of the white matter is significantly and positively correlated with anxiety scores on psychological tests (De Bellis et al., 2002b).

The difficulty dealing with uncertainty underlying much of the tendency to worry is directly associated with an intolerance for ambiguity. Clients with GAD tend to select threatening interpretations of ambiguous stimuli (Mathews & Mackintosh, 2000). Therapy should be directed toward helping clients develop tolerance for ambiguity and reevaluating the usefulness of worry.

Clients with GAD can learn to lessen the tendency to fuel worry by understanding how the brain circuits related to dealing with ambiguity need to be activated to inhibit the overactivity of the amygdala. By itself, the amygdala cannot tolerate ambiguity. One way to highlight this difficulty is by the "still face" paradigm described in Chapter 3. A child younger than 18 months of age cannot tolerate a neutral (ambiguous) face because the OFC, which deals with ambiguity, has not yet fully developed. Underdevelopment of the OFC, as occurs with insecure attachment or child abuse, would cause clients to have cognitive features that impair affect regulation in stressful situations, such as a slowed response to disengage from negative stimuli and attention to the hint of threat. Such clients tend to overestimate negative outcomes to neutral stimuli and to expect that negative events are more likely to occur than positive events.

NEUROSCIENCE

The amygdala is more responsive to fearful faces than to angry faces because there is an inherent ambiguity in fearful faces. Since the amygdala plays a major role in the resolution of predictive uncertainty associated with fearful faces, surprised faces also elicit ambiguous stimuli and activate the amygdala. Surprised faces are emotionally ambiguous. When those surprised faces are interpreted as positive, there is increased ventromedial prefrontal cortex (vmPFC) activity. There is decreased vmPFC activity when surprised faces are seen as negative (Kim, Somerville, Johnstone, Alexander, & Whalen, 2003). The vmPFC is located just above the OFC and associated with pure affect regulation and less with social functions than the OFC. But in general, the vmPFC subsumes the OFC. Surprised faces and the other emotionally ambiguous situations set up a competition between the vmPFC and the amygdala. The role of the vmPFC in resolving emotional ambiguity represents top-down regulation of the amygdala (Quirk & Beer, 2006).

To explain how to deal effectively with worry, point out that parts of the brain can be trained to tone down worry while another part of the brain that helps people deal with ambiguity and uncertainty, the OFC and anterior cingulate cortex (ACC), can be kindled. As I noted earlier, the OFC can help tone down the amygdala from overresponding when people feel anxious for no reason. When it is working well, the OFC negotiates through the ambiguities of life, the gray areas—essentially the uncertainties. For its part, the ACC is a conflict mediator and helps reconcile situations that are seemingly in opposition.

To help clients learn to neutralize the tendency to worry, you may introduce a variety of cognitive exposure exercises that can challenge the OFC to develop the capacity to appreciate ambiguity in life. For fears of personal inadequacy that impede risk taking and making mistakes, challenge clients to admit a personal mistake to someone and then not try to explain it away. A real challenge for clients with a high degree of self-consciousness could be to express an opinion on a subject in which they have limited knowledge. Because clients tend to think of themselves as perfectionists, ask them to complete a task in a less-than-perfect fashion. The key to this technique is for clients to resist the temptation to complete the task later to "make it right." By learning how to deal with ambiguity, clients build a stronger OFC. Accordingly, your work with clients can offer exposure to and development of an appreciation for ambiguity.

NEUROSCIENCE

Clients with GAD have also been shown to have weaker-than-normal white matter connections between those areas of the brain that regulate emotion, including the prefrontal and cingulate cortex (ACC) and the panic button, the amygdala (Nitschke et al., 2009). The primary white matter tract that connects these brain regions is called the uncinate fasciculus; it helps people distinguish truly worrisome situations from mild annoyances.

When the OFC and ACC are not well developed, clients tend to be overwhelmed by emotion. Finding it difficult to believe that they can feel upset or sad without falling apart, they overthink, which serves as a form of cognitive avoidance that fuels more uneasiness and more worry. These circuits can be strengthened with use in the same way a muscle is built by flexing and heavy lifting.

NEUROSCIENCE

In the brains of people with GAD, the circuits between the basolateral amygdala (which should be linked to the occipital, temporal, and frontal lobes) and the centromedial amygdala (which normally is linked to the subcortical areas, the thalamus, brain stem, and cerebellum) are muddled.

Also, the basolateral amygdala is less connected to all of its normal targets, and the centromedial amygdala is less connected with its normal targets and more connected with the basolateral amygdala. Meanwhile the amygdala is more connected to the cortical executive control network, which underlies the obsessive worries.

An area of the brain called the bed nucleus of the stria terminalis (BNST) is referred to as the extended amygdala. The BNST is also associated with GAD and the symptoms of free-floating anxiety, and contributes to a diffuse arousal underlying anxiety.

Clients with GAD tend to have a reduced orienting response to novel stimuli. A well-functioning orienting response is critical to react quickly and appropriately to novel situations, but the response habituates more slowly in clients with GAD, limiting their adaptability (Grawe, 2007). They continue to be hypervigilant, scanning their environment for potential danger, avoiding rather than approaching stressful situations. As they overread the potential stress and overrespond to it, they experience intense anticipatory anxiety, tying up their cognitive resources in ruminative preoccupation with personal concerns and worrying.

The amygdala functions as an orienting subsystem for the rest of the brain, alerting other systems that it is important to gather information and learn from situations. It serves as part of an integrative system that crosses categorical boundaries, such as emotion, motivation, vigilance, attention, and cognition (Whalen, Kim, Neta, & Davis, 2013). When the connectivity of this system is muddled, the process of tolerating uncertainty and ambiguity is impaired. As a result, the person is tormented with free-floating anxiety.

Because one of the major problems underlying the tendency to worry is the inability to deal with uncertainty, clients with GAD must be challenged to tolerate ambiguity. Without helping the client to increase the tension through exposure to ambiguity, the opportunity for neuroplasticity is lost. Instead, you may be seduced into reassuring clients to maintain the alliance. In such cases, your reassurance that all will be okay ironically serves to support clients' worry loop. They continue to be tremendously anxious if they cannot determine with certainty that everything will be all right. If you help clients avoid even a slight doubt and the most remote possibility that something may go wrong, their worry loop cranks up, fueling worries that will perpetuate other worries.

You may point out to clients that facing ambiguity and uncertainty is unavoidable. Since much of life is, in fact, uncertain, clients cannot be totally sure how things will work out or what they may encounter in the future. There is a great opportunity to worry if they cannot accept ambiguity and uncertainty. From this perspective, not being able to appreciate ambiguity means not being able to appreciate life.

Since GAD is due in part to intolerance for ambiguity, therapy necessarily includes exposure to ambiguity and uncertainty. One way to teach clients to bolster their OFC and ACC is to describe how ambiguity can become tolerable by exposure. Consistent with this goal, a CBT method called flooding the worry circuit, which helps clients learn to tolerate uncertainty, is useful. This method, which involves scheduling worrying time, helps to build the OFC through exposure to ambiguity.

Eventually clients learn to accept that there are no answers or outcomes for which to feel certain. Clients may wonder if this strategy will fuel even more worries. Actually, it offers clients time to develop the skills to learn that the worries are harmless.

CLIENT EDUCATION

Try the technique called the worry hour. Carry around a notebook or pad. As worries occur to you throughout the day, write them down. Then, perhaps between 5 and 6 AM each day, open the notebook and devote an entire hour to feasting on all these worries. You will become numb to the worries and bored. This technique will give your orbitofrontal cortex and anterior cingulate cortex time to learn that ambiguity is inherent in the texture and richness of life.

The goal is for clients to expose themselves to worries without trying to solve them. Only in rare cases can people who use this technique fill up the entire hour without strong encouragement to do so. You can ask clients to observe the worries uncritically and label them as merely worrisome thoughts. This technique, borrowed from the contemplative traditions, promotes detachment from the feelings of anxiety and anxious thoughts. In ACT, this technique is referred to as transforming thought "fusion" to thought "diffusion." When anxious thoughts are fused with the feelings of anxiety, such as illustrated in the statement "Oh, that thought makes me anxious," it is difficult to separate the thought from the feeling. Teaching clients to label anxious thoughts as such allows them to put distance between the feeling and the thought: They learn to tell themselves "Oh, that is an anxious *thought*." This technique shows that people do not need to embrace worrisome thoughts; instead, they are noticed for what they are, merely thoughts. It can be useful to point out the truism that clients have millions of thoughts that float by but they do not latch on to them because they know that as they daydream. They are merely fleeting images, ideas, and concepts that are part of their imagination. These thoughts flit in and out of consciousness unless they elicit an emotional charge. Only when they fuse with emotion, overactivating the amygdala, perhaps highjacking the PFC, do they generate anxious thoughts. You may suggest that the bad habit of fusing anxious feelings with thoughts occurs when clients "take the bait" to explore the possibility that a thought may be a signal of real danger. Because almost everything is in the remotest way plausible, anxious thoughts tend to stir up yet further anxious thoughts.

The process of labeling affective states reduces anxiety and negative affect. Labeling allows clients to detach from the affect of an anxious thought and to notice it as a mere thought. Accordingly, labeling has been associated with one of the talents of activity in the right ventrolateral prefrontal cortex(R-VLPFC), which allows clients to stand back and observe the thought (Lieberman et al., 2007). There is a significant difference between labeling thoughts such as "That is an anxiety-provoking thought" versus "This makes me anxious!" A further step toward detachment can include externalizing. Here, you can encourage clients to ask themselves "What would another person in this situation say, and how is s/he right?" Other methods of detachment can include looking into the future by encouraging clients to ask "How will I sensibly view this situation in six months?"

Some of the methods of appreciating ambiguity involve enlarging the perspective. For example, developing a sense of humor, especially about oneself, is probably one of the best psychological skills that clients can learn from you. Of course, this skill does not develop overnight. This is something you can model, showing clients that since you do not take yourself too seriously, neither do they need to. One step in this direction is to ask "What is funny about this?"

Deborah's Worry Loop

Deborah came to see me because she was tired of "worrying about anything and everything." She said that "as soon as I solve one problem, another occurs to me. It's like there are endless things to worry about, and I'm tired of it."

She went on to report that she had been a worrier as long as she could remember. Her mother, too, was a chronic worrier. "Maybe it's a worry gene that I inherited from her. Oh my God! Do you think that is possible?"

I explained that genes do not express themselves with that degree of specificity and that what she does in life has a great influence on turning on or off genes.

"Well, anyway," she said, "my dad tried to calm my mom down by trying to solve every problem . . ."

"Maybe trying to solve each problem makes your problem with worrying worse."

"Yeah, right," she said sarcastically. "Do you want my brain to explode?"

She gave me a great segue to describe how the job of her OFC is to deal with and appreciate the ambiguities in life. When her OFC is not doing its job, those ambiguities can fuel worries.

"So, you're saying I've got brain damage?"

"No, but you can exercise that part of your brain so that it can deal effectively with ambiguity."

I went on to describe how exposing herself to uncertainty, instead of trying to reassure herself that each worry should not be a concern, will help build her brain's capacity to neutralize to worry. To accomplish this, I introduced the worry hour. I told her to carry a pad of paper in her purse throughout the day so that when worries occur to her, she could write them down.

I added that, though she will write down things to worry about throughout the day, she can tell herself that she will give the worry enough time to do it justice later. Then between 5 and 6 AM each day, she should take out the pad with all the worries that she had collected that day and devote the entire hour to worrying about them.

At first, she thought that I was joking. "Why would I overload my brain? Do you want me to have a nervous breakdown?"

I explained that her brain will learn to let go of trying to solve problems that don't need to be solved. The exercise will give her brain an opportunity to learn to appreciate the shades of gray in life. It took a few weeks before Deborah could keep her worries only on paper until the allotted hour. Then, to her amazement, she had difficulty filling up that hour with "worry time." She said, "It gets boring after a while."

"To make the process really work," I replied, "you need to do it even when you really don't want to, especially when you find yourself so bored that you wonder 'what's the point anymore?' I'm asking you to try to worry when you feel that you have no more energy for worry."

I went on to tell her about the paradox that occurs when, for example, I ask her to get "pink elephants" out of her mind. The harder she tries, the more pink elephants she sees. By allowing pink elephants to drift into her mind, however, they soon drift *out* of her mind. With the worrying time exercise, not only did her worries drift away, but her OFC learned to appreciate ambiguity, the uncertainty of life.

Given that worrying is essentially an effort to reassure oneself that everything will be okay, it can be helpful to suggest that clients practice making a decision without reassurance. It is the reassurance efforts, either by clients themselves through worrying or through well-meaning friends or even you, that can fuel the worrying habit, which paradoxically inhibits the OFC from developing. Finally, because anxiety is partly based on future-oriented fears, helping clients learn to focus on the present and appreciate its nuances can neutralize anxiety. The effort to focus attention on a target of observation (sensations, thoughts, or emotions) and maintain awareness in the present moment will help clients learn that sensations, thoughts, and emotions are transient.

NEUROSCIENCE

The regulation of fear and negative affect involves the dorsolateral PFC (DLPFC), which is involved in the effortful manipulation or interpretation of a stimulus. The vlPFC and medial prefrontal cortex (mPFC) play a role in the selection of emotional interpretations and top-down modulation of the emotional meaning of the stimulus (Phelps, 2009). This cognitive regulation of fear involves DLPFC inhibition of the amygdala through the vmPFC, which mediates the inhibition of fear.

The concept of acceptance is particularly helpful to teach clients with the goal of lowering the anxiety level. There is much in life that people have no control over. Clients can gain control, however, over how they respond to anxiety symptoms. By accepting some of the symptoms, clients ironically diminish their intensity. I often tell clients that a dramatic example of how this works is illustrated in the approach taken by chronic pain programs. Chronic pain sufferers are no longer asked to try to ignore the pain or to try to get it out of their minds. Rather, they are now asked to observe and accept the pain. Many clients ask, "Why wouldn't a person who suffers from chronic pain try to do everything they can to get away from it?" The answer is that people suffering from pain expend an enormous amount of energy attempting to avoid the pain. They also tend to become anxious in response to the pain that they are trying to evade. Neurochemicals related to anxiety and stress tend to increase the pain. By turning toward the pain and accepting it, sufferers typically do not experience the pain at a level 10 on a 1 to 10 scale; perhaps it slides down to a level 4 or 6, with gradations in the pain. Putting anxiety in the same perspective, clients need not experience anxiety in the extreme, at level 10. By accepting the sensations, clients can find anxiety more tolerable and manageable.

You can help clients boost the approach networks of the left PFC (L-PFC) by encouraging them to recognize and appreciate that their behavior is in conflict with their values and goals. These insights work to motivate clients to make behavioral changes necessary to resolve discrepancies between approaching goals and avoiding them. If cognitive dissonance is kindled in therapy through an approach consistent with Rogerian/motivational interviewing and ACT, it can help leverage movement away from an avoidant and defensive posture to self-enhancing behaviors consistent with client values (Hayes, Strosahl, & Wilson, 1999; Miller & Rollnick, 2002).

In recent years, acceptance-based therapy models have become popular. Since people with GAD tend to react negatively to internal experiences and use worry as a way to avoid those experiences, it is useful to help clients to accept and observe rather than avoid internal experiences (Roemer & Orsillo, 2005). Through mindfulness-based strategies that include approach and acceptance, clients can learn to detach from anxiety while still acting in accordance with their values (Hayes et al., 1999; Kabat-Zinn, 2003).

During the last few decades, the therapeutic modalities have increasingly adopted mindfulness-based approaches. Most mental health programs feature mindfulness approaches for specific disorders, such as borderline personality disorder within the DBT modality (Linehan, 1993). At the University of California–Los Angeles, mindfulness was added to CBT in the treatment of obsessive-compulsive disorder (Baxter et al., 1992). Mindfulness and CBT were combined in the treatment of depression (Teasdale et al., 2002). One of the pioneers of this approach, Jon Kabat-Zinn, has utilized mindfulness for general medical problems, such as chronic pain (Kabat-Zinn, 2003).

NEUROSCIENCE

With the increased focus on what mindfulness practice imaging studies have shown that the association between mindfulness and the brain has indicated that long-term meditators show increased thickness of the mPFC and also enlargement of the right insula (Lazar et al., 2005). The mPFC has been associated with self-observation and mindfulness meditation (Cahn & Polich, 2006). The increased thickness of the mPFC is consistent with reports of improved affect regulation, observance, and attention while the increased thickness of the right insula corresponds to heightened awareness of the meditator's own body.

One of the reasons why the mindfulness approach has been applied to these disorders is its effectiveness with anxiety reduction. The process of labeling your emotions reduces anxiety through the relationship between PFC regions, which tame the amygdala by neural emotional regulation pathways.

Clients can be taught the steps of effectively dealing with GAD by using the phrase "get real" and the mnemonic REAL.

R—for relaxation. This includes techniques such as deep breathing, stretching, self-hypnosis, meditation, and prayer, used to activate the parasympathetic nervous system and increase vagal tone.

E—for exposure. Clients schedule an hour of worry time, allowing focused exposure to all their worries and giving their OFC a chance to work on developing the ability of dealing with the ambiguities inherent in life.

A—for acceptance. Since there is no ultimate certainty with much of life, acceptance allows worries to fade into the texture of normal living.

L—for labeling. When clients have an anxious thought, they can label it as just "an anxious thought," thereby detaching themselves from the feeling of anxiety.

Chapter 6

FOCALIZED ANXIETY

Autostress disorders that become fixated on a particular situation or stimulus can transform into phobias and panic disorder. The intense attention focused on the specific object or stressor, such as crossing a bridge, as is the case with phobias, or on physiological sensations, as is the case with panic disorder, generate fear and avoidance. The stress system works overtime to fuel behaviors to avoid what is feared.

As Franklin Delano Roosevelt said in his first inaugural speech in 1933, "The only thing we have to fear, is fear itself." Although he was talking about the consequences of the Great Depression, those words can certainly be applied to describe how focused fear, including of the sensations of the stress system, can feed anxiety.

FACING FEAR AND AVOIDANCE

Exteroceptive fear relates to stimuli outside of the body, such as fear of a spider or a bridge. Interoceptive fear relates to stimuli inside the body, such as a rapid heartbeat. Exteroceptive fear occurs when a client overreacts to feared objects or situations. In social phobia, exteroceptive fear occurs while a person stands in front of a group of people. Then interoceptive fear—a dry mouth, sweating, and butterflies in the stomach—signals that the person was right to fear public speaking.

As clients respond to either exteroceptive or interoceptive fear with avoidance, the stress symptoms are the very symptoms that they try to avoid. For example, at the beginning of a panic attack, clients react with heightened fear to a change in heart rate, stomach discomfort, dizziness, or some other body sensations. Unable to tolerate those sensations, the amygdala kicks in the sympathetic nervous system, which ironically intensifies more fear by hijacking the prefrontal cortex (PFC), resulting in unrealistic and catastrophic thoughts, such as that clients may be having a heart attack. Clients call 911, paramedics pick them up, and although they doubt cardiac arrest is the problem, they must rush the clients to the emergency room to ensure that they are medically clear. This scenario plays

129

out hundreds of times each year in every medical center. When I am on call for the hospital and I encounter a frightened patient, I explain what happened, then I invite him or her to my anxiety class to learn techniques to circumvent these terrifying experiences.

Acceptance and normalization of those bodily sensations necessarily involve exposure to them. The therapeutic practice of exposure enjoys a long and well-researched history. As a standard element of all evidenced-based approaches to anxiety disorders, it involves repeated systematic confrontation of feared and avoided stimuli. In interoceptive exposure, you encourage clients to intentionally induce the very unpleasant physical sensations they so fear while simultaneously withholding attempts at preventing or dampening those sensations. The critical benefit of interoceptive and in vivo exposure is that clients fully engage the panic sensations.

What if those sensations occur without psychological stress? Fear of those sensations can create anxiety. A wide variety of medical conditions, medications, dietary imbalances, and environmental exposure situations cause symptoms that ramp up the stress system. The symptoms of stress do not occur necessarily because clients are "stressed" in response but because of the biological chain of reactions associated with these conditions. The next box contains a small selection of conditions that create anxiety-like symptoms.

NEUROSCIENCE

Neurological Conditions
- Asthma
- Complex partial seizures
- Head injuries
- Hyperventilation
- Pulmonary abnormalities
- Vestibular dysfunctions

Cardiovascular Conditions
- High blood pressure
- Mitral valve prolapse
- Chronic obstructive pulmonary disease
- Lung cancer
- Toxic exposure
- Exposure to environmental toxins (hydrocarbons, mercury, carbon dioxide)

Dietary Deficiencies
- Calcium
- Magnesium

- Potassium
- Vitamin B12

Medical Conditions
- Adrenal tumor
- Cushing's disease
- Hypoglycemia
- Hypothyroidism
- Menière's disease
- Parathyroid disease
- Postconcussion syndrome

Endocrine Problems
- Cushing's syndrome
- Hyperthyroidism
- Hypoglycemia
- Menopause
- Pheochromocytoma
- Premenstrual syndrome

Medication and Drugs
- Alcohol (after a few hours of withdrawal)
- Antihistamines
- Benzodiazepines (a few hours of withdrawal depending on the half-life of the medication)
- Caffeine
- Calcium channel blockers
- Cocaine
- Monoamine oxidase inhibitors
- Marijuana (after several hours of withdrawal)
- Theophylline

The salient point here is that clients can react to symptoms of these conditions with fear that those sensations "mean" that something ominous will occur. That fear can overactivate the stress system and, if not put in perspective, can fuel an anxiety disorder that will have a life of its own long after the condition dissipates. In other words, it is unnecessary to determine the etiology of the symptoms in order to ameliorate anxiety for the conditions may have cleared long ago. For example, David was a toll taker on the Golden Gate Bridge. He typically did not wear a mask, and as a result he was exposed to hydrocarbons. He also began to suffer from respiratory problems for which he began taking an over-the-counter brand of pseudoephedrine. Soon he began feeling not only free-floating anxiety but also panic attacks, even when he was not working. He thought that he was "going crazy." Much of his attention was directed toward trying to avoid "triggering" the sensations of shortness of breath, rapid heartbeat, and dizziness. So he avoided stairways and exercise for fear of bringing on those sensations. After the Golden Gate Bridge laid off all toll takers, David started a new job that did not expose him to hydrocarbons. His allergies also cleared because he moved to a town with a low pollen count, so he quit taking antihistamines. However, he continued to have panic attacks. His focus on those sensations ramped up his stress system to be hypervigilant and overreactive to any sensation resembling the ones he so feared.

Since an overreactive stress system can focus attention onto what is feared, it can be the major factor in the development of an anxiety disorder. When the physiological sensations feel like the stress system is signaling danger, the hijacked PFC interprets those feelings to mean that something terrible is soon to happen. Helping clients put the anxiety-like symptoms in perspective can prevent anxiety outcomes.

When explaining the discomfort to clients, it is important to acknowledge how phobias and panic develop. Because the amygdala serves as a sort of smoke alarm for danger, it alerts the rest of the brain to prepare the body to protect itself by triggering avoidant behaviors. This is especially true if the fear is focused on a situation, object, or body sensations that he fears are dangerous. For example, the overwhelming feelings of fear and avoidance of the physical sensations fuel panic. The amygdala sets off a chain of events by signaling the hypothalamus to release corticotrophin-releasing hormone (CRH), which signals the pituitary to release adrenocorticotropic hormone (ACTH) to tell the adrenal glands to release adrenaline. Then, if the stressful situation persists, the adrenals will release cortisol.

This hypothalamic-pituitary-adrenal (HPA) axis is by no means the only part of the stress response system. It is, however, the best known. The amygdala also maintains projections to the locus coeruleus (LC), which releases the neurotransmitter norepinephrine (NE). The release of NE from the LC can itself trigger the HPA axis (Aston-Jones, Valentino, Van Bockstaele, & Meyerson, 1994). NE seems to maintain a preferential relationship with the right prefrontal cortex (R-PFC) and plays a major role in phobias and panic and other anxiety disorders. The greater the release of NE, the greater the activity in the R-PFC and the less activity in the left prefrontal cortex (L-PFC) (van der Kolk, Burbridge, & Suzuki, 1997; Southwick et al., 2005). This relative imbalance puts clients in an overwhelming predicament because the excessive rise in NE generates more global feelings of fear. But they have less capacity for verbal explanation for those feelings, because there is less activity in their verbally expressive L-PFC (Kent, Coplan, Mawlawi, Martinez, & Browne, 2005).

Excessive release of NE as occurs with stress engages the alpha1 and beta adrenoreceptors, which impairs PFC functions and disinhibits the amygdala. In this case, the amygdala can serve to hijack the PFC and take it "off-line," which can promote irrational thoughts and behavior, such as fearing enclosed spaces or meeting new people, or can cause clients to call an ambulance because of panic that they are having a heart attack when their heart pumps fast.

Fear and avoidance of what is feared fuel the stress system to self-perpetuate so that an autostress disorder develops. Clients hyperfocus on what is feared and avoid it at all costs. When you explain this sequence to clients, they may look at you in disbelief when you suggest that a principal aspect of therapy is the avoidance of avoidant behaviors. It is not only counterintuitive to approach what you fear; for decades well-meaning therapists have assumed that they were helping clients by identifying "triggers" to anxiety and then devising ways for clients to avoid those triggers. These countertherapeutic efforts actually make anxiety worse by supporting behaviors that kindle the autostress dynamics leading to anxiety disorders.

There are many forms of avoidance. Escape behaviors involve clients removing themselves from anxiety-provoking situations, such as walking away from strangers at social gatherings. Avoidant behaviors involve doing things to keep away from anxiety-provoking situations, such as not going to the social gathering at all. Procrastinating involves putting off to the last minute the anxiety-provoking situation, such as sitting in the car until they cannot delay any longer going into the building where the social gathering is taking place. Safety behaviors represent ways that clients fool themselves into believing that they are safe. For example, they may keep one tablet of lorazepam (Ativan) in a pocket, "just in case," even though they may not have taken any for over a year. Just the thought that the medication is available paradoxically gives clients comfort while at the same time subtly reminding them that they have a latent anxiety disorder that may rear its ugly head anytime.

CLIENT EDUCATION

Anxiety is associated with overactivity of your right prefrontal cortex and underactivity of your left prefrontal cortex. Avoiding what makes you anxious ironically makes your right prefrontal cortex even more active. As a consequence, it creates more anxiety. Even though it doesn't feel right immediately, facing your fears will eventually decrease them. Facing your fears will help the balance between the activities in the two sides of the brain.

All these forms of avoidance result in overactivity of the R-PFC, which is associated with anxiety disorders. Given that avoidant behaviors are promoted by the R-PFC and that it is generally overactivated in clients with anxiety disorders, it is important to explain how avoidance serves to kindle even more R-PFC activity. You may add that avoidance tends to sensitize the amygdala over the long term to overreact to stress. By explaining this paradox, you can help clients understand that what feels immediately safe and self-protective eventually makes anxiety worse.

Despite the fact that insight alone is not enough to change maladaptive behavior, it is useful to ask clients "Why is avoidance so hard to resist?" Here it can be productive to use a motivational interviewing approach to acknowledge with clients that avoidance works to reduce fear over the very short term. When you ask clients how they feel over the long term they typically will respond that they felt terrible.

The more clients avoid, the harder it is to resist avoiding because avoidance becomes habit. There is also a superficial logic to avoidance when clients ask, "Why wouldn't I avoid something that makes me anxious?" It can be particularly tricky to explore avoidant behavior with clients who have a codependent support system from which they receive some secondary gain, such as extra care, because people around them feel sympathy.

Here, too, a brain-based explanation helps reveal the superficial logic of avoidance. By explaining that brain systems associated with anxiety are activated with avoidance, you can give clients a tangible reason *not* to avoid. And if you can meet with family members along with clients, you may be able to form an alliance to help support clients learn how to resist the tendency toward avoidance.

Incremental Exposure and Approach Behavior

Exposure is fundamental to the treatment of anxiety. Since exposure is the opposite of avoidance, it is also associated with approach behaviors. As such, exposure kindles the L-PFC. Given that there is a right-hemisphere bias in general for anxiety disorders, anxious clients tend to feel overwhelmed with the "totality" of their concerns and have trouble identifying the details processed by the left hemisphere. One way to illustrate this asymmetry is to explain how some people feel speechless when frightened due to underactivation of the left frontal lobe and of Broca's area within the lobe (Rauch, Shin, Whalen, & Pitman, 1998).

As I explained in Chapter 1, the L-PFC is associated not only with approach behaviors but also with positive emotions. The L-PFC is also capable of calming the amygdala, unlike the R-PFC. Since the L-PFC is detail oriented, in contrast to the R-PFC, which is oriented to the total gestalt, you can suggest that clients focus and engage in discrete details in the form of specific behaviors through an incremental approach. In other words, by breaking down behaviors into doable small chunks, clients can gain ground achieving goals, feeling good about accomplishments, all while activating the L-PFC.

One of the reasons that the flooding technique employed in the early 1970s failed with many clients was because it did not fully utilize the talents of the L-PFC. Because the left hemisphere processes details, flooding tended to skew activity to the R-PFC. The exposure exercises must, therefore, generate semitolerable steps slightly out of clients' comfort zone.

CLIENT EDUCATION

To chip away at your anxiety, you must break down your goals into doable chunks, then incrementally step just outside of your comfort zone to kick-start your left prefrontal cortex so that it can calm your amygdala.

There are reasons that incremental exposure works to rewire the brain. As I described in Chapter 1, neuroplasticity requires moderate activation and the inverse U-shape curve. In other words, a little anxiety provides the neurochemical fuel to rewire the brain.

The benefit of a graduated and moderate degree of anxiety occurs when consolidating memory. NE and epinephrine (adrenaline) play central roles in the amygdala encoding and consolidating implicit memories. A moderate level of these catecholamines maximizes the middle of the inverted U and is optimal for learning new skills, such as how to defuse a panic attack before it starts. Too little NE, such as occurs with boredom where no attention is generated, results in little or no consolidation of new learning about how to deal with fear. Too much activation, as would be the case with the perception of a catastrophic situation, narrows attention to the fear.

To teach clients the importance of getting out of their comfort zone using moderate and incremental steps, it can be helpful to describe the "neurochemical switch" as the mechanism for the inverted U. You can illustrate how challenges rewire the brain through a moderate increase in the level of NE because of its high affinity for the alpha2A receptors, which results in alert wakefulness and also at times a moderate level of anxiety. In other words, getting even incrementally out of the comfort zone facilitates people's PFC to regulate behavior and suppresses overactivity of the amygdala.

NEUROSCIENCE

The excessive elevation of NE triggers a cascade of other PFC-impairing factors and increases in cortisol. These neurochemical factors ramp up anxiety by overactivating the amygdala and further releasing NE through the locus coeruleus, dopamine via the ventral tegmental area, and acetylcholine via the dorsolateral tegmental nucleus. All these factors further dampen the PFC's capacity for problem-solving and rational behavior. Consequently, clients are prone to heightened startle responses, vigilance, insomnia, flashbacks, intrusive memories, and an increase of further fear conditioning.

The medial PFC (mPFC) plays a role in inhibiting the activity of the amygdala. Specifically, the connection between the infra-limbic cortex

(continued)

(continued)

(IL), a subregion of the ventromedial PFC (vmPFC), and intercalated cells (ITCs) within the amygdala comprises a pathway for inhibition to occur. The ITCs are inhibitory neurons that connect to the basal nucleus B, the lateral nucleus LA, and the central nucleus CE. Thus, during recall of extinction, the conditioned stimulus–related responses in the IL region lead to ITC excitation, which in turn inhibits communication between the LA (where fear memories are stored) and the CE (the output of the fear response) (Quirk, Russo, Barron, & Lebron, 2000). In fact, researchers have stimulated the IL region of the vmPFC, resulting in decreased excitability of the neurons in the CE and the decreased expression of conditioned fear (Quirk, Likhtik, Pelletier, & Paré, 2003). If there is communication between the LA (where fear memories are stored) and the CE (which is involved in the expression of fear), the expression of fear is inhibited. Finally, some researchers have suggested that projections from the vmPFC and the LA region of the amygdala may play a role in the inhibition of fear during extinction (Rosenkranz, Moore, & Grace, 2003).

In an article titled "A Call to Action: Overcoming Anxiety through Active Coping," LeDoux and Gorman (2001) described the pathway for active coping involving the LA, which projects to the B, which in turn projects to the striatum to convey the reinforcing nature of action.

CLIENT EDUCATION

I know you feel like you're not ready to take the first step to get out of your comfort zone, but not feeling ready provides the fuel to rewire your brain so that you can enlarge your comfort zone by taking these steps.

NEUROSCIENCE

It has been believed that extinction does not erase or undo anxiety. After extinction, a conditional fear can return through a range of circumstances including the simple passage of time via spontaneous recovery, exposure to the unconditioned stimulus, or exposure to the conditioned stimulus in a novel context. The recovery or reappearance of fear indicates that extinction training actually involves new learning via the mPFC, hippocampus, and amygdala to inhibit the expression of conditioned fear rather than eliminating its underlying representation (Phelps, 2009).

One of the neuromechanisms for exposure provided by the stress response system occurs through the involvement of beta endorphin (BE) and its anxiolytic effects. BE has been long known to be released into the bloodstream from various endocrine sources in response to stress. It appears that there are higher concentrations of BE in the morning than the evening. As an endogenously produced opioid compound with analgesic properties, BE is activated in response to physical pain, temperature change, conditioned fear, and even social conflict.

BE is co-released with ACTH but is initially blocked by ATCH at the common receptor sites. The positive effects from exposure result in part from the fact that the more rapidly decaying ACTH is displaced by the delayed BE anxiolytic effects several minutes after the exposure (Carr, 1998).

Acute and controllable stress appears to activate the opioid systems; nonopioid systems appear to be activated by intense, chronic, sustained, and uncontrollable stress. The key is the *perception* of stress; uncontrollable stress not only relates to predominantly nonopioid systems but also increased passivity and helpless behavior as well as greater levels of anxiety (Henry, 1992). The key to effective therapy is to help clients stay with exposure to the feared situation long enough for BE to have its therapeutic effect.

NEUROSCIENCE

The stress-induced release of BE occurs in both the development of the avoidance response and its treatment by exposure therapy (Carr, 1998). More specifically, the stress-induced anxiolytic response provides a potent reinforcing mechanism that is the basis for operant conditioning of the avoidance responses. For its part, exposure behaviorally induces an increase in the stress-induced anxiolytic BE response. Exposure disrupts and extinguishes the contingent relationship between avoidance and the stress-induced reinforcer by establishing a new contingent relationship between a coping response associated with the feared situation and the stress-inducing anxiolytic BE response. Because BE disassociates to binding sites more slowly than ACTH, if clients stay in the exposure situation long enough, over a period of time, they will become habituated to the fear-inducing situation.

Speeding Up the Slow Track

When describing the brain-based dynamics of anxiety to clients, two factors can illustrate how anxiety can feel so overwhelming and out of their control. As I noted in Chapters 3 and 4, there are two routes to the amygdala, the fast track and the slow tracks. The fast track is so named because it occurs before the slow track and activates the amygdala before the cortex. This means that clients can feel fear before consciously knowing why. The slow track is so named because information is sent to the cortex before going to the amygdala. This means that clients think before feeling emotion. In most clients with anxiety disorders, their fast track is on too often and their slow track rarely works. They need to slow down their fast track and speed up their slow track.

Another way to conceptualize this dilemma is to recognize that bottom-up processes are dominant for clients with anxiety disorders. The interaction between the bottom-up activation, from the amygdala, and top down, from the PFC, are skewed so heavily toward bottom-up reactions that clients feel anxiety so intensely that the functioning of their top-down control system is overridden (LeDoux, & Gorman, 2001). Activation of the PFC plays a central role in the regulation of amygdala output, keeping bottom-up processes in check (Bishop, 2007). The importance of the interaction between the amygdala and the PFC as well as the structural and functional connectivity between them represents a better predictor of anxiety than the activity of either region alone (Kim & Whalen, 2009).

NEUROSCIENCE

Successful top-down control over anxiety is associated with increased cortical thickness of the vmPFC. Affect labeling—that is, putting emotions into words—is associated with diminished amygdala and greater ventrolateral PFC (vlPFC) activity and increased thickness of the vmPFC (Lieberman et al., 2007). The top-down emotional regulation involves interactions between the PFC (both dorsolateral PFC [dlPFC] and mPFC) and the anterior cingulate cortex (ACC) influence over subcortical areas, especially the amygdala.

Speeding up the slow tract to exert better top-down control over anxiety and the associated hyperactivity of the amygdala involves activating the cortex and hippocampus and the thinking and explicit memory capabilities. Cognitive-oriented therapies have attempted to do just that without explaining the brain systems involved. For example, many cognitive approaches have identified "thinking errors," including black-and-white thinking, polarization, and catastrophication. The common factor among these errors is the globalized thinking associated with R-PFC.

One way to help clients remember brain-based methods to speed up the slow track and specifically the L-PFC ways of thinking is to help them conceptualize layers of thought. These layers include automatic thoughts, assumptions, and core beliefs that are associated with approaching fears, not avoiding them. Automatic thoughts represent the most superficial thinking layer of the slow track. You can explain automatic thoughts as the first thought to pop up when people encounter stressful experiences. To some degree, automatic thoughts are fueled by implicit memory bias because the fast track to the amygdala occurs just before automatic thoughts, so that fear-based feeling states can immediately color thoughts. A way to help the client understand how this happens is to describe how his amygdala can hijack his prefrontal cortex when the automatic thought seeks to confirm an unrealistic fear. On the other hand, in an attempt to speed up the slow track at the automatic thought level, he can interrupt the fast track impulse with a pause so as to help his cortex catch up and to become aware of the present moment, and realistically appraise the situation with the left PFC being engaged by asking himself, "what is really happening and what can I do that is constructive instead of avoiding?" In anger management programs, the "time out" technique is one of the first things that attendees learn. In this case, you are introducing a time gap to allow clients' PFC to form realistic, nonhijacked thoughts. Similarly, this time lag technique actually represents an opportunity for the slow track to catch up to the fast track, which promotes realistic thought appraisal before reacting with immediate fear.

Another way to help clients change their formation of automatic thoughts is to reduce the polarity in how they frame situations. Instead of asking clients to shift to a totally positive automatic thought free of anxiety, ask for a neutral thought, which acknowledges some anxiety while it defuses the intolerable anxiety.

CLIENT EDUCATION

Practice pausing for a moment to reflect first on what actually is happening. Then ask yourself what you can do that is practical and a step toward rather than away from the immediate fear.

The next layer of the slow track to help clients learn to speed up involves assumptions that they have developed. Assumptions function as their personalized theories around how they deal with certain situations. Clients with social phobia, for example, may assume that every time they meet a new person, they will self-sabotage the interaction so that the other person will go away, shocked by the client's ineptitude. Negative assumptions such as these can fuel the worry track with self-perpetuating beliefs that avoidant and/or withdrawal behaviors are reasonable.

Like automatic thoughts, assumptions can be reasonably reframed by encouraging clients to acknowledge some difficulty with stress. For example, instead of asking clients to tell themselves that they are no longer socially awkward, a more realistic theorem is that they are "learning how to become more socially fluid. The more I practice, the more I improve. There will be rough spots, but I will become smoother with practice."

With a shift toward approach cognitions, assumptions can be constructive in that they lead to a can-do attitude. Assumptions followed by actual behavior that steps toward fears and acting as if they can handle the situation despite the fact that fears are still there will in time lead to less fear.

You can describe the next layer as a deeper level of the slow track, which involves core beliefs. These are the ways that clients describe themselves. Core beliefs are existential life descriptors in which people frame themselves, such as having a disability. It is at this level that clients describe the prognosis for themselves. If they think of themselves as irreparably damaged by unfortunate victim life experiences, then there is little hope for a positive future. If, however, you can help clients reconstruct a narrative that they are durable survivors, the prognosis likely will be more positive.

A shift to the core belief of being survivors helps frame clients' past as having required action and approach behaviors. So too will a viable future necessitate actively meeting the challenges ahead. The core belief in being survivors carries with it a sense of healthy optimism that is associated with confronting fears and doing what had to be done to survive.

Your effort to help clients depathologize their experiences and to explain the symptoms of their anxiety from a brain-based perspective can help them understand that the solutions are tangible. Understanding that the brain is not hardwired with disability but softwired by experience can help motivate clients to rewire core beliefs.

Each of these layers of the slow track represents ways that the cortex can be organized as clients adjust to challenges in the world. To help clients learn to speed up the slow track at each layer, you can encourage them to shift their thinking from a global/passive (R-PFC) mode to a detail/action (L-PFC) mode to develop new thoughts.

Albert Bandura, the grandfather of social modeling theory, has long maintained that people who believed in their ability to succeed is the most important factor that prevents anxiety disorders (Bandura, 1997). If clients fear that they are unable to cope with anxiety in what they assume to be a potentially threatening situation, their anxiety increases. When clients develop self-efficacy, their anxiety decreases. In other words, when clients believe that they are able to deal with the situation, their anxiety level goes down. When they observe and accept the physical sensations and thoughts that arise, their sense of mastery over them makes anxiety fade.

I often describe the two-factor theory of emotion, or Schacter–Singer theory (1962), which states that emotion is based on two factors: physiological arousal and cognitive label. Schacter and Singer conducted well-known studies that involved administering epinephrine (adrenaline) to subjects who were led to believe that they were either in a positive (controllable) or negative (uncontrollable) situation. Those who believed that they were in an uncontrollable situation experienced increased anxiety from the epinephrine. Those who were led to believe that they were in a controllable situation reported great pleasure. The point is that a shot of adrenaline does not necessarily lead to anxiety. It is all in how people interpret the sensations from a top-down perspective. If they interpret the physical sensations positively, or at least as a neutral experience, they will not be plagued by anxiety.

Clients with panic disorder are phobic about their own bodily sensations and constantly monitor the body for any physical sensation that might "warn" them that an attack is on the way. They try to make sure nothing terrible happens by avoiding anything that might stir up those bodily sensations, such as jogging or running up the stairs.

Since panic attacks can seemingly come out of the blue, they occur when clients feel the physical sensations they fear. To control the conditions in which these sensations occur, clients avoid what they believe leads to the sensations and assume that they gain temporary control. Clients nevertheless fear that those physical sensations always seem to be around the next corner.

PHOBIAS

Phobias bind the anxiety onto a specific type of stress trigger. Clients can generate intense fears of specific objects, situations, or environments. For example, the most common phobias include fear of flying, meeting new people, crossing bridges, driving, being in large crowds, heights, and enclosures. There are a number of different variations of social phobias involving excessive anxiety in specific situations, such as meeting new people or being in a room with strangers.

Consistent with the effort to normalize client experience, you can help them frame the stress response in such a way that it becomes tangible and more easily managed. To this end, it can be helpful to note that the most common fear is public speaking. As with all types of anxiety, for social phobia, avoidance is paradoxical and self-reinforcing because it works only in the short term. The more clients avoid social situations, the greater their phobia becomes. Because clients avoid social situations and afford themselves little opportunity for the amygdala to habituate to such situations, the fears will grow. In some ways this concept is counterintuitive; clients feel "better" immediately after avoiding the people because they can present challenging and often confusing situations.

The primary way to overcome social phobia is to practice social exposure that rewires the brain to gradually increase tolerance to social situations. As clients learn how to stop avoiding such situations and instead incrementally expose themselves to them, they rewire their social brain networks.

CLIENT EDUCATION

You have many social brain circuits that have been dormant. As with muscles that have atrophied, working out in the beginning is painful, but the pain soon goes away. Social brain networks thrive on positive social interaction. Once you get started, they will wake up. Not only will you find it easier to be with people, but you also will find it enjoyable.

With repeated exposure, clients eventually lose their fear and become more comfortable in social situations. As they see themselves function better in the social arena practicing social skills, they will be more likely to continue practicing because they gradually become more comfortable doing so.

As mentioned, the fear of public speaking is common. You can invite clients to dispel the illusion that there are perfect people by modeling imperfection yourself. This can free up clients to acknowledge the truism that we all are simply trying to do our best. If it is public speaking that clients fear, it can also be reassuring to know that they need not present themselves as flawless speakers. You can remind clients that people enjoy listening to real human beings who can present information while not trying to be perfect.

I describe how I learned to confront my fear of public speaking. As a student in college and even in graduate school, I found myself becoming anxious when speaking in front of large groups of people. Like most people, I feared saying something stupid. Worse was the fear that someone would see that I was nervous when I spoke. Over the years as I managed very large groups of people in the mental health system, I had to speak with authority and at times had to field very hotly contested discussions. Now I speak to hundreds of people in presentations.

Josh came to see me because he was concerned that he would not be able to get through an upcoming family wedding without being the subject of scorn and residual gossip for years to come. He reported that over the preceding few years, he had become progressively more self-conscious in social situations. His solution was to pull back and "gather strength" so that eventually he could become strong enough mentally and emotionally to deal with the stress of the complexities inherent in communicating with other people. So he avoided people, especially groups. He did not understand why his efforts to gather strength by pulling back did not result in any increase to his self-confidence. Instead, his self-confidence in social situations seemed to be eroding.

By the time he finally sought help, he was worried that the people at work had tagged him as a social misfit. He was obsessed with the fear that they thought him expendable if the company were to downsize, as it had done twice in the last few years. His social phobia was far greater than a fear of just one family gathering.

One of my first goals was to help him understand that his avoidance of social situations actually made his social anxiety worse. Paradoxically, avoidance made his amygdala more alert to anxiety-provoking social cues. The solution was to put his efforts in the opposite direction of what "felt right": namely, social exposure. To rewire his brain, he had to do what he did not feel like doing, which involved spending more time with people, not less time.

Years before he became socially isolated, he had gone to the gym on a regular basis and had lifted weights. This gave me a wonderful opportunity to use body building as an analogy to explain brain building. A want-to-be body builder cannot bench press 250 pounds on the first day, but building muscle mass does not happen overnight. It takes many workouts stretched over a long period of time.

"Can't you just give me a pill?" Josh asked, clearly irritated that he was hearing not only what he expected but also what he didn't want to hear.

"If you want to rewire your brain so that you won't have anxiety in social situations, going without antianxiety medication will be the best route. Besides, preparation for the wedding will present as an opportunity. Your work situation will only improve as your social skills do, and those skills do not come in pill form. Your toned-up physique didn't come from a pill either. It came from your body building workout." I asked him to describe his workout routine. Toward the end of the period when he went to the gym, he lifted weights three times a week for 1 hour, depending on which part of his body he was emphasizing that day.

"Ah, then you weren't just working on one muscle group?"

"Oh, no. I had to work different groups. And I'd also add a little more weight each time."

"Just like a good workout for the brain. We want your brain to rewire so that you are versatile, not capable just in one social situation, such as spending a few hours at a wedding."

"Oh, great. What did I get myself into? Maybe I shouldn't have opened my mouth."

I gave him a sly look.

"You're right. I guess I set my own trap."

"And it's a good one at that."

With my guidance over the next few months, Josh put himself in a variety of social situations, careful to incrementally increase the social challenge each time and extend the amount of time he stayed in the social situation. Well before the wedding, he found himself in the break room at work. One of his coworkers said, "Welcome back. We wondered if you thought that you were too good for us."

"Kinda the opposite," Josh said with a laugh.

PANIC DISORDER

Panic disorder afflicts women at a rate of 2 to 1 over men (Kessler, Chiu, Ruscio, Shear, & Walters, 2006). Women tend to experience a higher incidence of agoraphobia, more catastrophic thoughts associated with panic attacks, and more physiological sensations, especially respiration-related symptoms such as difficulty breathing, feeling faint, and feeling smothered (Sheikh, Leskin, & Klein, 2002).

Panic disorder is one of the most dramatic and frightening types of anxiety disorders because clients tend to experience bursts of seemingly uncontrollable physical and psychological symptoms that usually occur out of the blue, without any apparent cause, spurring on intense fear. The physical symptoms can include a racing heart, shortness of breath, and chest pain; the psychological symptoms can include a fear of dying, having a heart attack, or going crazy. Each of these symptoms independently can fuel a panic attack if clients fear that they mean that something catastrophic is about to occur. These physical sensations can intensify when clients overreact with fearful thoughts, such as "I can't breathe, I must be dying!" Then more physical sensations occur, which fuel even more fearful thoughts, such as "I'm having a heart attack!"

During a panic attack, clients can feel overwhelming rushes of anxiety that come in surges. The attacks also occur periodically so that clients never know when they will occur again. Panic attacks are so called because that is what they feel like. They seem to just happen, with clients having no control over them. A panic attack by itself doesn't mean that a person has panic disorder. The key to whether one or even a few panic attacks becomes a panic disorder is fear that the symptoms of stress mean something more ominous is occurring. This pattern of overreacting tends to fuel neuroplasticity and repeated panic attacks.

Panic disorder can occur with other anxiety disorders. As many as 50% of people with panic disorder have generalized anxiety disorder (GAD), phobias, and obsessive-compulsive disorder (OCD) as well as depression. If clients suffer from panic disorder and also depression, they may be less motivated to try new skills, and when they do accomplish some positive changes, they may tend to appraise them negatively. Also, because depression generally lowers physiological arousal, clients might not make adequate use of interoceptive exposure exercises (discussed below). For these reasons, dealing with depression through behavior activation (see Chapter 9) simultaneously with learning how to deal with anxiety will activate the L-PFC and deemphasize activation in the R-PFC.

It is not just people who suffer from panic disorder and posttraumatic stress disorder (PTSD) who respond with fear to bodily sensations such as rapid heartbeat and shortness of breath. So do people with GAD. By necessity, therapy must induce some of the physical sensations associated with anxiety and panic so that clients can habituate to them and neutralize their negative effects.

It is important to make clear to clients that the physical sensations that precede panic attacks do not *cause* the attacks. The overreaction to those physical sensations is actually what causes the attacks. To illustrate how overreaction to bodily sensations can trigger a cascade of events that result in a panic attack, it can be useful to ask what happens when clients climb a few flights of stairs and find that their heartbeat quickens.

Some people with panic disorder avoid exercise as a way to avoid heart palpitations and sweating because they fear triggering a panic attack. However, researchers have demonstrated that people do not experience a panic attack while exercising (Anthony, Roth Ledley, Liss, & Swinson, 2006). Exercise, in fact, has been shown to be an effective treatment for panic disorder. Smits, Powers, Berry, and Otto (2007) recommend that workout sessions of moderate to high intensity should last up to 30 minutes and should be completed approximately two to four times a week, for at least 4 weeks. Exercise not only provides interoceptive exposure but neurochemical changes to alleviate anxiety

CLIENT EDUCATION

Do your physical sensations ever include shortness of breath, rapid heartbeat, sweating, headaches, or nausea? Each one of these physical sensations is but a minor symptom of stress. Overreacting to those symptoms can tumble you into a panic attack.

During the last 40 years, most anxiety researchers have adopted the view that panic disorders are in part the result of excessive attention to benign physical sensations. The catastrophic misinterpretation of these body sensations stoke up the sympathetic nervous system. The fact that clients tend to gravitate to these misinterpretations led to the concept of anxiety sensitivity, which describes the fear of a catastrophic outcome from these physical sensations (Schmidt & Woolaway-Bickel, 2006). Anxiety sensitivity is widely considered a cognitive risk factor for panic disorder (Smits, Powers, Cho, & Telch, 2004; Wen & Zinbarg, 2007). Clients with panic disorder believe that having panic attacks has long-range catastrophic implications for health. This fear further heightens the negative expectations and the supersensitivity to benign physical sensations that may signal a panic attack.

The short-term solution provided by avoidant behaviors creates a long-term anxiety problem because the amygdala becomes oversensitized to minor sensations. For its part, the hijacked PFC narrows attention to warning signals that are really false alarms. It is important to address how "safety" behaviors, such as carrying around a bottle of benzodiazepines, actually can prevent the panic symptoms from extinguishing.

Exposure exercises should be broad based so that they help clients extinguish multiple conditioned stimuli that can serve as cues instead of dealing with each cue one at a time. In other words, to optimize the extinction of panic cues, it is best if you help clients vary the contexts in which exposure is carried out.

One of the cognitive strategies embraced by cognitive-behavioral therapists is to help clients reevaluate the cost of panic. For example, you may teach the client to say "If I have panic symptoms, what's so bad about that? When was the last time I died from panic?" In other words, by asking questions that have a hint of absurdity, clients can do two things: identify erroneous beliefs by examining evidence that does not support them and also distance themselves from those erroneous beliefs.

Biological and psychological factors act synergistically to increase client vulnerability to fear more episodes of physiological arousal, which contribute to more false alarms. These false alarms tend to be learned alarms that are classically conditioned. As such, they sharpen the focus on the bodily sensations, which then increases the likelihood that these sensations will become cues for possible learned alarms in the future (Barlow, & Craske, 2007).

It is important to convey to clients that panic attacks are triggered by sensations that are merely false alarms, not signs of some greater problem. Reacting to these sensations as something more ominous than *false* alarms will trigger the fight-or-flight response, during which time clients will feel an intense need to flee from something terrible. Because they do not know what that terrible thing might be, they may become convinced that they need to get to an emergency room, for fear of having a heart attack.

By providing some basic education on the stress systems, including the sympathetic nervous system and the hypothalamic-pituitary-adrenal axis (HPA), you can help clients understand how the functions of these systems offer perfectly natural reactions to a real threat and put the sensations in perspective. These stress systems

were indispensable when our ancestors faced predators. They underwent immediate physiological changes to prepare themselves to fight or take flight. Their
bodies pumped with adrenaline to make their hearts beat rapidly, causing blood
to flow to their extremities to ready them for action. Their breathing became rapid
and shallow to quickly oxygenate their blood, they perspired to cool their over-
heated bodies, and their muscles tensed to brace for quick movements. Their attention narrowed to focus solely on the danger and prevent distraction.

Humans still have this fight-or-flight mechanism to cope with real emergencies.
But for clients who suffer from panic disorder, these physical sensations are triggered by false alarms when there is no reason to fight or flee. Clients must learn
that they have developed a bad habit of thinking or feeling that danger exists where
it does not and, most important, that they have a tendency to misread physical
symptoms, such as dry mouth, nausea, and dizziness, as cause for alarm.

CLIENT EDUCATION

Your bodily sensations are not the cause for alarm. Real danger is. Keep
your stress system available for the rare times when you really need it.
Don't let your body be the boy who cried wolf.

It is important to help clients differentiate between false alarms and real
alarms. False alarms are learned (conditioned) alarms. When clients try to avoid
all potential frightening bodily sensations, those sensations become learned
alarms that become more resistant to extinction. The paradox occurs when clients try to avoid physical sensations. When they try really hard not to feel the
sensations, they feel them even more.

One of the basic principles used in many chronic pain programs is to teach
people afflicted with chronic pain to stop trying to avoid or block out the physical
sensations of pain. Instead they are asked to observe and accept the pain. This can
be especially frightening if clients have been traumatized by debilitating pain. They
wonder why they must face terrible pain when they have had too much of it already.
The paradoxical answer is that accepting the pain actually causes it to fade. This is
the first step toward making chronic pain tolerable. The same principle applies to
the physical sensations associated with panic. Although clients want desperately to
stop feeling those sensations, they must instead observe and accept them.

The fundamental lesson for clients to learn is that the more they fear the
physical sensations that they have associated with panic, the more they become
hypervigilant about them. Then, when even normal bodily sensations occur,
they too become alarming. Clients can break this vicious cycle at any point by
recognizing the physical sensations as normal bodily sensations that they can
embrace instead of needing to avoid. By shifting away from the all-or-nothing
intolerance and instead accepting random variations of sensations, clients can
defuse panic attacks before they begin.

Clients need to be taught that the only way out of this panic dilemma is to habituate to those physical sensations so they do not trigger false alarms resulting in panic attacks. The behavior therapy technique called interoceptive exposure is an evidence-based practice that helps clients habituate to their own bodily sensations, so that they no longer trigger panic.

Interoceptive exposure involves teaching clients to systematically desensitize themselves to those very physical sensations they find intolerable so that they can habituate to them. During interoceptive exposure experiences, you can invite clients to speed up their slow track by restructuring their thinking, using positive self-talk and narratives, while intermittently embracing the physical sensations. By developing new automatic thoughts and assumptions during interoceptive exposure exercises, clients gain confidence and learn to ride out those physical sensations, so they eventually become part of a richly textured and interesting life.

The therapeutic practice of exposure enjoys a long and well-researched history. As a standard element of all approaches to anxiety disorders, exposure involves repeated systematic confrontation of feared and avoided stimuli. In interoceptive exposure, you encourage clients to intentionally induce the very unpleasant panic-like physical sensations they so fear while simultaneously withholding attempts at preventing or dampening those sensations. The critical benefit of interoceptive and in vivo exposure is that clients fully engage the panic sensations.

The goal is not to eliminate the physical sensations but to normalize them, which will make them more manageable. People without panic disorder experience random physical sensations, such as rapid heartbeat and shortness of breath, as innocuous.

The interoceptive exercises include inducing these physical sensations:

- Overbreathing, generally referred to as hyperventilation. One way to induce overbreathing is to ask clients to run in place.
- Because some clients fear not getting enough air, you may ask the client to hold his breath.
- Many clients fear getting dizzy. One way to induce the experience is by spinning in a chair.
- Putting the head between the legs and then sitting up standing up quickly from lying on the floor are methods to induce light-headedness.
- Shaking the head from side to side is another method to induce dizziness.
- An often-noted sensation of discomfort is having a lump in the throat. Clients with panic disorder may become hyperalert to any difficulty swallowing. You may ask them to swallow quickly or swallow very slowly.
- Muscle tension is often a major symptom of stress and thereby triggers panic. Tensing the body helps clients recognize that muscle tension is a normal symptom of stress, not a cause for panic.
- Standing up quickly from lying on the floor.

Of all the interoceptive exposure exercises, overbreathing produces many of the physiological sensations associated with panic. Overbreathing sometimes leads to light-headedness, a rapid heartbeat, and racing thoughts. As an interoceptive exercise it can show how clients can unlink hyperventilation and panic. To teach clients how to habituate to overbreathing, invite them to participate with you by breathing quickly for 1½ minutes. Alternatively, you can both breathe through a straw for 1 minute, or try holding your noses while breathing through the straw while trying to get as much air as you can.

Brain-based therapy for people with panic disorder necessarily ought to include all of the next three interventions simultaneously:

1.　Desensitizing the amygdala by avoiding avoidance
2.　Interoceptive exposure exercises so clients can learn to embrace their own bodily sensations
3.　Speeding up the slow track by getting the L-PFC involved

Clients can be taught the crucial steps in beating panic disorder by using the mnemonic BEAT.

B—for body. The word can remind them that when they feel symptoms in their body, such as their heart racing or breathing too fast, they should just ride it out.

E—for exposure. They can remind themselves that through the interoceptive exposure exercises, they can regain tolerance to the variations in bodily sensations and say to themselves "This is not a heart attack but just bodily sensations that I have felt many times before. Besides, when is the last time I died from a panic attack? I can befriend my own body!" These shifts in perspective eventually help them to habituate to those sensations.

A—for the amygdala with its fast and slow tracks. Clients can remind themselves that their fast track can learn to slow down as their slow track learns to speed up. Their slow track involves their cortex, which is responsible for thinking.

T—for thinking. Clients can remind themselves that what they think is happening has a dramatic effect on what they feel is happening. When those thoughts are realistic, the slow track to their amygdala speeds up, which calms it down.

Chapter 7

POSTTRAUMATIC STRESS DISORDER

Throughout history people have been traumatized by natural and human-made disasters. Yet posttraumatic stress disorder (PTSD) was not recognized as a psychological disorder until 1980, partly due to Vietnam veterans finally receiving attention for the horrors of war that they experienced. Previously war-time trauma had been simply labeled "shell shock" or "war fatigue," but little was done to remedy these conditions beyond pulling the soldier out of combat. PTSD has garnered considerable attention over the past 25 years with the Afghan and Iraq wars. Yet trauma from rape and other types of assault have always occurred in overwhelming numbers.

Because of the dramatic increase in the numbers of people finally recognized as suffering from PTSD, the mental health community has been searching for well-researched approaches to providing effective psychotherapy. The US Department of Defense, the Veterans Administration, the Australian Centre for Posttraumatic Mental Health, and the Kaiser Permanente Medical Centers have all produced guidelines for PTSD. This chapter presents new insights gained from neuroscience, evidence-based practice, and memory research that can contribute to the brain-based common denominators among all the approaches as well as how to present the information to clients.

Overall, there are three phases to a brain-based therapy approach applied to PTSD. Briefly, these phases are as follows:

1. *Stabilization.* The stabilization phase is employed immediately after a traumatic event. You can provide psychological first aid to stabilize, calm, and orient victims of traumatic events. Given that only a relatively small percentage of those who experience traumatic events develop PTSD, a major effort is made to minimize the vulnerability to move from Acute Stress Disorder (diagnosed right after the traumatic event) to develop PTSD.

2. *Integration*. Since one of the hallmarks of PTSD is the dysregulation and fragmentation of memory systems, therapy during phase 2 involves the integration of the dysregulated implicit and explicit memory systems. Integration of implicit memory cues within the explicit memory system is critical for the development of affect regulation and a sense of a coherent sense of self.

3. *Posttraumatic growth*. The final phase involves the movement toward long-term recovery with greater resiliency. Growth also is based on developing a sense of meaning and direction in life.

This chapter is organized a little differently from the preceding chapters because with trauma there are opportunities to intervene immediately after the event(s) to prevent greater impairment. We discuss each phase in sequence because of the time factor and the phases of intervention. Finally, the mnemonic SAFE is recommended as a method by which to teach clients to remember the important steps that contribute to the sustained feeling of safety.

PHASE 1: STABILIZATION

Immediately after a traumatic event, victims should be offered interventions that stabilize, calm, and minimize their risks of future impairment. During the first month after the event, the symptoms of acute stress disorder (ASD) typically are the same as PTSD. Since most people do recover and do not develop PTSD, the purpose of Phase 1, therefore, is to provide preventive steps to avoid the development of PTSD. The four steps to the phase 1 approach include: (1) support, (2) assessment, (3) education, and (4) goal setting.

Support

Victims need an opportunity to feel accepted, understood, and comforted. Your calm and reassuring presence helps prevent them from being isolated with confusing feelings, such as hyperarousal and reexperiencing the trauma. Victims' responses will reflect their attachment style, described in Chapter 2. If insecurely attached, your attempts to provide empathetic support may be complicated by a less receptive response. Whatever the degree of resistance, helping them avoid isolation will provide a social buffer.

Since a significant risk factor for subsequent vulnerability for PTSD is lack of social support following a traumatic event (Bowler, Mergler, Huel, & Cone, 1994; Ozer, Best, Lipsey, & Weiss, 2003; Solomon, Mikulincer, & Avitzur, 1998), one of your initial concerns should include a comprehensive review of victims' social support systems. They can be informed that initial support activates the social brain networks, which help reduce immediate distress in response to the trauma.

In addition to these factors, the quality of social support is a critical factor in determining people's vulnerability to developing PTSD. The neurodynamics of social support are based on the same factors explained in Chapter 1, including oxytocin, which activates the parasympathetic nervous system and other social brain networks, including the social engagement system, mirror neurons, and so on. Increasing social support also serves to normalize daily activities. Although traumatized clients tend to feel detached from other people, the maxim "Fake it until you make it" should be the order of the day, along with "One day at a time." By receiving empathetic support, clients will feel less isolated and anxious, knowing that there is someone who understands and cares.

CLIENT EDUCATION

You may feel like isolating yourself now because you feel alone. It is quite common after a traumatic event. However, when people isolate themselves, they get worse and feel even more alone. You don't have to tell others all the gory details. In fact, this is not a good time to do that. Parts of your brain that activate when you are with people also buffer the pain that you must be feeling right now. When those brain areas shut down from lack of use, you feel more pain.

Assessment

An assessment of victims' overall functioning level should be multilevel. Because suicide potential is increased in people who have been traumatized, risk factors such as suicide potential and lethality must addressed. Up to 33% of people treated in an outpatient setting with PTSD have been reported to have engaged in self-harm behaviors (Zlotnick, Mattia, & Zimmerman, 1999). The risk goes up if victims suffer from all the symptoms of ASD. If so, it is advisable to increase the frequency of sessions and to call in other providers if risks of self-harm are evident.

The assessment should avoid needless and premature diagnosis. Despite the high numbers of people who experience or witness trauma, not all of them eventually suffer from PTSD. In fact, only 9% of those exposed to a traumatic stressor develop PTSD (Breslau, Davis, Andreski, Federman, & Anthony, 1998).

Although the estimated lifetime prevalence of having experienced a trauma is as high as 81.7% (Sledjeski et al., 2008), the lifetime prevalence of PTSD is dramatically lower at 6.7% (Kessler, Chiu, Demler, & Walters, 2005). Women and girls are nearly twice as likely to meet the criteria for PTSD. This gender difference in prevalence rates has not been accounted for by corresponding rates of exposure to trauma (Kessler, Chiu, Ruscio, Shear, & Walters, 1995).

Common posttrauma, main symptoms include:

- *Reexperiencing symptoms*, such as flashbacks, nightmares, recurrent and intrusive recollections of the event including sensations, images, thoughts, or perceptions.

- *Avoidance symptoms*, including thoughts, feelings, or conversations associated with the trauma. Avoidance also includes numbing. One possible extreme of avoidance involves disassociation. Allen (2001) describes a "continuum of deattachment" to disassociation which includes:
  - *Mild detachment*, involving an altered sense of self and a breakdown in the person's ability to notice outside events.
  - *Moderate detachment*, involving an experience of unreality extending to feelings of depersonalization and derealization.
  - *Extreme detachment*, ranging from a state of unresponsiveness to catatonia.
  - *Hyperarousal symptoms*, including difficulty falling or staying asleep and difficulty concentrating during the daytime. Clients tend to be hypervigilant and/or have an exaggerated startle response with possibly an anger problem or at least irritability.

Clients who have been chronically traumatized and have shut down and dissociated have difficulty feeling their bodies and differentiating emotions; and they feel like empty shells. They typically have less right insula activity. Whereas, those clients in a state of dramatic hyperarousal have an increase in activation of the right insula. People who have experienced trauma and developed PTSD either feel too much or not enough emotion. The challenge is to help them get back into the range of tolerance, to dynamic equilibrium.

Several risk factors need to be assessed. For example, if clients have a dissociative experience, referred to as peritraumatic dissociation, during or after the traumatic event, their likelihood of having a future PTSD response is increased (Candel & Merckelbach, 2004).

Sleep and diet must be assessed and stabilized. If clients are sleep deprived, the next day's levels of cortisol, adrenaline, and norepinephrine (NE) will tend to be elevated. As described later in this chapter, these neurochemical elevations increase people's vulnerability to develop PTSD. Substance abuse should be assessed and abstinence achieved. It is not uncommon for those who have been traumatized to self-medicate. You can warn clients that the direct result of substance abuse posttrauma is paradoxically an intensification of symptoms and a greater likelihood of developing PTSD.

Education

By validating clients' feelings, you both depathologize and reassure them that these feelings are indeed common after trauma. Also, when you offer information about typical initial symptoms following traumatic events, clients are warned that these symptoms may occur and are common reactions to having been traumatized. Because clients are forewarned, they respond less intensely to those expected symptoms. Victims who are not forewarned of these symptoms become alarmed by them and overreact, thinking that they must be worse off than the professionals thought.

Goal Setting

Because of the abrupt shock from the trauma, the foundational factors for a healthy brain described in Chapter 2 by the mnemonic SEEDS are typically destabilized. In the first phase posttrauma, stabilizing the SEEDS factors take primacy importance. Clients should be strongly advised not to isolate themselves from family and friends. Initially, increasing social support should not be directed toward talking about the details of the traumatic event. In fact, clients should be told that getting into the details too soon is ill advised. Later, with your help, the details of the actual event will be explored and put into perspective (Phase 2). You can use the phrase from Alcoholics Anonymous, "Fake it until you make it," to help encourage clients to normalize their social contacts.

Clients should be strongly advised to avoid using drugs and/or alcohol because both will intensify their symptoms. Dietary information should be explored in depth. Rather than simply asking "How is your diet?" it is critical to take a complete inventory of what clients actually are eating on a regular basis. For example, clients should be advised to minimize simple carbohydrates and excessive caffeine. Since insomnia and nightmares are common, sleep hygiene recommendations should be offered to maximize sleep potential. Daily exercise will decrease clients' stress neurochemistry and result in better sleep latency. Therefore, exercise, especially in the late afternoon, should be a routine recommendation; not only does it provide an anxiolytic and antidepressant effect, but when practiced in the 3-to-6-hour window before bedtime, it promotes deeper sleep.

Support for the concept of the Phase 1 focus on stabilization comes from a variety of studies on neurodynamics and neurochemistry. For example, clients can be informed that immediately following the traumatic incident, several adaptive initial neural reactions occur. Without these response systems, our species would not have survived and evolved. PTSD develops when these systems do not deactivate after the danger subsides. Rather, the systems can continue to be activated on a chronic basis without any effort to stabilize. The initial goal is to help those systems deactivate.

Clients generally are comforted to learn that it is quite normal for trauma to heighten amygdala activity, which prepares people to respond even more quickly should danger occur again. However, the orbitofrontal cortex (OFC), which normally inhibits amygdala overactivity, can itself be inhibited. When amygdala hyperactivity is not inhibited by the OFC immediately after a trauma, clients' alarm system is ramped up to veer on the side of false positives. The amygdala, as described in Chapter 2, maintains more extensive connections going up to the OFC than those coming back down from the medial prefrontal cortex (mPFC). Immediately posttrauma, the amygdala takes advantage of these bottom-up connections and prepares clients' brains to be hyperalert for more danger, making them prone to false positives for danger. The ramped-up amygdala activity occurs even when clients are resting, which makes them feeling on edge, jittery, and hypervigilant.

NEUROSCIENCE

While there is less activity in the OFC, there is enhanced dendritic aborization in the amygdala (Vyas, Bernal, & Chattarji, 2003; Vyas, Mitra, Rao, & Chattarji, 2002). Overall, there is a positive relationship between the degree of amygdala activity and anxiety symptom severity. The hyperarousal and increased tendency toward the startle response are further illustrated by increased blood flow in the amygdala, reflecting overactivity in people with PTSD (Pissiota et al., 2002; Semple et al., 2000). Correspondingly, there is reduced gray matter volume in the mPFC (Carrion et al., 2001; DeBellis et al., 2002a). The reduction in the mPFC represents an impaired ability to inhibit the hyperarousal generated by the amygdala.

Consistent with these findings, there tends to be a failure to activate the anterior cingulate cortex (ACC), which is associated with diminished mPFC activity in response to traumatic memories. Studies utilizing positron emission tomography (PET) scans to measure patterns of neural activity associated with traumatic images and sounds have shown decreased activity in the left prefrontal cortex (L-PFC) and ACC (Bremner et al., 1999).

Given that the ACC is important in monitoring emotional experience and that there is generally greater intensity of negative emotions associated with PTSD, these deficits represent a failure of the ACC to exert appropriate top-down inhibition. Also, since, as noted in Chapter 1, the L-PFC is associated with positive emotion, there is a breakdown in the capacity to maintain positive emotion. This picture, coupled with the studies showing increased amygdala and right- (R-) PFC activity (associated with negative emotion, avoidance, and withdrawal), reflects a failure to inhibit negative emotion.

You can explain that your efforts beginning in Phase 1 are directed toward shoring up clients' OFCs and their ability to dampen the hyperarousal and reexperiencing that occur due to amygdala overactivity. Additionally, clients can put more emphasis on the L-PFC than the R-PFC by working on concrete goals. The initial support, education, and establishment of concrete goals help shore up the OFC, providing structure and immediate context to the efforts to stabilize emotions and prevent the development of PTSD. The emphasis on approach behaviors through taking actual steps emphasizes the L-PFC over the tendency to withdraw associated with the R-PFC.

Many clients are curious and quite receptive to learn about neurochemistry and how to change it without having to depend on medication. Several neurochemical factors impair the PFC's capacity to inhibit amygdala overactivity. These include elevation of NE, increases in cortisol and its interactions with catecholines, and increased cytokines.

NEUROSCIENCE

NE plays a major role in the pathophysiology of developing and maintaining PTSD. There is a normal cycle of cortisol production for most people, with increased production beginning around 5:00 AM and a drop around 4:00 PM. Variations from this natural cycle are seen as problematic. High cortisol levels in the evening 1 month after the trauma increases the chances that clients will move from ASD to PTSD.

The more months that have elapsed since the trauma, the lower the morning cortisol and adrenocorticotropic hormone (ACTH) levels, including a drop in daily volume. If the chronic stressor is still present, there tends to be a rise in evening levels with an overall increase in daily output. If the threat is physical, there tends to be a flat output of cortisol. Finally, if the stressor is social, such as with a divorce, there is an increase in output, including in the morning.

There is also the case of hypocortisolism, which involves low cortisol in the morning. A meta-analysis of 107 studies on hypocortisolism in the morning found greater concentrations in the evening (Miller, Chen, & Zhou, 2007). This is especially the case if the person was subjected to pain. In such cases, there is a flatter diurnal rhythm and a higher daily volume of cortisol output.

The amygdala triggers elevated levels of NE through its rich connections with the locus coeruleus (LC), which is the primary source of NE in the brain. Because elevations in NE have been associated with the development of PTSD, some trauma victims have been given beta blockers, such as propranolol, immediately after the trauma. Compared to controls, these clients are less prone to develop PTSD. In other words, the prescription of a beta blocker is essentially prophylactic because high levels of NE prime the amygdala into overactivity. With less activity in the amygdala, there is a reduction in the release of NE, and less traumatic memory is encoded.

Levels of NE, both peripherally (throughout the body) and centrally (within the brain). typically are elevated posttrauma. High levels of NE are associated with the symptoms of hyperarousal and reexperiencing (flashbacks) (O'Donnell, Hegadoren, & Coupland, 2004; Southwick et al., 2005). NE also contributes to the development and maintenance of intrusive thoughts and nightmares (Cahill, 1997). Typically, in children with PTSD, NE increases over time.

High levels of NE ramp up anxiety by unleashing the amygdala and further triggering even more release through the LC. Additionally, the ventral tegmental area releases increased levels of dopamine (DA), and the dorsolateral tegmental nucleus releases increased levels of acetylcholine (ACh). All these factors further dampen the PFC's capacity for problem solving and rational behavior.

Consequently, there is a heightened tendency toward startle response, vigilance, insomnia, flashbacks, intrusive memories, and increased fear conditioning.

Cortisol and cytokines are the other two major players in the neurochemistry of PTSD. Elevations in cortisol in the evening are more reliable predictors of later PTSD than measures of cortisol during other times of the day. Also, elevations of proinflammatory cytokines, such as interleukin- (IL-) 6, soon after the trauma are also predictive of PTSD development 6 months later and are significantly correlated with high evening cortisol levels.

NEUROSCIENCE

Elevated IL-6 (an anti-inflammatory cytokine) contributes to disrupting the hypothalamic-pituitary-adrenal axis (HPA) axis (Chrousos et al.,1995). Several studies have examined the immune system function of adults with PTSD and found increased levels of pro-inflammatory cytokines circulating or in their cerebrospinal fluid (Baker et al., 2001; Rohleder, Joksimovic, Wolf, & Kirschbaum, 2004).

The secretion of IL-6 inflammatory cytokines can be triggered by activating beta adenoreceptors by the increases in NE. Inflammation can also occur through the hyperactivity of other systems of acute stress, including the CRH/Phistamine axis, and promote the acute phase reaction driven by the combination of elevated cortisol and IL-6 (Elenkov, Iezzoni, Daly, Harris, & Chrousos, 2005). For example, children who experienced trauma tend to have elevated IL-6 and evening cortisol, which makes them more likely to develop PTSD than children who experienced trauma and did not have those elevated levels (Papanicolaou et al., 2005).

All these factors combined demonstrate that the stabilization intent of Phase 1 is critical as a preventive measure for the development of PTSD. In other words, minimizing high levels of NE, cortisol, and inflammatory cytokines stabilizes traumatized people. Accordingly, the PFC is then better able to inhibit amygdala overactivity, and the person's potential to develop PTSD is reduced.

With these factors in mind, it is important to note that the once-standard psychological intervention called critical incident debriefing (CID) employed just after trauma is largely considered countertherapeutic today. CID actually conflicts with the principal goal of Phase 1: Stabilization. The key point is that memory consolidation takes time, and heightening stress neurochemistry by a premature review of the traumatic details accelerates the encoding of the traumatic memory. By getting into the details of the trauma too early, clients code into memory more frightening imagery than otherwise would occur. Too early exposure heightens amygdala reactivity, which spikes levels of NE and codes more implicit memory. Specifically, the higher the levels of NE and cortisol, the greater the chances of traumatic memory consolidation. Clients can be informed that instead of raising stress neurochemistry, the therapeutic effort during Phase 1 should be directed toward stabilization. By lowering elevated stress chemistry, Phase 1 aims for less traumatic memory to be encoded.

NEUROSCIENCE

The ACC is activated when people try to reconcile incongruent conditions, as compared to congruent or neutral conditions. And the dorsal ACC is believed to be associated with the resolution of conflict on cognitive tasks (Drevets & Raiche, 1998).

Individuals with PTSD show an increased activation of the dorsal ACC when exposed to combat-related words (Shin et al., 2001). Also found is decreased activation of the rostral ACC when PSTD participants are exposed to trauma-related stimuli. This decreased activation of the rostral ACC could be related to an inability to down-regulate amygdala response. Thus, there is an attentional bias to threat and hypervigilance.

CLIENT EDUCATION

Exercise is one of the easiest methods to decrease the levels of cortisol and cytokines. Brisk walking is one of the easiest ways to get exercise. It can be done anywhere and anytime. If done in the late afternoon, when stress chemistry is abnormally high and when there should be a natural lowering of stress neurochemistry, you gain an overall sleep benefit because low levels of stress chemistry promote sleep later in the night.

PHASE 2: MEMORY INTEGRATION

Many international consensus panels, such as the Institute of Medicine (IOM) in the United States, the National Institute of Clinical Excellence (NICE) in the United Kingdom, the American Psychological Association (APA), and the International Society for Traumatic Stress Studies (ISTSS), have made recommendations regarding what type of therapeutic approach to employ with people who have been traumatized. The consensus is that exposure therapy combined with some other form of cognitive-behavioral therapy (CBT) is the most effective. The IOM added that there is inadequate evidence to verify the efficiency of psychopharmacotherapy for PTSD. In fact, the NICE (2004) states: "Drug treatments for post-traumatic stress disorder should not be used as a routine first-line treatment for adults (in general use or by specialist mental health professionals) in preference to a trauma-focused psychological therapy." The consensus panels also recommend against the use of psychological debriefing (individual or group). For example, the ISTSS guidelines state: "There is no evidence to suggest that a single-session individual psychological debriefing is effective in the prevention of post-traumatic stress disorder (PTSD) symptoms shortly after a traumatic event or in the prevention of longer-term psychological sequel. The current evidence suggests that individual psychological debriefing should not be used" (Foa et al., 2009, p. 540). The point here is that while debriefing *right after* the trauma is countertherapeutic, exposure later is part of phase two.

Although the ISTSS states that there is strong evidence for the use of CBT in preventing chronic PTSD among people who experienced most traumas, the evidence is not strong for traumas with interpersonal violence, including rape. The ISTSS recommends that CBT be applied after a period of monitoring and support.

Clients with PTSD tend to suffer from fragmented senses of self. Fragmentation results in the loss of a cohesive experience of time, whereby the past traumatic event can instantaneously surge into the present, hijacking clients' sense of safety in the here and now. Emotions become fragmented from cognition, so that people feel too overwhelmed to put their emotional experience into context. To address the memory fragmentation, clients can be informed that memory integration will help them gain a sense of self and ability to regulate affect.

The therapeutic reconsolidation of the memory forms the foundation for clients to regain a sense of self and their capacity to regulate affect. Clients can be told that the once-elevated stress hormones have stabilized to a new (albeit elevated) baseline, and the second phase of therapy involves exposure and integration of the fragmented and dysregulated memory systems. This integration is fundamental for clients with PTSD because it is the dysregulation of these memory systems that contributes to a major part of the disorder. Specifically, implicit memory (emotional and sensory memory) is extremely out of sync with explicit memory (context and conscious understanding). One way to explain this dilemma is to ask if clients with PTSD experience surges in anxious feelings triggered by sights, sounds, smells, and the like that immediately trigger panic symptoms. The explicit memory system, which is driven by the cortex and hippocampus, is overwhelmed by the onslaught of dysregulated anxious feelings and emotions. During therapy in Phase 2, clients will learn to rebuild a capacity to regulate emotion and integrate the implicit and explicit memory systems.

Memory integration is facilitated by acceptance, through which clients learn that in the here and now there is safety. Based on the safety of the present they can make plans to move ahead with a viable future. Successful accomplishment of the integration necessitates four steps:

1. You must assess clients' current state of explicit memory system functioning to determine the pace and the extent to which integration is possible.
2. You help clients identify the cues that trigger flashbacks.
3. You prime integration by orchestrating a safe emergency during a therapeutic window that applies to the implicit memory cues.
4. You teach clients to use multiple channels of processing, including somatic grounding, in order to integrate their experiences.

Assessing Explicit Memory Capacity

It is best to begin memory system integration by assessing clients' *capacity* for integration. Without an understanding of the degree of explicit memory impairment and capacities, you may run the risk of expecting clients to integrate the memory systems at a faster or slower speed than they are able to do successfully. The amount of explicit memory impairment plays a large role in the degree to which clients may suffer from PTSD.

Most clients with PTSD who are not brain injured typically remember that the traumatic event happened but describe blank periods or gaps in the details of what occurred. Their recollection of these details is often vague, unclear, and disorganized (Harvey & Byant, 1999). These symptoms are largely related to the different effects of explicit and implicit memories and specifically to the activity of the hippocampus and the amygdala.

Consistent with reports of explicit memory deficits, clients with PTSD often have declarative and autobiographical memory problems. For example, inpatient adolescents who had experienced trauma were reported to have reduced autobiographical memory; the degree of memory loss was correlated with the number and severity of traumatic events (de Decker, Hermans, Raes, & Eelen, 2003). Similarly, semantic memory deficits were found in adult veterans with PTSD compared to controls (Yehuda, Boisoneau, Lowy, & Giller, 1995).

NEUROSCIENCE

Especially marked by the thousands of returning war veterans with traumatic brain injury (TBI), mental health providers have tried to determine the degree to which the veterans also suffer from PTSD. The symptoms of TBI and PTSD follow a slightly different course. To begin with, the diagnosis of TBI is made partly on posttraumatic amnesia (PTA), the length of time patients are unable to store into memory any details about the traumatic incident. If the PTA range is between 5 to 24 hours (mild to moderate PTA), the ASD is comparable to non-TBI samples (Harvey & Bryant, 1998a).

However, implicit memories may be present even though explicit memories are not, because the hippocampus needed a consolidation period and it was perturbed (Joseph & Masterson, 1999). Often patients with TBI who are assessed after trauma, then 6 weeks later, show no PTSD symptoms. But months later, PTSD symptoms are evident in both TBI and non-TBI groups (Bryant & Harvey, 1998).

The co-occurrence of a TBI and a psychologically traumatic event that caused the TBI can increase the implicit memory of the event while

(continued)

(*continued*)

undermining the explicit memory. Such a co-occurrence could increase the risk for heightened PTSD symptoms because cognitive representation of the trauma is impaired. This impairment of the explicit memory system increases with the severity of the TBI.

Post Traumatic Amnesia (PTA) generally involves some disorientation and inability to store and retrieve new information. With mild TBI, there typically are some islands of memory within the PTA period. The duration of PTA can be assessed over a 3-day period using a measure, which involves memory and orientation, such as the Westmead PTA Scale and the Galveston Orientation and Amnesia Test, to categorize the severity of the TBI (Shores et al., 1998; Sohlberg & Mateer, 1989).

Shortly after the TBI occurs, it is difficult to determine whether it will affect the development of PTSD. But at 3 months posttrauma, there are often no differences between TBI and non-TBI groups in the PTSD symptom profile (Jones, Harvey, & Brewin, 2005). Although the presence of a TBI influences the temporal distribution of emotional symptoms, it does not guarantee protection against ASD/PTSD (Bryant & Harvey, 1998).

Overall, the degree of impairment from TBI results from an extended PTA and impairment in explicit, not implicit, memory. The explicit memory system is largely dependent on a viable hippocampus while the implicit (emotional) memory system is amygdala driven. Thus, explicit memory is significantly vulnerable to disruptions from a TBI because the hippocampus needs time to consolidate explicit memory. In contrast, implicit memory may not be impaired because fragmentary sensations can be encoded immediately during the trauma, even in the absence of consistent consciousness.

Of course, most people who suffer from PTSD have not had a TBI, but those people who do illustrate that there are varying degrees of impairment of the explicit memory system. It is advisable to carefully assess explicit capacity and impairment in preparation for plans to integrate memory systems to what clients can tolerate without retraumatization and at what pace to orchestrate the integration of the memory systems.

The degree to which explicit memory is impaired is related to the degree to which the hippocampus and the PFC are impaired. Other brain regions associated with PTSD also can place limits on therapy as well as slow its pace. Over the past 15 years, neuroimaging studies involving PTSD symptom provocation have identified some consistent findings, including reduced activity in the left hemisphere, dorsolateral PFC (DLPFC), hippocampus, and Broca's area. Also, these studies have shown increased activation in the parahippocampal gyrus, posterior cingulate, and amygdala (Bremner, 2002; Nutt & Malizia, 2004; Rauch et al., 1998).

Since the early 1990s, there have been consistent reports of damage to the hippocampus among PTSD patients. This damage, assumed to have resulted from excessive cortisol, is also associated with verbal memory deficits (Bremner, Krystal, Southwick, & Charney, 1995). Also, the decreased activity in Broca's area appears to correspond to difficulty in coherently expressing a verbal narrative of the traumatic event (Hull, 2002). And the dysfunction of the DLPFC may be associated with problems in working memory, language, cognition, and integration of verbal expression with emotions.

Working memory deficits associated with PTSD reflect significantly less activation of the left dorsolateral prefrontal cortex (Clark et al., 2003). Consistent with asymmetry, clients with a childhood history of abuse tend to use their left hemispheres when thinking about neutral memories. When they recall early upsetting memories, they use their right hemispheres (Teicher et al. 2003). People without an abuse history tend to have a more integrated and bilateral response to recalling both neutral and traumatic memories. The left hemispheres of many adults who were abused as children appear developmentally arrested, especially the left frontal lobes (van der Kolk, et al., 1997).

The most dramatic memory deficits correspond to reductions in hippocampal volume. Magnetic resonance imaging– (MRI-) based measurements of hippocampal volume have shown reduced volumes for combat-related PTSD and PTSD related to childhood physical and sexual abuse (Bremner et al., 1995; Bremner et al., 1997). High levels of cortisol are associated with a range of separate neuroanatomical effects on the hippocampus, including impairment of synaptic plasticity, inhibition of neurogenesis, and ultimately neuronal death (Sapolsky, 2003). Clients who learn about these impairments can be encouraged to know that they are thought to be potentially reversible (Sapolsky, 2003).

NEUROSCIENCE

The structural integrity of specific areas of the brain associated with PTSD have been measured by a variety of methods. Two areas of the brain of particular interest have been the ACC and the hippocampus.

With regard to the hippocampus, a 23% reduction of N-acetyl aspartate (NAA) has been found bilaterally in the hippocampal region. Also noted has been a 26% reduction in choline in the right hippocampus relative to controls (Schuff et al., 2001). The reduction in NAA in the absence of loss of hippocampal volume in PTSD may reflect metabolic impairments or neuronal loss in the presence of glial proliferation.

(continued)

(continued)

> Overall, the studies of NAA/creatine indicate reduced neuronal integrity in the hippocampus. The reduced volumes, especially in the ACC, are associated with changes in NAA, which is a measure of neural integrity. For example, one study found lower NAA/creatine ratios in the ACC of children and adolescents with PTSD (Shin, Rauch, & Pitman, 2005).
>
> One way to measure the relative activity or inactivity of various areas of the brain is by changes in cerebral blood flow (CBF). Consistent with structural imaging studies, it appears that there is less activity in the mPFC, which includes the ACC. These areas of the brain, when not activated, essentially allow amygdala overactivity. Alternatively, when appropriately activated, the amygdala can be kept in check. Specifically, PET studies of regional CBF (rCBF) in the PFC have found decreased activation of the PFC, including the subcallosal cortex, as well as failure to activate the ACC (Bremner et al., 1999).

CLIENT EDUCATION

You may have experienced some memory problems caused by the extreme stress. As we work together, your memory will improve for positive events while the negative memories will become more tolerable.

The aversive effects of high stress do not occur with moderate stress because different types of receptors in the hippocampus. At low to moderate levels of stress, there is a heavy occupancy of mineralocorticoid receptors in the hippocampus. The classic memory impairment appears to be associated with high levels of stress and occupancy of cortisol receptors.

The traditional model that PTSD results in hippocampal volume reductions was complicated by reports that traumatized children had not suffered from hippocampal shrinkage (DeBellis et al., 1999; Karl et al., 2006). However, although the reduction in hippocampal volume does not appear right after the trauma, it does appear with the passage of time. The hippocampal size differences between adults and children with PTSD appear to reflect gradual damage to the structure of the hippocampus that may not be evident until postpubertal development and that chronic PTSD that persists into adulthood (Gilbertson et al., 2002).

The passage of time also affects hippocampal asymmetry. For example, in contrast to people without PTSD who have hippocampal asymmetry, with the left larger than the right, adults who experienced childhood abuse have been reported to have near symmetry. Adult PTSD may disrupt normal asymmetrical hippocampal development. Hippocampal volume reduction occurs at some time between childhood and adulthood, and those reductions are associated with severity of PTSD symptoms (Woon & Hedges, 2008).

The failure to find reductions in hippocampal volume in traumatized children, although reductions have been found in adults with PTSD, raised the question of whether smaller hippocampal volumes represent a predisposing factor instead of a cause of PTSD.

Given that only roughly 11% to 18% of the people who experience a life-threatening trauma develop PTSD, researchers have long searched for factors that increase the risk. By the late 1990s, one factor that began to be explored is the premorbid size of the hippocampus: The hippocampus, and specifically its skill at registering explicit memory, including context, time sequencing, and somatic organization, is impoverished in people with PTSD. Also critical is the thermostat function of the hippocampus via its cortisol receptors. When it is working well, the hippocampus can act to turn down the release of cortisol.

To assess the premorbid integrity of the hippocampus, researchers took monozygotic twin brothers, one of whom had combat-related PTSD and the other who never went to war. Both had smaller hippocampal volumes. Thus, the vulnerability hypothesis may be viable as a possible partial explanation for risk. It appears that both the vulnerability hypothesis and the cortisol-cascade hypothesis are correct (Gilbertson et al., 2002).

The development of PTSD after trauma in people with a small hippocampus before trauma represents a diminished ability to turn off the production of cortisol and the overall stress response. This impairment represents a breakdown in the "thermostat function" described in Chapter 3.

Meanwhile, the amygdala responds to the increase in cortisol by ramping up its activity. People who have ramped-up amygdala activity along with simultaneous impairment of the hippocampus thermostat function are prone to hypervigilance and increased false positives for danger.

Although it is common that clients with PTSD have experienced some impairment to their hippocampus and their explicit memory system leading to a diminished ability to defuse anxiety, the hippocampus can be rebuilt. Both physical and cognitive exercises help rebuild the hippocampus.

CLIENT EDUCATION

Although the part of your brain that lays down memories may be temporarily impaired, it can be rebuilt by both aerobic exercise and cognitive exercise.

NEUROSCIENCE

By the mid-1990s, there were reports that victims of trauma and chronic stress experience wide variations in cortisol levels. Some combat veterans, Holocaust survivors, and other trauma victims actually have reduced cortisol secretion, referred to as hypocortisolism, as well as other abnormal HPA activity (Gunnar & Vazquez, 2001; Yehuda et al., 1995, 1998). The most robust evidence comes from patients who experienced chronic and intractable PTSD.

Although PTSD generally has been associated with hyperactivity of the HPA axis, it can lead secondarily to reduced cortisol levels through a negative feedback process (Yehuda et al., 1998). A meta-analysis of 107 studies on morning hypocortisolism found that the dysregulation in cortisol reflected greater concentrations of afternoon/evening cortisol (especially if the person was subjected to shame), a flatter diurnal rhythm, and a higher daily volume of cortisol output (Miller, Chen, & Zhou, 2007). These findings suggest that chronic stress is accompanied by a dysregulated pattern of cortisol secretion with lower-than-normal morning output and higher-than-normal secretion across the rest of the day into the evening, as well as an overall flattened diurnal rhythm.

CLIENT EDUCATION

With the dysregulation of cortisol, especially the elevation in the evening, insomnia is a common symptom. One quick way to lower cortisol and improve sleep is through exercise in the late afternoon or early evening.

A 2007 IOM thorough review of all the psychotherapy research for PTSD requested by the Veterans Administration discovered that few treatments had very clear empirical support. This included eye movement desensitization and reprocessing (EMDR), group therapy, hypnotherapy, eclectic therapy, and CBT without exposure. On the other hand, the study found efficacy in the use of therapies applying the use of exposure as occurs with prolonged exposure (PE) and cognitive processing therapy (CPT) (Foa et al., 2009).

Many variations of the exposure paradigm have been explored. For example, imaginal exposure exposes clients to memory of the trauma in structured, guided imagery format. Trauma exposure helps clients to reduce anxiety associated with trauma memory through extinction of conditioned fear while organizing the memory into a coherent narrative. This process eventually calms an overactive amygdala.

It is generally believed that someone with PTSD needs a minimum of 12 therapy sessions, no matter the technique used. The CBT approach starts with psychoeducation, anxiety management, and coping skills. A minimum of 4 to 6 imaginal exposure sessions, with a temporary increase of anxiety and reexperiencing of symptoms, is also expected. Simultaneously, the therapist promotes the cognitive processing of trauma memory and combines associated meaning, which involves beliefs that build on self-efficiency. Actual in vivo situational exposure, as in CBT and PE, targets avoidance of trauma-related situations. Finally, interoceptive exposure targets "fear of fear," or somatic phobia, as employed in treatment for panic disorder.

Though the use of medications in treatment of PTSD has been controversial, especially the use of benzodiazepines, one drug actually increases neuroplasticity: D-cycloserine (DCS). DCS is an antibiotic used in higher doses to treat tuberculosis. It has been shown to bind to N-methyl-D-aspartate (NMDA) receptors. Use of this drug promotes and speeds up exposure effects of neuroplasticity within the amygdala through the NMDA receptors. Treatment with DCS is most efficacious prior to or immediately following exposure (Ledgerwood, Richardson, & Cranney, 2003). When DCS has been used, fewer sessions are required to successfully treat social phobia (Davis, Ressler, Rothbaum, & Richardson, 2006).

Integrating Memory Systems

Once you have assessed the degree of dysregulation among memory systems, you can help clients integrate them by building up from clients' current functioning level. The methods you use to help clients integrate the implicit and explicit memory systems need to go beyond theoretical perspectives of the past to develop a robust brain-based therapy.

Memory of trauma can be stored in explicit memory as verbally accessible memories (VAMs) on the conscious memory level, which comprises the narrative memory of the trauma and implicit memory as situationally accessible memories (SAMs), which are largely nonconscious sensations. Whereas explicit-memory VAMs can be accessed in therapy through deliberate recall, implicit-memory SAMs are accessible only through cues that activate the nonconscious network (Brewin, 2005).

Explicit memories of the trauma comprise the verbal description of the past, the context of the event(s), and the chronology. It is this memory system that, although it may be impaired, needs to be rebuilt so clients can use its abilities of context and time to integrate implicit memory of the trauma, which tends to have a timeless quality. Brewin 2005 note:

> These memories are available for verbal communication with others, but the amount of information they contain is restricted because they only record what has been consistently attended to. Diversion of attention to the immediate source of threat and the effects of high levels of arousal greatly restrict the volume of information that can be registered during the event itself. (pp. 139)

Traumatized clients use their explicit memory systems to evaluate the trauma, both when it is happening and afterward, and to ask themselves how the event could have been prevented or what the potential consequences and implications of the experience are. Brewin 2005 refer to the emotions that accompany VAM (explicit) system memories as "secondary emotions" because they were not experienced at the time of the trauma itself. They are directed at the past, such as regret or anger about careless risks taken, or to the future, such as sadness at the loss of cherished plans and hopelessness at the thought of not finding fulfillment. These secondary emotions involve guilt and shame over the perceived failure of not preventing the event.

Largely amygdala driven, the implicit system, by contrast, contains information that has been obtained from lower-level processing of the traumatic scene, information that includes sights, sounds, and bodily sensations, such as the changes in heart rate, temperature, or pain that were too briefly apprehended to be bound together in conscious memory required for the explicit system. The implicit system triggers the flashbacks that occur involuntarily by situational reminders of the trauma.

Because the amygdala orchestrates a wide spectrum of neurochemical and autonomic reactions to stress, the state-based implicit memories are associated with specific breathing patterns, muscle tensions, gastrointestinal sensations, heart rate, and so on. One or all of these sensations can serve as the implicit cue for a flashback. As in therapy with people with panic disorders, interoceptive exposure exercises serve as evidence-based practices.

CLIENT EDUCATION

Flashbacks do not usually happen out of nowhere. Rather, they may be triggered by the same bodily sensations that you felt during or right after the trauma. Our job together is to help you learn to make friends with those sensations so that they do not trigger a flashback. To help you reown your body, we can induce the very sensations that you find frightening so that when they occur randomly, they will not trigger panic.

The interplay between explicit and implicit systems is influenced by the intensity of emotion. Since explicit memories are highly dependent on the hippocampal-PFC memory system, during periods of intense emotion, they can be superseded by amygdala-driven implicit memories. In such situations, the implicit system can drive the explicit system to encode fear-based memory.

Since the implicit memory system is largely nonconscious and can involve the fast track to the amygdala, sensory information, such as smells or sounds, go directly to the amygdala from the thalamus. High levels of stress overactivate the amygdala and elevate levels of cortisol, NE, and cytokines, which result in impairments to the hippocampus, PFC, and explicit memory system that they make possible.

During periods of intense emotion driven by traumatic experiences, hippocampal processing of information underlying explicit memory tends to be reduced, and formation of implicit memories is increased due to heightened amygdala reactivity. The increase in implicit memories and the decrease in explicit memories correspond to increased trauma reminders in the form of flashbacks triggered by sights, sounds, and smells that are experienced by a sense of timeless threat.

Nonhippocampally-dependent implicit memories appear to be more resistant to change and the passage of time than explicit memories, which are far more vulnerable to modification over time. Thus, implicit memories are not restricted to verbally coded memories and are more extensive. Because they are difficult to communicate to a therapist, they are also difficult to update by a purely verbally based approach. Flashbacks, for example, are spontaneous and difficult to control because it is difficult to regulate exposure to sights, smells, sounds, and the like that act to trigger flashbacks. The emotions triggered have been referred to as "primary emotions," consisting of fear, helplessness, and horror (Brewin, 2005). The more complex and extended the traumatic experience, the more clients tend to experience a range of emotions.

Priming Integration

Because the cues for flashbacks are essentially fragmented implicit memories that occur sporadically, they are difficult to access and must be orchestrated to occur. This deliberate orchestration of implicit memory cues is referred to as exposure. It is through well-managed exposure that therapy can build the explicit memory system so that the implicit memory cues can be better regulated.

Emotional engagement with traumatic memories is a critical part of recovery (Zoellner, Fitzgibbons, & Foa, 2001) as well as engagement of the traumatic memory cues that serve to maintain PTSD symptoms. From a practical perspective, exposure may necessitate imagery-based memories. This can include writing or reading about the trauma or role playing (Taylor, 2004).

Given that clients with PTSD engage in automatic dysfunctional information processing, helping them understand this automatic processing and reframe and recontextualize their symptoms will restore a sense of healthy self-organization.

In therapy, you can lead clients to deliberately maintain attention on the content of the flashbacks by no longer trying to suppress them. In this way, the memories encoded in the SAM system become reconsolidated in the VAM system. Through this exposure process, the indelible qualities of the SAM images and sensations thus become linked with the spatial and temporal context of the VAM system. Consolidation in the VAM system occurs when SAMs are triggered and are put into the context of time and place so that clients can remind themselves that they are now safe and the trauma or threat is in the past. Clients can feel secure in the present with a sense of safety that the trauma and danger are behind them.

The exposure of the implicit memory SAMs and reconsolidation process with the explicit memory VAMs must be repeated multiple times, not only because there generally exists a lot of information in the SAM system to be re-encoded but also because neuroplasticity necessitates repetition. Rehearsing the newly consolidated VAM memories repeatedly will promote easier access to the SAM memories. The integrated VAM and SAM memories compete with the old SAM memories of the trauma by putting those memories in perspective in the here and now. This process turns down the activation of the sympathetic nervous system through the VAM system network in the PFC and hippocampus, which functions to put the brakes on the HPA axis by inhibiting the amygdala overactivity.

CLIENT EDUCATION

As you slowly expose yourself to the frightening implicit memory cues that trigger flashbacks, you can bring them under control. You can activate the triggers while we simultaneously bring meaning, context, and realistic thoughts into mind so that you will be better able to live without fear that the frightening feelings and nightmares will continue.

The interaction between the SAM and VAM systems promoted through exposure and cognitive restructuring processes results in CBF changes during retrieval of traumatic memories before and after psychotherapy (Peres et al., 2007). The narrative organization of explicit memory is modified by associated experiences of emotional context and the state of consciousness during the recall process.

The therapeutic integration of SAMs and VAMs is consistent with the Expert Consensus Guidelines series of treatment for PTSD (1999), which states that exposure-based therapy is the treatment of choice for intrusive thoughts, flashbacks, trauma-related fears, and avoidance. Generally, the therapeutic approaches to PTSD combine cognitive (explicit memory) restructuring methods with exposure. Exposure to the traumatic memories occurs through a well-constructed process that incorporates the emotional content (Brewin, 2005; Littrell, 1998).

Therapeutic attention should be on the fragmented SAM-related flashback memories, sometimes referred to as "hot spots." Hot spots are brief moments when emotions are particularly intense and correspond to flashbacks. These hot spots are important points of focus in exposure therapy rather than the entire event (Ehlers & Clark, 2000).

From the perspective of a dual-memory system, hot spots may correspond to moments where there is maximal functioning separation between visuospatial and verbal processing (Brewin, 2005). This separation can lead to a large discrepancy between the contents of the respective memory systems (VAM and SAM). These are moments that provide retrieval cues that need recording into verbal memory so that they do not trigger flashbacks.

For example, if the client is a combat war veteran and flashbacks are triggered by implicit memory cues such as loud popping sounds that resemble gunfire or by the smell of gunpowder, he may experience flashbacks at a Fourth of July fireworks display or by hearing a car backfiring. Therapy during Phase 2 involves your effort to orchestrate his exposure to stimuli as similar as possible to gunfire or loud popping noises within 30 minutes of each session. During the sessions, you and the client co-construct a forward-looking adaptive narrative that provides context and meaning so that when the implicit memory stimulus is detected, autonomic arousal is tempered along with the overactivity of the amygdala.

CLIENT EDUCATION

Every time you go through this exercise, it will get easier. Your brain will rewire its connections between the higher parts of your brain, including your cortex and hippocampus, so that they can put the brakes on the panic button, the amygdala.

Sustained conscious attention to these implicit SAM memories promotes integration with the VAM system, which strengthens coping skills enhanced by PFC inhibitory control over the amygdala, ultimately diminishing flashbacks. This restructuring and integration of the memory systems through the development of a new narrative combines memories of successful self-efficacy prior to the trauma and constructive lessons learned after the trauma.

The reinterpretation and reconsolidation of traumatic memories, accomplished through exposure and cognitive restructuring, can alleviate some of the distressing PTSD symptoms by challenging the nature of the representations of the traumatic event (Peres, McFarlane, Nasello, & Moores, 2008). The affective shift combined with new explicit, hippocampally driven memories (VAMs) allows the traumatic and fragmented memories (SAMs) to transform into integrated emotional and cognitive memories that can be more easily managed and available for narrative expression. In other words, when uncomfortable feelings come up, instead of reverting to flashbacks laced with panic feelings, clients can stay in the present and calm themselves. Just as dreams can be thought of as a weather vane of daily life, nightmares can similarly fade away.

CLIENT EDUCATION

Through this process of memory consolidation, what had triggered flashbacks and panic feelings can begin to fade away. Those panic feelings will lose their timelessness and be placed where they belong, in the past.

Inverted U and the Therapeutic Window

Integration of implicit and explicit memory (SAMs and VAMs) arousal levels must be therapeutically managed to be consistent with the dynamics of the inverted U, aiding neuroplasticity. For example, if arousal levels are too low, traumatic images are not accessed. If arousal levels are too high, clients can begin to dissociate or become so overwhelmed with the traumatic memory that they lose contact with immediate surroundings. Since hippocampal and PFC networks can become impaired, clients will reexperience the trauma. Effective therapy involves strengthening those networks, carefully integrating SAM information with the VAM system (Brewin, 2005). The integration orchestrated with a moderate level of activation to expand the width of the therapeutic window.

NEUROSCIENCE

The capacity for relatively clear information processing in clients suffering from PTSD can be impaired by the difficulty in controlling trauma-related thoughts following trauma-related cues. However, there is less support for the concept that PTSD involves increased susceptibility to intentional forgetting or suppressing of trauma-related material (Constans, 2005). Rather, unwanted processing of emotional memories may reflect a cognitive gating deficit. Here, the PFC cannot adequately regulate the amygdala.

During an emotional event, the amygdala links episodic memory to the emotions triggered by the event. Over time, relevant information about the event is extracted from episodic memory into semantic memory and stored in the cortex. With PTSD, there is a breakdown in the extraction process of memory transfer and integration. When clients with PTSD try to minimize consequences of this failure, flashbacks break through the defenses of avoidance and numbing.

Recovery requires reestablishment of these failed processes in integration. You can explain that there is an opportunity for recovery because memory reconsolidation occurs every time a memory is retrieved. The memory trace goes through another period of consolidation in the therapeutic context of the safe emergency. Pharmacological adjuncts to this process are beta-adrenergic antagonists (i.e., propranolol) that block reconsolidation of implicit fear-based memories by indirectly influencing protein synthesis in the amygdala (Debiec & LeDoux, 2004).

This reconsolidation is particularly relevant when working with trauma. The so-called window of tolerance represents the degree to which people can remain receptive to new input and learn from therapy. Therefore, therapy should focus on helping clients stay within the top boundary of the window of tolerance. This perspective is consistent with the Yerkes-Dodson learning curve and the need for moderate arousal. From a neurotransmitter perspective, this accesses the NMDA glutamate receptors and the alpha2A NE receptors, thus facilitating neuroplasticity. The window of tolerance serves as a range that must expand through incremental exposure, always exceeding what clients think may be possible.

NEUROSCIENCE

Therapy necessitates optimizing moderate levels of NE, which access the alpha2 autoreceptors that provide a braking function for NE. When NE is released by the presynaptic neuron, it makes contact with both post- and presynaptic neurons. While the contact with postsynaptic neurons can trigger an action potential, NE interlocks with the alpha2 autoreceptor on the presynapatic neuron, which released the NE, initially where it acts to slow down the release of NE.

Generally the checks and balances work fine unless people are overwhelmed by anxiety and/or trauma. Then this system gets destabilized. If people then consume too much caffeine, they experience excessive anxiety. This happens if the alpha2 presynaptic NE autoreceptor is agonized (blocked), so that the braking action does not occur. The stimulant yohombine and caffeine are alpha2 agonists. When people with PTSD consume excessive amounts of yohombine or caffeine, they may experience excessive NE, which may precipitate panic attacks.

For a variety of reasons, certain people may be more vulnerable to even minor fluctuations in brain chemistry. For example, people may have hyposensitive alpha2 NE autoreceptors that are insensitive to excessive NE and do not act to shut it down. As a result of the insensitivity, NE is not shut down but is rather increased.

CLIENT EDUCATION

After you have suffered trauma, your brain chemistry can be imbalanced in the direction of maintaining superalertness. Even minor changes in your diet can trigger alarm when there is no danger.

Considering the often-delicate and dysregulated neurochemistry and the hyperactivity of the amygdala, work in the therapeutic window necessitates gradual exposure. An incremental approach works best so that the traumatic implicit memories can be dealt with in smaller units and from less distressing to more distressing. The Subjective Units of Distress Scale (SUDS) approach, often used in CBT, allows you and clients an opportunity to break down the levels of distress into doable chunks.

Clients need to gradually move out of their comfort levels and should be told that a moderate degree of anxiety is most productive. Waiting to feel comfortable is counterproductive. The more distinctive the newly consolidated explicit memories and insights are while they are fused with a moderate degree of anxiety, the more likely that the trauma flashbacks will diminish in intensity.

Traumatic memories are vulnerable to being triggered and reexperienced in flashbacks because they are fragmented and disorganized. The integration of the implicit and explicit making those memories makes them coherent and better structured to reduce the risk of unwanted intrusions (Ehlers & Clark, 2000). Essentially, when traumatic memories are reactivated through exposure and reconsolidation by incorporating them into more accurate information, they become less distressing and more easily managed.

It is not enough to offer clients incremental exposure exercises from a CBT-connectionist perspective, which aims merely to connect the disconnected memory systems. A constructivist perspective goes beyond the connectionist model, helping clients envision a future with meaning. Generally, therapeutic approaches that attempt to integrate implicit and explicit memories of traumatic experiences by constructing an adaptive narrative by necessity evokes implicit memories through exposure, in vivo or imagery. Yet Chris Brewin (2005) notes some limitations with holding to simply a CBT view:

> "All these therapeutic approaches reflect the essentially rationalist assump-tions of classical cognitive behavioral therapy, in which patients are seen as possessing inaccurate or otherwise faulty memories or beliefs that have to be corrected. The basic concept of memory transformation is, however, shared by alternative approaches that are more constructivist than ration-alist. For example, it has been suggested that the function of eliciting a detailed verbal or written account of a horrific experience is to assist the person in turning "traumatic memories" into "narrative memories." In this formulation raw sensory data that need to be interpreted and anchored within a personal narrative framework that provides them with meaning. This approach is not rationalist in that the new narrative account does not need to be "correct" but simply to provide a coherent and acceptable ac-count in the individual's own terms. (p. 276)

Overall memories cannot be simply corrected. Therapy must instead promote the construction of alternative memories. Newly constructed memories then compete with the original memories for control of behavior and attention with the emphasis on "self"-organization described in Chapter 1.

REM, Non-REM, and Memory

Sleep disturbances are quite common with clients suffering from PTSD. Typi-cally there is an alternation of sleep architecture (the stages of sleep) with the lighter levels of sleep (stages 1 and 2) and rapid-eye-movement (REM) sleep (dream sleep) increased, and the deepest level of sleep (stage 4, which is represented by delta waves) decreased. This means that in addition to the loss of sleep due to insomnia, the sleep produced is of poor quality, and clients wake up feeling sleep deprived as well as fatigued.

Normally, during REM slee, there is a lack of input from the hippocampus to the cortex. Because little spatial and temporal coherence comes from the hippocampus, the cortex produces dreams and images that include weak associations, unpredictable juxtapositions of barely related objects, locations, and characters in often-illogical sequences. Dream images and plotlines float free in time and space.

In contrast to REM sleep, during non-REM sleep, there is a flow of information from the hippocampus to the cortex. This outflow of hippocampal information to the cortex may serve to reinforce old memories. During REM sleep, the blocking of hippocampal outflow helps prevent semantic associations from falling back into predictable, overlearned patterns and the formation of new memories (Stickgold, 2002).

NEUROSCIENCE

Using exposures with response prevention (ERPs) in electroencephalogram (EEG) studies, researchers have shown that patients with PTSD respond to a broader range of environmental stimuli for a longer period of time as if those stimuli were novel. They have an impaired ability to filter out irrelevant stimuli; they attend to more stimuli as if they had importance and relevance (Metzger, Gilbertson, & Orr, 2005). Their tendency toward poor habituation and lowered stress thresholds contributes to hyperactivity.

Despite Freud's contention that dreams are composed of day residue, dreams usually are composed of factoids from the day, not contextually accurate images or stories. However, people suffering from PTSD are the exception. PTSD clients have a breakdown of the normal blockade of hippocampal outflow to the cortex. Traumatic episodic memories are repetitively replayed in recurrent nightmares. This breakdown prevents the normal integration of the episodic memory and leads to PTSD (Stickgold, Hobson, Fosse, & Fosse, 2001).

Various factors account for this breakdown. People with PTSD generally experience fragmented sleep and may retain an inappropriate level of vigilance even while asleep. They also have been noted to have reduced time in REM sleep in part because of the increase in NE (Glaubman, Mikulincer, Porat, Wasserman, & Birger, 1990). These phenomena may be related to the increased levels of NE and adrenaline that are often associated with PTSD.

High levels of NE are of particular significance because in people without PTSD, the shift into REM sleep is marked by turning off NE and serotonin.

The failure to shut down NE in people with PTSD leads to a dissociated neuro-modulary state and incomplete entry to REM sleep. Instead of weak associations of REM sleep, there is a shift to strong associations that involves a replay of traumatic memories (Stickgold, 2002).

Sleep is critical for the consolidation of memory. While non-REM sleep is important for strengthening explicit memories, REM sleep is important for strengthening implicit memories (Plihal & Born, 1997). Information flows out of the hippocampus and into the cortex during non-REM sleep. In contrast, information flows from the cortex to the hippocampus during REM sleep (Buzsáki, 1996).

Semantic memory activates weak associations in REM sleep but strong associations in non-REM sleep (Stickgold et al., 2001). REM and non-REM sleep differ as well in neurotransmitter activation. Specifically, serotonin dominates in non-REM sleep (Portus et al., 1998) while ACh dominates during REM sleep (Kametani & Kawamura, 1990). The shift to REM sleep and processing memories in the cortex is dependent on the cessation of NE and serotonin. The failure to turn off NE during this shift plays a large role in producing a dysfunctional system.

One factor that contributes to PTSD is an inability to inhibit NE release during REM sleep. The increase of NE during sleep may break down the weak associations in the cortex necessary for the integration of traumatic memories into the narrative association networks. This failure to blockade hippocampal outflow and inappropriate increase of NE leads to the recurring reenactments of traumatic memories (Buzsáki, 1996; Stickgold, 2002).

As a result of the blocked integration, there is no feedback to the hippocampus, so it is starved of instructions to weaken the episodic memory of the traumas and their associated negative effect. This chain of events perpetuates self-sustaining nightmares, a condition of PTSD.

Somatic Therapies

A considerable amount of attention has been devoted to somatic-based therapies, including the so-called bilateral-reprocessing therapies, such as Eye Movement Desensitization and Reprocessing (EMDR); and the tapping therapy, such as the Emotional Freedom Technique (EFT), Sensorimotor Psychotherapy, and Somatic Experiencing. It is important to explore if there are common factors among these approaches that are efficacious from a brain-based therapy perspective.

In the context of the dynamics of REM sleep and its dysregulation during PTSD, several researchers have tried to make sense of the somatic therapies, such EMDR and EFT (Stickgold, 2002). Since the early 1990s, EMDR has gained considerable notoriety (Shapiro, 1995). First regarded as a curiosity, it has since grown to be accepted and practiced by a large number of trained therapists.

Early EMDR utilized bilateral eye movements as one of its principal methods, along with processing traumatic memories and rating symptoms with SUDS, as in many CBTs. Later EMDR therapists began to use bilateral knee slapping and alternating flicking lights or sounds to achieve bilateral activation. Some researchers and therapists have attained positive results with alternating finger tapping or the use of other stimuli (Bergmann, 1998). According to this perspective, bilateral shifts in attention are thought to allow the brain to resynchronize from being asymmetrical in functioning. This facilitation of bilateral stimulation primarily facilitates greater hemisphere interaction and inhibition of amygdala overactivity. Subsequent research has found that the bilateral movements are not a factor in the efficacy of the therapeutic method.

With EMDR, eye movements originally were thought of as essential to the processing of the traumatic memory (Shapiro, 2001). However, the importance of eye movements has not gained empirical support (Spates, Koch, Pagoto, Cusack, & Waller, 2009). In recent years, some EMDR therapists have moved from eye movements to other procedures, including asking the client to alternate finger tapping from right to left, claiming equivalent mechanisms to eye movements (Shapiro, 2001). Here, too, dismantling studies have not demonstrated that the bilateral movements affect symptom reduction (Cahill, Carrigan, & Frueh, 1999). The bottom line is that well-respected and well-designed outcome studies have found no advantage of EMDR over exposure therapy alone (Rothbaum, Astin, & Marsteller, 2005).

It appears that the somatic therapies disrupt the configuration of traumatic memories not through a specific theory-driven process but by common factors to help clients reconsolidate and integrate those memories. Like other non–somatic-based therapies, they offer clients a supportive relationship and incremental exposure to traumatic memories. The exposure process helps clients integrate traumatic thoughts and emotions. Another common factor among the eye movements, tapping, and other body movements is an expectancy set that something therapeutic will occur.

The somatic approaches also include attention to physical sensations orchestrated by the therapist. Stickgold (2002) has proposed that the underlying neurobiological mechanism of action of EMDR is the repetitive redirecting of attention that induces a state similar to that of REM sleep, which is optimally configured to support the cortical integration of traumatic memories into general semantic networks. This integration can then lead to a reduction in the strength of hippocampally mediated episodic memories of the traumatic event as well as the memories associated with the amygdala-dependent negative affect.

Somatic stimulation, whether induced by eye movements, bilateral stimulation, tapping, acupressure, or acupuncture, induce a shift in attention involving the orientation response (Sokolov, 1990). The orientation response may induce a REM-like state that facilitates the cortical integration of traumatic memories (Stickgold, 2002). This reorienting of attention can be triggered automatically when a sudden movement grabs client attention or intentionally when clients choose to look at an object. The reorienting of attention requires clients to release focus from one location so that it can shift to a new location. When you repeatedly reorient client attention from one location to another by the tapping or eye movements, you can produce shifts in required brain activation and neuromodulation similar to those produced during REM sleep.

NEUROSCIENCE

The reorientation of attention and the startle response produce shifts in regional brain activation and neuromodulation similar to those produced in REM sleep (Stickgold, 2002). Specifically, inducing the startle response leads to activation of brain stem circuits that also can initiate a state similar to REM sleep. Consistent with the initiation of REM sleep, the brain stem initiates a burst of pontogeniculoccipital (PGO) waves. Inducing the startle response leads to activation of brain stem circuits that can initiate a state similar to REM sleep.

These neurocircuits include those responsible for releasing, shifting, and then refocusing attention. They involve the ACC, which is significant for both sleep and PTSD, as well as the superior colliculus, which is activated by the PGO waves and control eye movements. Also, the cholinergic system increases while noradrenergic system decreases facilitate the release of attention prior to the shift (Clark, Geffen, & Geffen, 1987). Consistent with this model, EMDR has been shown to activate the ACC and the left frontal cortex (Levin, Lazrove, & van der Kolk, 1999). Additionally, EMDR has been found to decrease galvanic skin response (GSR), especially related to reducing adrenergic drive.

These constant reorienting shifts in attention, however they are achieved, activate the same neurocircuits that facilitate REM-like memory processing (Stickgold, 2002). The REM-like state facilitates the integration of traumatic memories into associative cortical networks without interference from hippocampal-mediated episodic recall. The integrated corticohippocorpal circuits induce a weakening of the traumatic episodic memory with its associated affect. This helps clients to see the significance and meaning of the traumatic event from a perspective that incorporates their entire lives and lessens the impairment that the trauma caused.

Through the use of somatic-type therapies that evoke the orienting response and its similarity with REM sleep, traumatic memories can be integrated through focused therapeutic effort. Unlike REM sleep, when PFC activity is largely inhibited (Hobson, Stickgold, & Pace-Schott, 1998), these approaches involve PFC activation through effort and focused attention. Through imaginal exposure, by holding an image in mind while engaging in somatic stimulation, the reconsolidation of implicit and explicit memories associated with the trauma will be biased by the current context of the safe emergency of the therapeutic relationship. By providing the safe emergency with moderated degrees of anxiety with the associated moderate level of NE, you can facilitate the optimal conditions for therapeutic neuroplasticity.

CLIENT EDUCATION

I am going to ask you to direct your attention to the specific movement while at the same time we go over the traumatic event and put it into the past. This will help you reset your brain so that it will no longer be stuck in the past and you can move ahead to enjoy a possible future.

PHASE 3: POSTTRAUMATIC GROWTH

After the integration of the implicit and explicit memories, Phase 3 involves working with clients to develop a viable sense of self-efficacy which has been referred to as an optimistic future and posttraumatic growth. There is a valuable potential for positive growth to occur after a trauma. Up to 50% of trauma victims report some sort of positive outcome posttrauma (Updegraff & Taylor, 2000).

Helping clients move beyond recovery to resilience involves their developing a sense of meaning in regard to having experienced traumatic events(s) (Tedeschi, 1999). Posttraumatic growth involves constructive changes in clients' sense of self, relationships, and philosophy of life.

Nowhere is the importance of meaning better illustrated than in one of the most inspiring books in our field, Victor Frankl's *Man's Search for Meaning* (2006). Despite suffering the horrors of Auschwitz and its aftermath, Frankl embraced a transcending sense of meaning by demonstrating how those who have been deeply traumatized can move on to wisdom and growth.

CLIENT EDUCATION

Many people who have been horribly traumatized have gone ahead to gain a deep sense of meaning and to enjoy a positive future.

Helping clients transcend the trauma to gain hope for a healthy future often involves learning about people who have done it. I often describe my Armenian grandparents and cousins, who lived through a horrific genocide, only to later thrive in the United States and France. Alternatively, I describe Victor Frankl's experiences. Whatever illustration is used, the principal point is that people do not need to feel damaged beyond hope.

Despite having experienced traumatic event(s), clients can gain from posttraumatic growth as they broaden their sense of self, relationships, and philosophy of life. This self-organization involves helping clients leap to a higher level of psychological organization as they acknowledge their connection to the world and depth of meaning. This enhanced sense of meaning of life is critical as clients try to make sense of and accept what happened.

The posttraumatic growth is part of the self-organizing process as they transcend the trauma to understand, with greater meaning and an acceptance of their relationship to the world. The changes in clients' sense of self help them acknowledge their connection to the world, acknowledge their vulnerability, and wake up from the illusion of invulnerability. This paradoxical understanding of human vulnerability and the acceptance of what has occurred gives clients better control and a sense of true strength. The changes to their relationships reflect an enhanced sense of relatedness to others. Being able to connect empathetically with others allows clients to deepen intimacy and true sharing of feelings and thoughts about what happened to them and about their aspirations for the future.

By encouraging clients to engage with you in a process of trying to make sense of what happened to them while acknowledging that an immediate explanation may not suffice, the PTSD symptoms can subside as clients take a wider look at their place in the world and try to derive meaning from that wider perspective. With much less focus on the emotional pain of the trauma than in Phase 2, Phase 3 offers clients the opportunity to reestablish a sense of connectivity with people and the world around them. Clients lose their old sense of self ("old me") and learn to see their new sense of self ("new me") as more appreciative of the interdependence of all parts of the world.

CLIENT EDUCATION

There is no turning back before the trauma to the old you. But the new you can be wiser and use the opportunity to become a deeper and more caring person.

Sandra Bloom (1998) noted that people who experience danger and/or trauma have a natural inclination to gather together for safety and healing. This natural human tendency can be promoted after a trauma to provide clients with a sense of social transformation afterward. The common purpose that responds to the trauma, such as a support or political group that seeks to repair the ills of society, can be a parallel healing for the individual. For example, Marc Klaas, father of abducted 12-year-old Polly Klaas, founded and directed an organization to educate people about child abduction. A mother who lost a daughter to a drunk driver formed Mothers Against Drunk Driving (MADD). Again, Victor Frankl not only survived Auschwitz but the years thereafter by expanding on a sense of meaning and commitment to others.

Increasing cognitive complexity and self-organization bolsters clients' stress-protective abilities (Tennen & Affleck, 1998). Self-complexity increases as you help clients expand the number of different perspectives they have of themselves. Optimally one of those perspectives is that their sense of self is complex enough to weather the stress.

In their book *Trauma and Transformation*, Tedeschi and Calhoun (1995) offer seven principles of growth after trauma:

1. Growth occurs when one's psychological schemas are changed by traumatic events. Old schemas are destroyed and replaced by new schemas. "I almost died! Why?"
2. Some assumptions are resistant to disconformation. These assumptions buffer us from initial distress from the trauma but reduce the possibilities for schema change and growth.
3. Positive evaluations of self must follow trauma for growth to occur. This reframing can be as basic as "I am a survivor."
4. Different types of events are likely to cause different types of growth, whether the events were caused by others or oneself.
5. Certain personality characteristics are related to the possibility for growth. For example, hardiness, optimism, and self-efficacy allow one to see growth within those perspectives.
6. Growth occurs when the trauma serves as a central pivotal change in one's life. It allows one to shift perspective to a new era.
7. Wisdom results from growth. Clients see what's possible and what is not, just like the Serenity Prayer.

SAFE

Clients can remember the important steps to regaining a sense of safety by using the mnemonic SAFE. The letters in the mnemonic correspond to

S—for sharing
A—for acceptance
F—for family/friends
E—for exposure

Clients must practice each of the aspects to regaining a sense of safety simultaneously.

Sharing

Clients can be told that it is quite common for people who have been traumatized to feel like no one understands. The more they keep all the confusing thoughts and feelings inside of themselves, the more confused they feel by those thoughts and feelings. You may tell them that sharing involves being open with significant others. As a result of doing so, clients will feel less alone and isolated. Sharing does not mean having to go into all the details of the trauma with everyone. Rather, sharing involves acknowledging with those who matter that clients had a traumatic experience and that they are in the process of recovering. It also involves airing what occurred with someone who can help put it all in perspective, such as a therapist. Clients can remind themselves that sharing also involves sharing aspirations for the future.

Acceptance

Often people who have been traumatized find it difficult to accept the fact that they have been traumatized. Avoidance symptoms so central to PTSD are partly related to this difficulty in accepting what happened because of the frightening feelings that come up. Unfortunately, avoidance serves only to increase the reactivity of the amygdala. Acceptance allows victims to move on.

Family and Friends

Clients can be told that not only is it common for people who have been traumatized to feel alone, but they often isolate themselves from family and friends. They can be told that the areas in their social brain networks deactivate when they withdraw, and when these networks deactivate, anxiety and depression increase. Being with family and friends allows those networks to activate and provide comfort, even when the topic or focus of getting together has nothing overtly to do with the trauma.

Exposure

Clients can be told that one of the most difficult things for people with PTSD to do is to confront the feelings and sensations that send them into panic. Yet when they avoid those triggers to panic, they occur more often. Paradoxically, the way to turn them off is to confront them. For example, if sounds that remind them of gunfire trigger a panic attack, eventually going to a fireworks display (and doing it often as possible) will help them habituate to the sounds that trigger an attack.

Many clients are confused by the increased feelings of stress and anxiety that continue to plague them long after the identified stressor or traumatic incident. Their brain responded by "priming" the neurocircuits that respond to danger. The primed system is sensitized to hyperrespond to stress (DeBellis, Hooper, & Sapia, 2005). The increase in sensitization that traumatized clients often feel contributes to hypervigilance and overresponsiveness to stress. Sensitized memories related to the trauma trigger flashbacks and rekindle fear neural networks, so that previously traumatized clients reexperience the danger long after it has passed.

NEUROSCIENCE

"Priming" is a term that involves the sensitization of the neurocircuits that make a response to repeated stress increase in magnitude via kindling the neurocircuits underlying the memories of the trauma. Hormones such as arginine and vasopressin and neurotransmitters such as the catecholamines act synergistically with CRH to activate neurocircuits to be ready for more danger. When the amygdala processes emotional stress, the HPA axis functions are enhanced through higher ACTH and higher 24-hour free cortisol concentrations.

> Increases in the level of stress enhance dendritic aborization in the amygdala (Vyas, Bernal, & Chattarji, 2003; Vyas, Mitra, Rao, & Chattarji, 2002). In other words, the amygdala grows in complexity through increased connections between neurons and can be activated more easily. Increased NE levels trigger the periaqueductal gray (PAG), which maintains a connection to the amygdala, causing the "freeze," and to dissociation from the psychic and physical stress of trauma (Murburg, 1997; van der Kolk, McFarlane, & Weisaeth, 1996).

For clients with PTSD, it is useful to normalize amygdala responses by explaining that from an evolutionary perspective it kept our species safe. When our ancestors encountered a life-threatening situation, they became hyperalert not only to that situation but to similar dangerous situations. That alarm system protected them in the future from anything remotely resembling the original danger. This meant that there has always been an increased chance for false positives. In other words, after a near-death experience, our ancestors became hypervigilant, perhaps a little jumpy, ready to bolt should the need arise. It has always been better to be safe than sorry. However, for clients with anxiety disorders, their alarm system is on high alert to ensure that the trauma does not happen again. With the new knowledge clients have gained from you, they can make this alert system work more effectively so that they can turn off the system when it is not needed.

CLIENT EDUCATION

Your alarm system is stuck in the on position. We can work together to turn it back to the ready as really needed position.

Chapter 8

OBSESSIVE-COMPULSIVE DISORDER

The concept and phenomenon of obsessive-compulsive disorder (OCD) has long been debated with regard to whether it is a form of anxiety or a separate disorder. Most recently with the fifth edition of the *Diagnostic and Statistical Manual of Mental Disorders* (DSM-5; 2013), OCD is not classified with anxiety disorders, and hoarding has been separated out of the OCD category. OCD includes unwanted intrusive thoughts that can range from annoying or frightening to repulsive. Because clients who are plagued by these thoughts find it next to impossible to get them out of their minds, the thoughts are considered "obsessive."

Obsessive thoughts can co-opt concerns, reactions, worries, and fears and blow concerns out of proportion. Clients with OCD lose the ability to judge the likelihood of their thoughts coming true. The more clients try to avoid these thoughts, the stronger and more uncomfortable they become. Because the thoughts are not easily dismissed, clients cannot readily follow the advice of family and friends to just think about something else.

Some common topics that trigger obsessive thoughts are listed next:

- Perfection, correctness, orderliness, exactness
- Cleanliness, germs, contamination
- Safety, security
- Need to save or collect things
- Immorality, sexuality, perversity
- Aggression, violence

Compulsive behaviors are often related in a logical way to obsessive thoughts. That is, a person with an obsessive fear of germs or contamination may engage in compulsive washing and housecleaning. Compulsive checking of locks on the doors and windows may follow obsessive thoughts about safety. Compulsive prayer might follow obsessive thoughts about immoral behavior. However, there are also cases in which there is no logical link between the obsession and the compulsion. This seems especially true with the compulsion to count things or repeat words or phrases until clients sense things are in order or feel "just right."

Up to 98% of people with OCD engage in behaviors (compulsions) to reduce discomfort from their obsessions (Foa et al., 1995). These compulsions are repetitive and/or ritualistic behaviors, often with the goal of reducing anxiety or discomfort. There are a wide variety of compulsions, often grouped into categories of cleaning, checking, ordering/arranging, counting, and repeating. Hoarding has been separated out in *DSM-5*. The most common compulsion reported by people with OCD is checking (Ruscio, Stein, Chiu, & Kessler, 2010).

Some common compulsions include excessive:

- Counting, praying, repeating words;
- Hand washing, bathing, grooming, housecleaning;
- Avoiding "contaminated" objects;
- Checking doors, windows, locks, stove, appliances, food;
- Retracing one's movements or driving route to ensure no one was hurt.

One characteristic of OCD is that the worry or fear often is for the safety of others. This pattern sometimes develops in a woman soon after having a child, with obsessive thoughts revolving around the child's safety. Of course, it is normal for parents to be concerned for their baby's health and safety. Most parents, especially those with young children, have near-constant thoughts about where the children are, whether they are fed, whether their homework is done, and so on. The difference between the typical concerns of parents and the concerns of clients with OCD has to do with how easily and frequently those fears get triggered, how uncomfortable clients get, how long the thoughts persist, and what clients do to calm themselves.

Clients with a compulsion to wash and clean have a belief of where germs may be hiding and/or a heightened sensitivity to contamination. They may avoid shaking hands with others and have developed clever ways to get in and out of public buildings without touching door handles. While it is actually a smart move to avoid touching door handles in public buildings and to wash one's hands, clients with this form of OCD may compulsively wash their arms and entire body after touching or believing they were contaminated. The self-cleansing can last for hours and sometimes require rigorous adherence to a specific ritualized sequence. Sometimes, if the ritual sequence is interrupted or not followed exactly, clients must start the entire sequence again from the beginning. Housecleaning rituals are common among clients with this type of OCD; initially they may downplay their OCD, saying they like their home to be orderly. This often includes frequent vacuuming and excessive cleaning of the kitchen or bathrooms.

Some clients repeatedly check stoves, irons, and locks on doors and windows. Sensible, onetime checking differs from feeling compelled to check three or more times before being satisfied that things are in order. During the initial check, clients have the anxious sense that they cannot stop checking until they have done it the special way that gives them a feeling of order. Another type of compulsion to check involves clients retracing driving routes to ensure that they have not harmed anyone during the drive. Clients may even watch the news to verify they did not cause an accident. Some clients may compulsively inspect their bodies to ensure no injuries, ticks, or diseases were acquired during the day. I have seen many clients who frequently visit doctors with obsessive fear that they are ill despite consistent reassurance that they are okay.

Repeating behaviors typically are done multiple times, until clients feel that the last repetition was done "just right" so as to reduce the sense of discomfort. Repeated activities may include buttoning and unbuttoning clothing, dressing and undressing, stepping in and out of a room, opening and closing doors or cabinets "the right number of times," or turning light switches on and off repeatedly until gaining a sense of order. Clients with counting compulsions may even regard certain numbers as good or bad. Objects or sequences that contain "bad" numbers need to be reorganized or repeated with only the "good" ones. Clients with a combined compulsion to wash and count feel the need to wash the "correct" number of times.

Counting and other thought rituals can be triggered by intrusive thoughts or images of harm, disaster, aggression, violence, sexual acts, or immoral or blasphemous behavior. The thought ritual is intended to undo or neutralize the intrusive thought so as to avoid contributing to harm. Thought rituals can take many forms, including prayer, asking forgiveness, striking a bargain with God, mentally saying the opposite of the dangerous thought, and thinking a "magical" phrase a particular number of times.

People suffering from OCD can be severely plagued by shame and embarrassment since their thoughts and behaviors can seem quite bizarre. Many people with OCD do not offer information about their shame and guilt in therapy until asked about it directly. Also, it is very uncommon for people to volunteer information about their odd thoughts or behaviors. Once the topic is opened, however, they generally find great relief in finally talking with a mental health professional.

Children who develop OCD before puberty generally are male. Motor tics are common, including Tourette's disorder. Adult-onset OCD tends to affect women more than men.

The most widely used OCD outcome measure is the Yale-Brown Obsessive-Compulsive Scale (Y-BOCS; Williams, Powers, & Foa, 2012). The Y-BOCS is a semistructured interview that usually takes 30 minutes to complete. It consists of a checklist of obsessions and compulsions and a 10-item severity scale. It is useful in pretreatment, and it helps in the planning of a therapeutic strategy with clients.

DESCRIBING THE OCD CIRCUIT

Many clients with OCD are particularly receptive to brain-based explanations. Although compulsive behaviors seem to temporarily reduce anxiety in the moment and help clients find relief, the behaviors keep OCD brain circuits activated and strong. Discuss in detail with clients how they can make use of this knowledge to weaken the OCD brain circuits while simultaneously strengthening healthier alternative circuits.

OCD involves habits that are very hard to break. A subcortical area of the brain called the basal ganglia and, specifically, the striatum serves many functions, including habit formation. When this area of the brain is disinhibited it is as if a filter or gate is broken, allowing obsessive thoughts and compulsions to flood through automatically. The striatum is composed of two parts, the caudate nucleus and putamen. The caudate nucleus serves as a gate for thoughts and emotions; the putamen serves as the gate movement.

When the caudate and putamen are unrestrained and are not doing their job of filtering out nuisance information, clients are bombarded by obsessions and compulsions. This unfiltered information rushes through the open gate to flood the orbitofrontal cortex (OFC), which responds by generating error messages: "This is wrong! This is wrong!" Then clients engage in compulsive behaviors to make things right.

The OFC is also hijacked by his hyperactive amygdala, though not to the extreme as with anxiety disorders. Key to implicit memory and the amygdala reacts to events and situations that are potentially dangerous and activates the fear circuit in the body. Though much less of a factor with OCD than other anxiety disorders, when extremely activated it signals the rest of the stress network, including the locus coeruleus, to release norepinephrine and the hypothalamus to secrete corticotropin-releasing hormone (CRH), which in turn triggers the pituitary gland to release adrenocorticotropic hormone (ACTH) in the bloodstream. This triggers the adrenal glands to release epinephrine (adrenaline) and norepinephrine. If the stress persists for longer than about 30 minutes, cortisol is released. All of this activity further excites the amygdala to keep the fear circuit going and to signal that something needs to be done to put things in order.

Although most clients with OCD generally do not have panic attacks, they anxiously obsess about things not feeling right. If they do not engage in the compulsive behavior, their fear circuit becomes hyperactive. When they engage in a compulsive behavior to turn off the fear network, they gain only temporary relief. By not learning to turn off the fear circuit naturally, they avoid discomfort by engaging in the compulsive behaviors, which, ironically, contributes to more obsessive thinking.

OCD involves hyperactivity in the relationship among the OFC, the basal ganglia, and the thalamus. Normally there is a dynamic balance between activation/disinhibition and inhibition, which is associated with the flexible, situation-appropriate initiation and termination of behavior. When this balance is impaired, OCD-like symptoms emerge.

Huntington's disease and Tourette's disorder are extreme neurological examples of a breakdown in the balance between activation and inhibition. They occur as a result of tonic imbalance skewed in favor of activation. Parkinson's disease, in contrast, is skewed in the direction of inhibition. Though OCD is not related to these neurological disorders, the point is that OCD is a breakdown in favor of the activation path, whereby automatic behaviors become difficult to inhibit. Because the OFC becomes hijacked into overactivation in the pathway, successful therapy necessarily involves kindling the attention and the inhibition pathway, which involves the dorsolateral prefrontal cortex (DLPFC). The DLPFC is involved in positive, goal-oriented, rational, and reflective behavior while the OFC is more involved in emotionally driven behavior.

NEUROSCIENCE

The activating circuits underlying OCD are associated with the ventral medial PFC, the striatum, and the dorsal thalamus. The route inhibiting OCD symptoms is associated with the DLPFC to the striatum. OFC hyperactivity (the ventral PFC) is one of the main causes of OCD (Baxter et al., 2000).

With OCD, the compulsions recruit inefficient striatum (caudate nucleus) in order to achieve that thalamic gating to neutralize obsession and anxiety. Overall, magnetic resonance imaging (MRI) studies of OCD have reported abnormalities in the OFC and anterior cingulate cortex (ACC) and in caudate activity (Baxter et al., 1987; Swedo et al., 1992).

NEUROSCIENCE

Based on research with patients with OCD who have engaged in cognitive-behavioral therapy (CBT), there tends to be decreased metabolism in the right caudate nucleus, a portion of the basal ganglia (Linden, 2006). Further, after exposure and response prevention, some clients show a significant decrease in thalamic metabolism along with a significant increase in the right ACC (Saxena et al., 2009).

There is evidence for a corticobasal ganglia circuit dysfunction in OCD. Specifically, there tends to be abnormal metabolic activity in the OFC, the ACC, and the caudate nucleus (the anterior part of the striatum, which is part of the subcortical area called the basal ganglia; Graybiel & Rauch, 2000).

For Tourette's disorder, which is associated with OCD, especially for prepubescent males, the putamen (posterior part of the striatum) seems to be implicated. The repetitive tics or actions are the predominant symptoms of what have been called the motor loop.

In support of the model, MRI and spectroscopy studies show reduced neuronal density in the striatum of people with OCD (Fitzgerald, Moore, Paulson, Stewart, & Rosenberg, 2000).

Clients are usually quite heartened to learn that there is a brain-based way to turn off the OCD circuit. They can learn to provide support for their beleaguered OFC so it can inhibit the overactivity of the amygdala and the fear network. Clients can teach their OFC to strengthen the connections to the amygdala to calm it down. Instead of being hijacked, the amygdala and the OFC can learn to regain control and shut down the fear network.

You may inform clients that the DLPFC can come to the aid of the OFC. The DLPFC, a major part of the brain's executive control center, is key to working memory skills and attention. Compulsive behavior occurs almost on autopilot; it is so habitual that afterward clients are troubled by it. By using the DLPFC to strengthen their attention skills, clients can break out of autopilot and gain an observational moment for the OFC to disengage its effort to try to solve a problem where there is no problem to solve.

NEUROSCIENCE

The idea that the striatum is involved in the pathophysiology of OCD has a long and interesting history. The idea was first proposed by Constantin von Economo, who described patients suffering from obsessions and compulsions following the great 1912 epidemic of viral encephalitis in Europe. More recently, Swedo and colleagues (1998) studied disorders precipitated by rheumatic fever caused by streptococcal infection. Such infections can lead to Sydenham's chorea, which is characterized by obsessions, compulsions, tics, and other OCD-like symptoms. The overall group of disorders has been referred to as pediatric autoimmune neuropsychiatric disorders associated with streptococcal infections (PANDAS). Their underlying pathophysiology is thought to involve an autoimmune-mediated attack precipitated by the strep infection (Swedo et al., 1998).

One of the healthy talents of the OFC is to appreciate ambiguity, the many shades of gray in life, and tolerate uncertainty. The support it gets from the DLPFC can free it from being hijacked and can help it develop these talents. Therapy, therefore, necessarily must include strengthening attention to the here-and-now and focus on rebuilding people's capacity to deal with uncertain thoughts and feelings that arise when they observe and reframe from their usual pattern of obsessions and compulsions.

Connections between the OFC and amygdala strengthen as clients learn how to tolerate discomfort through exposure. Meanwhile, therapy can help them to become relaxed instead of anxious and show them how to stop engaging in compulsive behaviors. The PFC and hippocampus process explicit memory, which involves recognizing that clients have engaged in the compulsive behavior many times before, only to feel compelled to do it again. When working optimally, the hippocampus can help balance out the activity of the amygdala. Since fear activates the amygdala, clients could be led to activate memories of OCD being wrong, despite their adrenaline-induced false alarms, and find out that "nothing bad happened the last time I ignored it." By ignoring the alarm, clients can strengthen the downward control connections between the OFC and the amygdala by the brake mechanism of the nonautopilot brain.

Teaching the Client to Neutralize Doubt

OCD has been called the doubting disease because clients who compulsively wash, for example, doubt the ability of the skin and body to block infection and doubt that one shower is enough. Checkers doubt that they turned off the stove. Doubt and uncertainty often lead to a spike in anxiety and the tendency to fall back into habit.

The acquisition and maintenance of procedural memories, or habits, form some of the core aspects of OCD. Specifically, the striatum is involved in the OCD circuit and habit formation, also referred to as the procedural type of implicit memory. When the striatum is stuck in the on position during a period of discomfort, it is as if a gate has been left open, which allows repetitive obsessions to flood the OFC and quickly trigger "automatic" compulsive behaviors by the striatum. When the striatum is not stuck in the habit, usually people do not need to give much thought to inhibit automatic behaviors. Overlearned procedural memories, such as riding a bike or driving a car, occur on autopilot so that we can talk to a friend about something totally unrelated to bicycle riding or driving a car. Once clients observe an automatic compulsive behavior (procedural memory) with the conscious mind, they are free to do something new.

To explain the connection between procedural memory and OCD, you may point out that when clients initiate normal hand washing, they follow a set routine:

1. Turn on the water.
2. Wet hands.
3. Soap hand.
4. Scrub for several seconds.
5. Rinse hands.
6. Turn off water.
7. Dry hands.

Often while clients are washing their hands, they do not focus on what they are doing. He could be thinking about a friend that he is going to visit. When he is done washing his hands, he can move on to the next behavior, such as brushing his teeth. Often with OCD, however, this compulsive behavior does not terminate, and clients may feel the need to wash their hands again, perhaps 10 times or for 10 minutes or when some other "magical" termination point is reached. The thought of germs triggers the amygdala, and the striatum gets stuck open. Client efforts to stop washing hands do not terminate this OCD loop until their amygdala feels satisfied that the danger has passed by washing the correct number of times, determined by the OFC cortex.

The problem-solving function of the OFC and striatum, the habit function of the results in hand washing to solve the obsession with dirtiness, until eventually the response is exhausted. Then clients finally feel that their hands are clean, and they can stop washing and go on to the next activity.

The important point to highlight with clients is that when they get stuck in one of these OFC loops, they need to use their DLPFC and hippocampus functions to break out and consciously take hold of the manual controls. Part of the challenge with OCD is that the amygdala and striatum are powerful and not comfortable being challenged. The OFC immediately begins to doubt whether clients should take the manual controls away from the automatic habits driven by the striatum or instead obey the amygdala's danger signal and let the striatum run on autopilot. Because clients are dealing with the autopilot, they can learn to consciously observe that OCD thoughts and feelings are false danger signals.

Remind clients of the phrase "Cells that fire together wire together." This can describe how the brain can rewire as they learn to break old (OCD) habits. By breaking out of autopilot through attention to the now and making connections between new noncompulsive behaviors while simultaneously exposing themselves to discomfort, clients can interrupt the OCD habit loop.

Specifically they can learn to override the overactivity of the amygdala and teach the striatum new habits that include productive thoughts and behaviors. This can be monitored by activating the DLPFC and hippocampus to exert their full executive control talents that recognize that obsessive thoughts and compulsive behaviors do not make sense. By weaving this executive control into memory, when OCD thoughts emerge, clients will be able to phase out the obsessions and compulsive behaviors.

If clients check the doors four times before leaving the house, ask them to check them only three times, then leave. Then ask if anything happened as a result of clients omitting the fourth check. Typically, clients will answer that their anxiety level shot up. At that point, encourage them to continue with this plan while noting that eventually their amygdala will "get bored" because nothing bad ever happens.

It is unfortunate that many young therapists are unfamiliar with Victor Frankl, because he foresaw and developed many concepts and therapeutic strategies employed today. Once such practice is called paradoxical intention, which bypasses the tendency to become obsessed with a thought by deliberately bringing it to the forefront of consciousness (Frankl, 1975).

As a sort of psychodynamic/existential form of confronting obsessive thinking, this approach foreshadowed the exposure-based CBT approaches used today.

With paradoxical intention, you encourage clients to wish for the things that they most fear, even to the point of exaggerating it until it seems humorous. Frankl viewed the element of humor as key. Since fighting against it only makes the obsession stronger, the way to break the obsessive cycle is to confront the obsession rather than resisting and engaging in compulsions. By facing and exaggerating it, the idea becomes absurd to clients.

Applying an Exposure Hierarchy

Like most approaches to alter forms of anxiety, exposure can be extremely uncomfortable. The effective therapeutic approach orchestrates a moderate degree of exposure to rewire client brains incrementally to achieve the maximum gain with tolerable discomfort. Many approaches use an exposure hierarchy chart that orders a list of triggers low on the Subjective Units of Distress Scale (SUDS) at the top of the page, progressing to triggers with the highest SUDS ratings at the bottom of the chart.

Exposure and Response Prevention

Over the course of 40 years, the principal CBT therapeutic approach to OCD has become what is known as exposure and response prevention (EX/RP). Sometimes the word "response" is replaced by the word "ritual" because not all responses are compulsions.

EX/RP has been used in a wide variety of formats and settings, including individual, group, and family therapy as well as in computer-based, self-help, and intensive programs (National Institute for Clinical Excellence, 2004).

The exposure sessions work best if they are frequent and last from 45 minutes to 2 hours. The initial goal is for clients to remain in the anxiety-provoking situation long enough to experience some reduction in anxiety and to realize that the feared disastrous consequences do not occur. With repeated exposures, clients' peak of distress and overall distress generally tend to decrease over the sessions.

Most approaches present exposure situations gradually so that clients experience only moderate levels of anxiety. A standard method of monitoring the level of anxiety is the SUDS scale.

The response/ritual prevention component requires that clients be instructed not to engage in the compulsions or rituals of any sort. Because clients believe that the rituals prevent the feared outcome, only by stopping the rituals do they learn that they do not protect them from obsessional concerns.

Much of the benefit of this approach is derived from clients gaining the ability to tolerate some discomfort. By monitoring the exposure hierarchy, clients can continually remind themselves of the need to persist.

Although clients have tried many times to resist engaging in compulsive behaviors, obsessive thoughts are more difficult to inhibit. Nevertheless, many clients with OCD have worked hard to limit the obsessive thinking and to avoid situations that will trigger them. They may try to distract themselves. When that fails, they use their compulsive ritual to terminate the obsession and the anxious/ uncomfortable feelings that go along with it.

ORDER

The word "order" is quite charged as it is paradoxical for clients with OCD. Ironically, clients' versions of order create OCD and the discordant feelings associated with it. You can teach clients to transform their old version of order into flexible and adaptive thoughts and behavior that shifts them from the rigid and maladaptive OCD habit. Since clients needs healthy order, not the disorder of OCD, you can help the remember how to rewire the brain so that OCD is wired out of their lives by introducing the mnemonic ORDER. Explain that the elements encoded in the mnemonic will help them remember how to put real order back into their life. The mnemonic ORDER contains methods that clients need to practice on a regular basis to rewire the brain.

The mnemonic ORDER represents these essential steps:

O—for observing. Instead of allowing themselves to engage in automatic obsessions and compulsive behaviors, ask clients to be mindful of what they are thinking and doing. By observing themselves begin to engage in obsessions and compulsions, they can break out of autopilot. This is the first step to detach from the OCD habit by becoming observers.

R—for reminding. Clients should remind themselves that they are obsessing and feel compelled to engage in the ritual because it is a symptom of the brain's OCD habit. Reminding themselves reveals the OCD obsessions for what they are, merely useless thoughts, and compulsive behaviors feeding the OCD.

D—for doing. By doing something different from habitual OCD compulsive behaviors, clients can establish new habits. The new behaviors should draw new and productive attention and interest that stimulates reward circuits.

E—for exposure. By exposing themselves to the situation or place that they find intolerable, clients allow themselves to tolerate discomfort and begin the process of habituation. This is the "E" part of ERP, which is one of the two principal approaches in the CBT approach to OCD.

R—for response prevention. By a concentrated effort to refrain from compulsive behaviors that make clients momentarily think they feel better, clients strengthen their inhibitory networks. This is the "R" and "P" part that complete the ERP CBT approach.

It is important to convey to clients that putting real ORDER back into their lives requires taking all of these steps together. Actively cultivating all the ORDER steps will help them rewire their brains so that OCD will not plague them. Clients will need to repeat the steps over and over again so that they maximize neuroplasticity. Let us take a closer look at each of the steps of the method enveloped in the mnemonic ORDER.

Observing

Since one of the principal features of OCD is a deeply entrenched habit, which by nature is automatic, the first step is to break out of autopilot. This requires that clients observe the mindless obsessional pattern by paying attention to what they are thinking and doing as if they were watching other people. By paying attention to how they obsess and compulsively behave, clients shake up the automatic obsessional thoughts and compulsive behaviors, and thus interrupt the OCD habit loop.

CLIENT EDUCATION

The first step in breaking out of your OCD habit is to observe what you are thinking and doing as if you are watching someone else. This will break you out of autopilot and interrupt your OCD habit. For example, say you are riding a bicycle. As soon as you observe how you are pedaling or keeping your balance, you start to wobble, which interrupts the smooth-riding habit, as if to cast doubt on it.

Observing activates the executive brain, and specifically the DCPFC. By observing, clients become "critics" of their own behavior, instead of mindlessly going from one obsessive thought to compulsive behavior. They stand back and observe themselves as if to say "Hey, wait a minute! What am I doing?"

By observing, clients afford themselves the opportunity to determine whether the obsessive thoughts are realistic. From the perspective of an observer of their own mental activity and behavior, they can immediately counter the automatic mindlessness of OCD, which breeds a narrowness in thinking and a locked-in brain pattern.

Like mindfulness, observing can help clients learn to become completely present in the here-and-now, to interrupt automatic habits. As clients become consciously present, they detach from obsessions about what might happen in the future if they do not engage in the compulsive behavior. Doing this allows clients to realistically appraise the current situation and ask themselves if they really need to repeat the same compulsive behaviors. By being mindfully observant of the present moment, clients take the first step to bringing ORDER back into life by detaching from the mindlessness of OCD.

Reminding

The reminding step requires that clients alert themselves that their thinking and behaviors are simply obsessional thinking and compulsive behaviors. You may suggest that when clients find themselves obsessing, they can say "This is my brain acting out its OCD habit that I am learning to break. My striatum is stuck on making it too easy to do my OCD habits. Constantly reminding myself of this habit is critical so that I can put things back in ORDER."

CLIENT EDUCATION

The reminding step activates your prefrontal cortex and hippocampus, your orbitofrontal cortex, which helps tame your amygdala. It says, in effect, "Hey, calm down! There's nothing to get alarmed about. This is just OCD!"

By reminding clients to label OCD for what it is, you can help them activate their left PFC, with all of its resources, using language to label what is going on at any one time, the left PFC also generates positive feelings. In contrast, when the right PFC is not balanced by as much activation from the left PFC, negative feelings such as anxiety can be generated.

CLIENT EDUCATION

Reminding yourself to label OCD obsessiveness and compulsive behaviors helps to free you from obsessional thinking and replace it with realistic thinking. In other words, instead of thinking that there may be a few more germs you didn't scrub off so you need to wash your hands one more time, you can relabel the situation by saying "If I didn't get all the germs out the last 10 times I washed my hands, they're not coming out. Besides, I'm cracking the skin in my hands so badly that germs can get lodged in the cracks. This is a good reason to quit washing my hands."

Labeling obsessions and compulsions as nothing more than symptoms of OCD rewires the brain because it strengthens the connections between the PFC and the amygdala, which had been overactivated and generating false alarms. This also helps the striatum to stop the bad habit and get ready to develop a new one. Labeling provides the striatum with training wheels so that it can get started filtering out nuisance thoughts so that clients will not suffer from OCD.

Doing

Learning to do something new instead of doing what they had compulsively done in the past is critical for neuroplasticity. For example, instead of washing hands for the 10th time, clients can take a walk or do some other pleasurable activity. The key here is for clients to engage in this new behavior long enough for them to establish a new, good habit. This new behavior must be more engaging than just a way of diverting attention from what clients feel compelled to do, which is the compulsive behavior. The new habit will develop if it captures client attention and interest instead of simply distracting clients briefly before they will resume the compulsive behavior.

With the new behavior capturing client attention, the PFC redirects brain resources and helps establish new wiring to support the efficiency of the new habit into the striatum. Rewiring functions best if the new behavior is practiced often enough that it becomes a new habit and replaces the old compulsive habit.

CLIENT EDUCATION

Develop a new habit to replace the OCD habit. For example, instead of checking the outside doors for the 8th time, check your flower beds to see how the new plants are growing. The attention that you devote to the new flower beds generates plans to fertilize them, water them more often, or add a few more flowers. As you drive away, reflect on what garden center to visit to buy new plants or fertilizer. This new habit shifts you from obsessing about whether you should drive back to check the doors the 9th time. Checking the plants each time you leave the house can become a ritual and a new habit that replaces the OCD habit.

The establishment of a new habit rewires the habit circuit, which includes the striatum, DLPFC, and the nucleus accumbens. When these brain areas are kindled with dopamine, the anticipation of pleasure is stimulated through activating the nucleus accumbens, and consequently the desire to do it again.

Engaging in the doing step will help clients establish a new behavior to replace the compulsive behaviors. This new behavior can be embellished by adding more details. For example, in regard to the garden, clients can notice how the leaves of the new plants are getting greener as they spend time fertilizing and watering.

Exposure

As with all efficacious approaches to anxiety disorders, exposure involves teaching clients to expose themselves to what they fear so that the tremendous discomfort eventually dissipates through habituation. It is important to point out that exposure to the discomfort of the situation is a critical element of the evidence-based treatment of OCD. It is essentially the opposite of avoidance, which promotes anxiety underlying the OCD and keeps the gate open so that the striatum can continue uninhibited on autopilot with compulsive behaviors to avoid feeling anxious. Although the compulsive behaviors serve only as short-term fixes, they fuel the long-term bad habit of OCD. You may point out that when clients who worry that they touched germs wash their hands, they feel immediate relief from anxiety, but the anxiety creeps back in, and clients wash their hands again to make that anxiety go away. This self-defeating avoidant behavior strengthens the compulsions that wire the brain to repeat the habit. Like with other anxiety disorders, confronting the fear with exposure weakens the bad habit of avoidant behavior. By exposing themselves to anxiety-provoking situations, whether it is using a public restroom or checking the doors only once as they leave for work, clients can create the conditions for long-term depression (LTD). With LTD, neurons that fire out of sync lose their link.

Clients who are taught to expose themselves to disturbing situations can take the critical step toward habituating to anxiety-provoking situations. In other words, by knowing that they do not die of a terrible infection after washing their hands only once, clients eventually can dampen the amygdala's overreactivity.

CLIENT EDUCATION

During exposure exercises, use realistic positive self-talk. This is essentially top-down control so that your prefrontal cortex tells your amygdala that there is nothing to get anxious about. Remind yourself that each time you didn't wash your hands more than once, nothing bad seemed to happen. By activating your prefrontal cortex in this way, you promote stronger downward connections from your prefrontal cortex to your amygdala. Remind yourself that the connections coming up from your amygdala to your cortex are stronger than the other way around. That is why you need to make a stronger effort to strengthen those connections going down, by reassuring positive self-talk and the involvement of your dorsolateral prefrontal cortex to stay present and make realistic decisions about your behaviors.

Response Prevention

Response prevention and exposure represent the two principal CBT approaches to evidenced-based practices for OCD. Also called ritual prevention, this step involves resisting the urge to engage in the compulsive ritual.

CLIENT EDUCATION

Response prevention follows the exposure step. Neuroplasticity requires a moderate degree of activation, often experienced as anxiety. This means that you want to use that anxiety and the stress chemistry associated with it to rewire your brain. You do not want to wait until you feel totally comfortable because you will lose this valuable opportunity. Response prevention works best when you feel some anxiety but do not engage in the old compulsive behavior. This may be a frightening thought, and you may think that I aim to torture you. But the fact is this: By not doing your old compulsive behavior during the exposure phase, you are doing the most important work in rewiring your brain.

OCD researchers recommend that clients spend at least 45 to 90 minutes in the uncomfortable feelings while not engaging in the old behavior. Clients need enough time to disengage from the old compulsive behavior to tolerate the discomfort and for LTD to occur in the striatum. This transition period of time allows the brain an opportunity to reorganize its resources to adjust to the reality that the client's worst fears did not occur when he or she did not engage in the old compulsive behavior.

Response prevention works to inhibit the compulsive response to an uncomfortable situation. By not engaging in the old compulsive behaviors, clients stop themselves from falling into the old OCD pattern. Clients should be told that it is quite natural to experience some anxiety, perhaps intense enough that they will feel like something will go terribly wrong if they do not do something to put things in order.

When using the ORDER method, clients need to know that there is no magic switch to flip. Repeating the ORDER sequence and conquering OCD takes consistent effort. Because OCD is a bad habit that is wired into the brain by repetition, clients will need to rewire the brain through repetition. Remind clients that the more cells fire together, the more they wire together. OCD had been strengthened every time clients followed an obsession with a compulsive behavior. Repeating the steps in the ORDER activates all the parts of the brain that need to be activated for clients to unlock the OCD disorder and wire in a new healthy ORDER. All the new connections between those parts of the brain strengthen each time the ORDER is repeated. Since efforts to employ the ORDER method will be tested by stress or even laziness, repetition of the ORDER is critical. Clients may be doing well for several months, seeing symptoms fade away. Then if clients experience major stress, such as a layoff from work, anxiety can trigger the old OCD behaviors. That is again where repeating the ORDER steps is all the more important.

HEALTH OBSESSIONS

I work within the largest full-service and integrated healthcare system in the United States and work closely with primary care physicians, dermatologists, cardiologists, and others. Often we discuss a group of patients who either obsess about or imagine a medical problem. These obsessions may center on a specific physical sensation or a wide variety of physical complaints.

Obsessions about health concerns can snowball from a minor physical problem to ideas about being seriously ill. If clients are worried about a particular physical sensation, even though it is not a symptom of a true medical problem, it can become a source of increasingly greater concern. The degree of worry clients devote to that sensation usually intensifies it. For example, if clients pay close attention to the mild symptoms of a headache, those symptoms can become more intense.

If clients have a tendency to obsess about stomach pain, they look out for any indication that stomach pain is on the way. Any stomach sensation turns on the alarm, and clients may say, "Oh no, here it comes!" This false alarm activates the amygdala and the fear circuit mechanisms, which increase anxiety by activating neurotransmitters such as norepinephrine and epinephrine (adrenaline), which increase the symptoms of a nervous stomach.

A similar sequence of sensations can occur when there is no initial stomach condition. If clients *believe* that they have a stomach condition, they will be extremely attentive to any sensation in the stomach. The point to raise with such clients is that everyone has stomach sensations, and clients will inevitably find stomach sensations if they look for them. To compound this obsessional search for stomach sensations, clients' fear circuits get activated. The resulting physical sensations intensify as the sympathetic nervous system arousal mechanisms become hyperactive. Because primary care physicians see so many patients seeking timely treatment, occasionally OCD patients who complain about physical sensations and/or factitious medical problems receive antianxiety or pain medication. Once benzodiazepines or synthetic opiates (both of which are addictive) are introduced, a vicious cycle occurs involving tolerance and withdrawal. The tolerance effect involves the need for higher doses to get the same anxiolytic or pain-reducing effect. During the withdrawal phase there is an increase in the very symptoms that clients find difficult to tolerate because of complex biochemical processes that involves the downward production of key neurotransmitters. As a result of this spiral, the anxiety or pain increases. Often the physicians increase the dosage to get the same anxiety or pain-reducing effect.

When symptoms do improve it is common for people to get so excited about their progress that they gravitate back to all-or-nothing thinking. Fueled by enthusiasm, they assume that they have been "cured" and that they are completely free of OCD. Once they have made this thinking error, they are at risk of experiencing minor setbacks with periods of disturbing anxiety, and they may fall back into their old pattern of obsessions and compulsive behaviors. What was once a little anxiety becomes an OCD. They assume that they are back to full-blown OCD, that all the progress they made is lost, and that they have to start all over again. Worse, some people think of themselves as incapable of making any long-term progress.

From a cognitive therapy point of view, you can encourage clients to identify their obsessions and compulsions as symptoms of OCD. Next you can invite them into a few behavioral experiences that disprove their errors in thinking about cause and effect.

Normally, a tonic balance between the neural systems that underlie the activation/disinhibition behavior programs allows for flexible, situation-appropriate initiation and inhibition of behavior. Not so for clients with OCD. For them, this balance is disrupted and skewed toward repetitive activation (Baxter et al., 2000).

NEUROSCIENCE

The neural systems involved in OCD involve the OFC, the basal ganglia, and the thalamus. Rewiring OCD symptoms and their abnormal cortico-ganglia circuit activity can be achieved by behavioral approaches in which clients are exposed systematically to the very stimuli that otherwise provoke the obsessions and compulsions (Baxter et al., 1992).

Finally, it is important to reiterate to clients that OCD hijacks the habit circuit. Normalizing it in this way not only makes it more tangible but also gives them hope that they can break the obsession compulsion habit. Just as old habits can be broken, new ones can develop, whatever their age. Using the ORDER technique can help break the OCD habit.

Chapter 9

DEPRESSION

M ajor depression is the fourth disorder worldwide in terms of disease burden. By 2030, it is expected to be the disorder with the highest cost of all psychological disorders in high-income countries (Mathers & Loncar, 2006).

Although prevalence rates for depression are somewhat lower for older adults, the prevalence for mild and minor depression is higher. On average, an episode of major depression lasts for 20 weeks and four episodes. The average relapse rate after recovery from the first major depressive episode is 20% to 30% in 3 years. After a person has suffered three or more episodes, the chance of relapse is 70% to 80%.

Depression can feel devastating and be a very lonely experience. Depressed clients typically do not feel like doing the very things that can serve to lift their depression. Worst yet, they do not know or are not convinced that the theory-driven approaches offered by therapists make sense. Brain-based explanations offer more substance and concrete explanation and serve as a route out of the chasm that depressed clients find themselves trapped in.

This chapter addresses how depressed clients can learn about the factors that contribute to depression and what to do about it. Through understanding how depression occurs and how to rewire the brain, clients can gain a road map. However, since there are many ways to become depressed, you must orchestrate a broad-based strategy to encourage clients to follow all the strategies simultaneously. Without such a plan, clients may say "I've tried that and it doesn't work."

GENDER AND DEPRESSION

Gender differences in depression occur only in postpubescence; the incidence of depression does not differ among prepubescent girls and boys. There are a variety of factors at play as to why this is the case, including variations in the levels of estrogen and progesterone. Drops in the level of estrogen effects serotonin. This is because estrogen works in conjunction with serotonin, influencing several stages of serotonin production, stimulating its secretion, transmission, and uptake in the body. Estrogen also inhibits the activity of

MAOs (monoamine oxidase), compounds which break down serotonin. When progesterone is low relative to estrogen, anxiety increases (Leibenluft, 1999; Northrup, 2001).

Another factor that may lead to more women being treated for depression is diagnostic confusion. Women outnumber men in the diagnosis of depression 2 to 1. However, men seek help less often. Unlike women, who more often report feelings of sadness, men repeat anger, irritability, and recklessness. Therefore, the diagnosis of depression in men can be written off as frustration and restlessness rather than a serious problem warranting intervention. Yet men outnumber women in suicide 4 to 1. After puberty, girls are three times more likely to become depressed.

One possible factor at play in the prevalence of depression among women may be genetics. Some women have a mutation in a gene called CREB1 associated with depression. CREB1 has a switch turned on by estrogen. Another factor may relate to the serotonin transporter gene (5-HTT), which is associated with women and depression. It is switched on by threats and stress.

Another hormone-related difference is reflected in medication response. Premenopausal women respond best to selective serotonin reuptake inhibitors (SSRIs), which seem to work best in the presence of estrogen (Kornstein et al., 2000). Men respond best to Wellbutrin and Tofranil, which target dopamine and norepinephrine. Apparently, in general men have a lesser deficit in their serotonergic neural circuits. Male brains make serotonin faster and generally have more available. Just like men, postmenopausal women respond best to non-serotonin medications.

Between 10% and 15% of mothers in the postpartum phase experience depression. Psychosocial factors increase the risk; it has been reported that mothers who receive little emotional support during pregnancy are more likely to develop postpartum depression (Nielsen Forman, Videbech, Hedegaard, Dalby Salvig, & Secher, 2000). They have been observed to touch their infants less on the second day after delivery (Ferber, 2004).

Estrogen can raise the level of cortisol, which is perhaps one of the reasons why there is an increased rate of depression in the postpartum period. Estrogen-boosting cortisol affects the level of serotonin. Also, estrogen and testosterone have opposite effects on gamma-aminobutyric acid (GABA). While testosterone stimulates GABA transmission, estrogen inhibits it. Testosterone, too, can boost the level of brain-derived neurotrophic factor (BDNF), and reduced BDNF is one potential causative factor of depression. Since testosterone boosts BDNF, this may explain one of the reasons why neurogenesis appears to decrease with advancing age.

ROLE OF INFLAMMATION

Many medical problems can create depressive symptoms. Drugs and alcohol also can cause depression. For example, benzodiazepines such as diazepam

(Valium), chlordiazepoxide (Librium), and lorazepam (Ativan) have side effects of depression. Some antihypertensives, including propranolol (Inderal), alpha-methyl-dopa (Aldomet), reserpine (Serpasil, Sandril), and clonidine (Catapres), cause depression. Often physicians who prescribe these medications do not have time to explain these side effects to their patients, due in part because of the economic forces of managed care and the fact that they have little training in the interface between medical problems and psychological problems. For that reason, you need to review clients' medication lists and provide guidance regarding what clients can do behaviorally to minimize risks and interactions.

Some illnesses both cause and are exacerbated by depression, including type 2 diabetes. There is a bidirectional relationship between depression and a variety of illnesses, which means that one accelerates the development of other. Major depression is associated with an increased risk for abdominal obesity, cardiovascular disease, and type 2 diabetes (Evans et al., 2005). Other illnesses, such as anemia, asthma, congestive heart failure, hepatitis, hypothyroidism, influenza, lupus, malnutrition, mononucleosis, multiple sclerosis, rheumatoid arthritis, syphilis, ulcerative colitis, and uremia, all lead to depressive symptoms and in turn less motivation to engage in behaviors that manage those illnesses.

CLIENT EDUCATION

Let us work together with your physician to treat your health problems and depression at the same time because they are interlinked. When your health improves, so will your depression, just as when your depression improves, so will your health.

Numerous studies have noted the association between depression and inflammation across the life cycle (Christian, Deichert, Gouin, Graham, & Kiecolt-Glaser, 2012). Multidirectional causal relationships occur among perceived stress, loneliness, depression, and inflammation (McDade, Hawkley, & Cacioppo, 2006). One of the many systemic routes to depression involves the stress-induced activation of the hypothalamic-pituitary-adrenal (HPA) axis that provokes the release of epinephrine (adrenaline) and NE, that stimulate the release of cytokines, which adversely affects the central nervous system, resulting in lethargy and withdrawal, which has been called "sickness behavior" (Dantzer & Kelley, 2007). The overall elevation of pro-inflammatory cytokines is associated with a depressive syndrome characterized by disturbances in mood, cognition, and neurovegetative behaviors that mimic major depression.

Inflammation can affect the brain through stimulation of peripheral afferent vagal nerves that innervate organs in the abdominal cavity (Konsman, Parnet, & Dantzer, 2002). Cytokine receptors, including those for interleukin 6 (IL-6), interleukin 1 (IL-1), and tumour necrosis factor (TNF-α) are also located in the brain. Reportedly IL-1 has significant effects on the hypothalamus and the hippocampus, which can play a role in sickness behavior (Bailey, Engler, Hunzeker, & Sheridan, 2003).

Another systemic route through which cytokines contribute to depression is by altering the levels of neurotransmitters, such as DA, NE, and serotonin, low levels of which have all been associated with depression. For example, elevated levels of cytokines reduce the availability of tryptophan, the amino acid precursor to serotonin synthesis (Schiepers, Wichers, & Maes, 2005). In other words, high levels of cytokines are associated with low levels of serotonin, and low levels are contributors to depression and anxiety.

The field of psychoneuroimmunology examines the interface among the immune system, the mind, and the brain. Indeed, it reveals that inflammation can have devastating effects on both mood and cognition. Inflammation can cause depressive cognitions and depressive moods on short- and long-term bases. Short-term inflammation, such as occurring postsurgery, dulls memory and moods in 7% to 26% of patients. Long-term inflammation can occur with chronic illnesses, such as type 2 diabetes and rheumatoid arthritis, both of which increase the enzyme indoleamine 2,3-dioxygenase (IDO), which is associated with inflammatory cytokines. Drugs that block IDO reveal the connection between inflammation and depression.

Although relative elevations in inflammatory cytokines are associated with depressed mood, not all cytokines are inherently destructive. Clients can be informed that cytokines are protein molecules that act as cellular messengers. If the levels cytokines are in the healthy range, they function as important parts of the immune system. Too little cytokine activity results in immunodeficiency, severe infection, and even death. Too much cytokine activity, or hyperarousal of inflammatory cytokines, can cause not only depression but can result in illness, tissue damage, or shock; in extreme cases, it can lead to death.

Stress can increase cytokines to abnormal levels, and significant elevations in cytokines can occur immediately after trauma. High cytokine levels can lower the concentration of various neurotransmitters which include, as noted above, serotonin, resulting in impaired cognitive processes, psychosis, anxiety, fearfulness, depression, and even thoughts of suicide. The spectrum of symptoms includes fatigue, social withdrawal, disturbances in mood, cognition, neurovegetative behaviors, and immobility, all of which appear very much like depression (Dantzer & Kelley, 2007). Although clients feel ill, less motivated, and less capable, lack of exercise and social engagement lead to more depression and still higher levels of cytokines and sickness behavior.

The biological link among depression, inflammation, and early life trauma or deprivation is related to the incidence of medical problems, such as diabetes and cardiovascular disease (Raison, Capuron, & Miller, 2006). Depressed patients with a history of early life trauma demonstrate significantly higher levels of the pro-inflammatory cytokines, such as IL-6, and activation of TNF-α (Pace et al., 2006).

CLIENT EDUCATION

Feeling ill makes you act ill. If you behave as if you are in fact ill, the feelings of depression will increase.

A variety of interventions can target stress, depression, and inflammation at the same time. Increasing social support has long been shown to buffer stress and help lift depression. As an illustration of the relationship to these factors with inflammation, social support also has been shown to lower levels of inflammation markers in circulating blood (Costanzo et al., 2005). Participation in religious organizations, which is a key source of social support for many people, has been shown to lower levels of IL-6 (Lutgendorf, Logan, Costanzo, & Lubaroff, 2004). Poor diet and no exercise are significantly associated with inflammation. Therefore, both factors need to be carefully monitored.

ANXIETY WITH DEPRESSION

Until recently, clients suffering from both anxiety and depression were understood as having two separate psychiatric disorders. The new emerging consensus acknowledges nonlinear and interconnected biopsychosocial processes.

Typically hyperactivation of the amygdala is associated with anxiety disorders. Yet an enlarged and hyperactive amygdala is also associated with depression (Drevets, 2001). Amygdala activation appears to normalize after successful treatment for depression. The high numbers of people who are both depressed and anxious probably reflect hyperactivity of the amygdala with people who are depressed. Instead of the old model of *DSM IV* whereby mental health providers diagnosed "comorbidities" of anxiety and depression as "two diagnoses on Axis 1," the developers of *DSM-5* opted for a spectrum approach, which acknowledges that a depressed person may also be anxious. The anxiety and depression need not be thought of as separate disorders but rather as part of a spectrum. In fact, some people become depressed if they are anxious. Anxiety can be understood as a risk factor for depression and is part of the reason why depressed clients have anxious implicit memory.

The link between anxiety and depression need not confuse clients. You can describe how chronic depression and anxiety can both be associated with increased levels of stress neurochemicals.

For at least 50 years, researchers have noted that many people with chronic major depression have associated elevated cortisol levels. Some people experience extreme dysregulation of their HPA axis, including structural changes in their brains and other parts of their bodies, such as enlargement of the pituitary and adrenal glands. The adrenal gland enlargement appears to result from hyper-secretion of adrenocorticotropic hormone (ACTH).

NEUROSCIENCE

In a healthy person, the HPA axis works well with the hypothalamus secreting corticotropic-releasing factor (CRF) and vasopressin (also known as antidiuretic hormone). For its part, vasopressin amplifies the effects of CRF, which stimulates the pituitary to secrete ACTH. The circulating ACTH acts on the adrenal cortex to induce the release of adrenaline and cortisol. Cortisol eventually exerts negative feedback effects via binding to glucocorticoid receptors in the pituitary and the hippocampus, resulting in down-regulation of HPA axis activity. Unfortunately, with many people with depression, this negative feedback process does not occur, despite high levels of cortisol.

The role of CRF in depression has received considerable attention because elevated CRF has long been found in depressed patients and in the cerebrospinal fluid (CSF) of depressed suicide victims (Arato et al., 1989). It is therefore no wonder that big pharma is actively developing drugs that target CRF.

The two CRF receptive subtypes, CRF1 and CRF2, have distinct neuroatomic and receptor pharmacology. The CRF1 subtype reportedly plays a central role in mediating depressive and anxious behaviors. Pharmacological research has shown that compounds that block this receptor may possess antidepressant and anxiolytic effects (Zobel et al., 2000).

Hypersecretion of CRF early in life, due to maternal deprivation of the baby or severe stress, may result in an altered set point for activity of the CRF neurons and of the HPA axis. These changes contribute to an overreaction to stress during adulthood as well as subsequent depression (Newport, Stowe, & Nemeroff, 2002).

Stress-induced depression can occur over a short period of time. The levels of DA, NE, and serotonin can drop for 90 minutes after stress. Lower DA is associated with psychomotor retardation and with decreased blood flow to the L-dorsolateral prefrontal cortex (DLPFC). It is important to note that the left PFC (L-PFC) can inhibit negative affect (Davidson & Irwin, 1999). Since greater L-PFC activation is associated with lowered amygdala activation, clients who are depressed as well as anxious can be told that efforts to activate their L-PFC through approach behaviors rather than withdrawal and avoidant behaviors will help alleviate both depression and anxiety.

CLIENT EDUCATION

When you are depressed, part of your brain called the left prefrontal cortex tends to be underactive. It can be activated by small and deliberate practical behaviors that will help calm your amygdala and lead to less anxiety and less depression.

Because of the amygdala's heightened sensitivity to cortisol, anxiety may be more likely during depression. The ramping up of cortisol can lead to increased amygdalar volume and anxiety (Sheline, Sanghavi, & Mintun, 1999). A more active amygdala can lead to norepinphrine and CRH dysregulation, which reduces serotonin while it increases the risk of depression as well as anxiety.

The relationship between depression and the amygdala cannot be overlooked. With more amygdala activation, the chances that memories will be encoded or anxiety or depressive stimuli will increase. When in particular moods, clients will recall memories that were encoded in those moods; these are referred to as state-based memories. When clients are depressed and anxious, they are more likely to recall memories laced with both anxiety and depression.

CLIENT EDUCATION

When you are depressed and/or anxious, you will more likely remember things that are depressing and anxiety provoking. This does not mean that nothing that happened in the past was positive. It just means that your amygdala and hippocampus are working together to recall depressed and anxiety-laced memories. When we work together to create positive mood states, you will have positive memories.

Memories that include a high emotional charge are more efficiently coded into memory than those that are emotionally neutral. These emotionally charged memories are facilitated by the basolateral amygdala and the release of the neurotransmitters NE and acetylcholine (Paré, 2003). During periods of depression with comorbid anxiety, the sustained activation of the amygdala can maintain the flow of anxious emotions, which results in attaching emotional significance to normally trivial events (Siegle, Steinhauer, Thase, Stenger, & Carter, 2002). Depressed clients therefore are more likely to remember trivial events and consider them important.

Cognition and Depression

Depression typically includes negativistic thinking that rejects and resists your suggestions and explanations for what clients are experiencing. While overly theoretical and esoteric explanations fail to describe how clients will find relief from depression, more practical and down-to-earth information will entice them to be receptive and to follow through with the suggestions you make. Clients with depression are distracted by, or in most cases overwhelmed with, the symptoms of depression. Therefore, the information and suggestions you provide must reach clients' current cognitive capacity.

For half a century there have been reports of explicit memory problems with depressed people. Much of the early theorizing about these memory deficits centered on the possibility that clients are distracted by internal stimuli. Yet structural reasons can account for the memory deficits, at least with a significant portion of chronically depressed people. Chronic depression has been found to play a significant role in the memory deficit. Some previously depressed people show hippocampal shrinkage in the range of 8% to 19%. There has been vigorous debate about the potential causes of the shrinkage; some researchers point to the cortisol increases from chronic depression and overactivation of the hippocampal cortisol receptors (Sapolsky, 2003). Excess of glutamate saturates the N-methyl-D-aspartate (NMDA) receptors and results in excitotoxicity. The hippocampal shrinkage can also be caused by blocked neurogenesis, which results in no regeneration of the hippocampus. Probably hippocampal atrophy is caused by all these factors.

NEUROSCIENCE

One of the most consistent neurological findings associated with major depression is a smaller hippocampus, relative to nondepressed people. (MacQueen et al., 2003; Sheline, Sanghavi, & Mintun, 1999). The subgenual region of the anterior cingulate cortex (ACC) also has been reported to have a smaller volume in depressed subjects compared to nondepressed people.

The ACC, which is positioned on the middle wall of each hemisphere just above the corpus callosum, is involved in a wide variety of cognitive and emotional functions. While its dorsal (top) portion is involved in cognitive functioning, its ventral (bottom) portion is involved in affective functioning. The affective component has extensive connections with a variety of subcortical areas, especially the amygdala. A part of the ACC (the subgenual ACC, which is also called Brodmann's area 25) is hyperactive and smaller in depressed people.

As noted above, severely stressed and depressed people tend to incur damage to their hippocampus. As a result, they tend to lose the ability to see the shades of gray and complexity inherent in most situations and tend to react in a black-and-white manner and overgeneralize (Viamontes & Beitman, 2006). This inability is based on faulty orthogonalization of information that ensures that new patterns do not interfere with the old and remain separable. Orthogonalization is aided by the availability of sufficient numbers of dentate gyrus neurons, neurons that, in healthy brains, are where neurogenesis occurs.

NEUROSCIENCE

Depression is also associated with impairment in the CA3 region of the hippocampus. This region is interconnected with other regions and is involved in "completing" previous encountered patterns when only parts of them are perceived. The tendency to complete patterns in an all-or-nothing, black-and-white way, to overgeneralize negativistically, is of major concern in therapy.

Explicit memory deficits can result not only in hippocampal atrophy but also in part the tendency to gravitate to extremes, presumably because of amygdala overactivity. The impairment of the areas around the hippocampus can also result in overgeneralizing. Specifically, the dentate gyrus facilitates orthogonalization of information, which involves ensuring that new patterns that are coded into memory do not interfere with old. The CA3 region also plays a role in this function, as it has many connections with other regions. Impairment in the dentate gyrus and CA3 results in black-and-white generalizations (Viamontes & Beitman, 2006).

Cognitive-behavioral Therapy (CBT) theorists have long identified black-and-white thinking as well as overgeneralization as contributing to depression. Here we find a clear interface between the psychological and neurodynamic explanations for depressive thinking. Cognitive effort to work on perception of the shades of gray as well as appreciating ambiguity strengthens this area through neuroplasticity.

Diet also can serve as a neuroprotective factor for the hippocampus. Specifically, omega-3 essential fatty acids play a part in limiting the devastating effects of cortisol on neurogenesis. Exercise reduces depression, in part by boosting BDNF and increasing serotonin, NE, and DA.

CLIENT EDUCATION

Because depression can impair your memory, you will need to maintain healthy habits to protect your hippocampus, the part of your brain involved in memory. Aerobic exercise, a balanced diet, and good-quality sleep are critical.

The role of the ACC, which is the front side of the gyrus just above the corpus callosum, appears to play a role in both cognition and affect. For many depressed people, the ACC may be difficult to activate. As a region of the brain that plays an important role in active engagement with conflicts, ambiguous situations, and the conscious experiencing of feelings, the ACC is important to help people negotiate difficult situations. Depressed clients tend to shut down when confronted with difficult situations. Research illustrates the importance of a variety of cognitive functions that are important to alleviate depression. Therapy that addresses depressed clients' tendencies to be overly critical presumably would contribute to less activity and more efficient neural firing in this area of the ACC. By providing this easing up of error detection, the PFC—the executive brain—would be better able to make practical decisions and generate existential insights that are more adaptable as well as realistic. These cognitive adjustments would be more productive if made by the L-PFC, emphasizing approach tendencies, instead of the right PFC (R-PFC) and its withdrawal tendencies.

The dorsal portion of the ACC is involved in cognition while the ventral portion is involved in affect. The ACC is a monitoring system that is activated when clients are faced with uncertain situations or demands that allow for multiple interpretations. It becomes active when clients assume something may go wrong. The ACC is chronically underactive in depressed people. Activity in the ACC increases when depression is lifted and in those clients who respond to medication (Mayberg 1999).

NEUROSCIENCE

Helen Mayberg of Emory University has shown that deep brain stimulation (DBS) at a specific site referred to as a depression switch can, at least for a short time, relieve people with otherwise intractable depression of their symptoms. Specifically, Brodmann's area 25 of the ACC has been implicated in chronic depression and is associated with error detection and social monitoring (Mayberg et al., 1999). Area 25 activates when people look at sad pictures. It is smaller but more active in depressed people and re-regulates after remission from depression. The ACC is wired into both top-down and bottom-up modules and plays an important role in processing fear, memory, error recognition, motivation, and sleep. Mayberg showed that electrodes implanted to inhibit area 25 produced dramatic results. Significantly depressed people found relief. These studies are consistent with other research that shows that reduced area 25 activity may mean more efficiency. Most critically, the PFC is "freed up" to provide improved executive functions (Mayberg, personal communication, 2006).

The ACC has been called a depression switch because it generally is considered a bridge between attention and emotion (Devinsky, Morrell, & Vogt, 1995). Decreased activity in the dorsal region of the ACC tends to be linked to impairment in attention and executive functions while the ventral region tends to be linked to emotional blunting, anhedonia, and reduced responsiveness. The dorsal part is connected to the DLPFC and executive functions such as working memory and decision making, while the rostral/ventral part is involved in emotions, as it is connected to the amygdala (Davidson, Pizzagalli, Nitschke, & Putnam, 2002).

People who are depressed tend to have excessive activity in the ventral part of the ACC. Those successfully treated tend to show increases in hippocampus and dorsal ACC activity in these regions, showing a decrease in rumination and an increase in optimism (Sharot, Riccardi, Raio, & Phelps, 2007). One initial step promoted by most therapeutic approaches counters mood-congruent bias with inquiry. In other words, you say, "Run that by me again. What specifically makes you feel bad about that?" Here the effort is to challenge the hippocampal record to provide a realistic, context-specific explicit memory to substantiate mood-congruent memories.

Davidson and colleagues (2002) identified two subtypes of depression that correspond to impairment in the ACC or the PFC. The ACC subtype is associated with those depressed clients who have resigned, do not perceive conflict between the demands in the environment and their state, and have lost the will to change. The PFC subtype perceives the conflict between the environment and their state but are unable to activate the PFC goal-oriented functions to facilitate change. The prognosis for the PFC subtype is better than for the ACC subtype (Mayberg, 1997).

The induction of sadness in healthy people activates the ventral ACC, along with the amygdala and the insula, in conjunction with a reduction of activity in the DLPFC. The improvement in symptoms of severely depressed people is associated with a reduction in blood flow to the subgenual ACC, insula, and orbitofrontal cortex (OFC) with corresponding increases in activating the DLPFC and dorsal ACC (Mayberg et al., 2005).

While applying CBT to treat depression, researchers used positron emission tomography (PET) to compare metabolic brain activity. They found that the reduction in depression was associated with a corresponding increase in metabolic activity in the hippocampus and the dorsal ACC. Simultaneously, there was a decrease in metabolic activity in the dorsal ventral PFC and medial prefrontal cortex (Goldapple et al., 2004).

SHIFTING TO ACTION

In popular culture, there is a cliché that when a person is feeling sad, anxious, or depressed, the way out is to "let those feelings run their course." Unfortunately, well-meaning therapists often tell clients to "go with your feelings, because emotions are wise." There is nothing wise about the emotions associated with depression; nor is there anything wise about the cognitions associated with depression. Part of the ill-conceived reasoning underlying this countertherapeutic advice stems from the early 20th-century belief that catharsis, "getting things out," was a major aspect of the therapeutic method. Catharsis as a psychological concept developed during Victorian Europe when more was felt than was discussed. Through talking about feelings, cathasis actually did serve as a critical step in the right direction. Unfortunately, more steps should have followed that initial opening. If depressed clients merely talked about feelings of depression, the depression would not only continue but could get worse. From a 21st-century perspective, the cathartic expression and "going with the feelings" of depression, as if they would run their course like a bad cold, eventually will be considered malpractice, because this approach leads to greater depression.

Clients need to understand that giving in to the symptoms of depression can fuel a downward spiral. A depressed mood is associated with a deactivated L-PFC and motivation circuit, which leads to less energy to fuel movement. The resulting psychomotor retardation leads to feeling even more sluggish, metabolically downregulated, and fatigued. As a result, clients can gain or lose weight and experience disturbed sleep. They may then experience anhedonia, which can demotivate them to maintain social ties and make them feel that there is nothing to gain by making the effort to engage in life. The social withdrawal leads to less pleasure and more rumination on the futility of any effort. When combined, the feelings of worthlessness and loneliness ultimately can lead to thoughts of death.

NEUROSCIENCE

Many clients state that they derive enjoyment from only a limited number of activities. They report feeling stuck in bad habits because of limitations that they assume to be hardwired. You can help them understand that the development of positive habits and the appreciation of pleasure is soft wired. From this explanation, clients can build the motivation to engage in a wider range of gratifying experiences. To this end, you can explain that the sum total of rewarding experiences modifies their medium spiny (MS) neurons and responsiveness to opportunities for immediate gratification. The mechanisms underlying these rewarding experiences involve the nucleus accumbens that indicate the value of reward opportunities through their firing rate. The faster the firing rate, the greater the anticipated reward. The MS neurons tally the amount of DA released in the nucleus accumbens over time; this tally provides a measure of the number and value of opportunities clients encountered recently.

> MS neurons have special dynamic receptors, referred to as D2 receptors, which change in responsiveness when DA hits them, making then fire more readily and harder to turn off (Dong et al., 2006). The total value of the opportunity that clients recently experienced gets translated into the strength or excitability of the MS neurons (Trafton & Gifford, 2008). As clients push themselves to encounter more rewarding opportunities, the more difficult it is to turn off these neurons. This means that it becomes easier for clients to derive pleasure from a wider variety of activities.

As I noted in Chapter 1, hemispheric affect asymmetry is among the most important discoveries in neuroscience with particular relevance to anxiety, depression, and therapy. The evidence from neurology associated with strokes reveals that people with a left-side stroke often experience a catastrophic effect and become very depressed. Some wonder why they should make the effort to go on living. In contrast, a right-side stroke results in a laissez-faire effect; patients demonstrate more acceptance of their condition and much less depression. They may regard the stroke as merely an inconvenience.

What left- and right-side strokes show is how hemispheric dominance shifts to the nonaffected side, so that a left-side stroke leads to right-hemisphere dominance and vice versa. The salient point with respect to depression is that too much right-hemisphere activity and not enough left-hemisphere activity contributes to depression.

Consistent with the reports from neurology are studies using a variety of imaging instruments to show that depression is associated with the relative inhibition of the L-PFC and relative activation of the R-PFC (Davidson, et al., 2002). The L-PFC is associated with positive emotions and is action oriented, while the R-PFC is associated with negative emotions and is passive and withdrawal oriented.

From a psychological perspective, this asymmetry has profound relevance to therapy with depressed clients. Instead of putting details into context, depressed clients are overwhelmed by a global and negative perspective and tend to withdraw from others. In an effort to rebalance the ratio of activity in the two hemispheres, the use of language, making interpretive sense of events, and generating a positive narrative promote optimistic emotions that are all products of robust left-hemispheric functioning.

The reestablishment of pleasurable activities is the common aim of all psychotherapeutic approaches to depression (Jacobson, Martell, & Dimidjian, 2001). This approach lies at the heart of the behavior activation technique. From a brain-based perspective, behavior activation activates the L-PFC.

CLIENT EDUCATION

Depression is associated with the underactivation of your left prefrontal cortex and the overactivation of your right prefrontal cortex. This means that you probably feel like withdrawing and isolating yourself. If you go with those feelings, you will feel even more depressed and activate your right prefrontal cortex even more. The solution to this dilemma is to activate your left prefrontal cortex. This occurs when you approach and engage in active behaviors when you least feel like it.

To rebalance the two sides of your brain, let us work together to get your left hemisphere reactivated. Since it is associated with positive emotions, this will help you lift out of depression. Since your left hemisphere also is associated with doing things while your right hemisphere is associated with avoidance and withdrawal, you will need to fight the pull to withdraw and do what you do not feel like doing.

NEUROSCIENCE

The right DLPFC (R-DLPFC) is associated with avoidance/withdrawal behaviors while the L-DLPFC is associated with approach behaviors. The L-OFC is associated with positive emotions while the R-OFC is associated with negative emotions.

Consistent with the affect asymmetry literature, it is common that there is decreased blood flow to the L-PFC in depressed patients (Bremner, 2002). Also noted have been functional abnormalities in the amygdala, hippocampus, basal ganglia, and cingulate cortex (Sheline, 2003). Significant enlargements have been noted the amygdala (Van Elst, Woermann, Lemieux, & Trimble, 2000).

Originally conceived as a distinct approach, behavioral activation (also referred to as activity scheduling) consists of the systematic structuring in pleasant activities and an increase in positive social interactions. It also involves teaching clients techniques to monitor mood and daily activities, then understand the connection between them (Lewinsohn et al., 1976). CBT for depression combined cognitive restructuring and behavioral activation (Beck et al., 1979).

CLIENT EDUCATION

If you do what you feel like doing, you will feel more depressed. Withdrawal and passivity will fuel your depression.

Much of the success of psychotherapy is dependent on client motivation. From a brain-based perspective, the nucleus accumbens and the amygdala, which are in close proximity, play a significant role in the motivational system. The nucleus accumbens integrates incoming sensory information, evaluates emotional memory from the amygdala, and influences decisions made by the PFC regarding motivated behavior ("go" or "stop" behavior) (Hoebel, Rada, Mark, & Pothos, 1999). If clients feel that the result of behavior is positive, those synapses mediated by DA are strengthened, and the associated motivation to engage in that behavior again is increased.

When clients want to understand why engaging in productive behaviors will help lift their depression, it can be useful to describe the effort-driven reward circuit in the brain (Lambert, 2008). This system underlies why the behavior activation technique, which involves engaging in productive behaviors, helps lift depression. Neurologically this network is referred to as the nucleus accumbens-striatal PFC because when the nucleus accumbens, the striatum, and the PFC all work together, mood becomes positive and pleasure is high. The nucleus accumbens is widely regarded as one of the brain's principal pleasure centers. When this area is activated by DA, clients anticipate pleasure and will more likely try to replicate that behavior again. When the striatum is also activated through the DA network, movement toward positive habits can be formed. Finally the PFC generates executive functions, such as planning and orchestrating motivation.

It can be very useful to inform clients that when they fail to engage in rewarding activities, there is less activity in the nucleus accumbens, which results in a corresponding loss of pleasure. When clients fail to move their bodies, there is a drop in activity in their striatums, which results in psychomotor retardation (essentially a fancy way to say movement is sluggish). And when clients are less attentive to the here and now and engage in less planning for the future, there is a drop in PFC activity, resulting in poor concentration, which some clients describe as a sort of brain fog.

The effort-driven reward circuit is critical for the lifting of depression (Lambert, 2008). The nucleus accumbens is a peanut-size structure positioned between the striatum, which is involved in movement, and the amygdala which is involved in emotional memory. As such it is involved in the interface between our emotions and our actions. It is also connected to our PFC, which controls problem solving, planning, and decision-making. It evolved to keep us engaged in behaviors critical for our survival, including eating and sex. Because it is a pleasure center, it is also involved in addictive behaviors.

The effort-driven reward network connects movement, emotion, and thinking. In depression there is less activity in this network. Specifically, when a client is depressed he loses a sense of pleasure, in part because his accumbens is deactivated. When his movement is sluggish, his striatum is barely activated. And when clients make little effort to concentrate, there seems to be less activity in the PFC.

To help lift depression, the effort-driven reward circuit needs to be revved up (Lambert, 2008). "Kindling" represents the process where neural systems are activated by use and follow-through. Just as a campfire is lighted first by lighting twigs before adding logs, clients can learn to kindle the effort-driven reward circuit by engaging in incrementally productive activities, as is the case with behavioral activation. Kindling this reward circuit raises the levels of DA and serotonin, resulting in an increase in positive feelings. Clients reap the rewards of their productive behavior and boost their self-control and self-esteem.

Some depressed clients understand and agree with the model conceptually but argue that they do not know where to start. It is useful to explain that clients can activate the PFC when they plan an activity. The striatum activates as they move to perform the activity. The nucleus accumbens activates when they anticipate pleasure of doing the activity prior to the next time.

CLIENT EDUCATION

To rev up your brain circuits to lift your depression, initially you will need to do some things you do not feel like doing.

The striatal neural circuit is involved in the acquisition of both positive and negative habits, including addiction. The anticipation of pleasure involves the release of DA from an area deep within the brain called the ventrotegmental area (VTA). When DA reaches the nucleus accumbens, clients will experience pleasure, and the PFC will begin to plan how they can perform the same behavior.

CLIENT EDUCATION

Just as no exercise can lead to the atrophy of your muscles and feeling weak, the lack of productive behavior can lead to losing the brain circuits that help you feel like doing things that make you feel better.

For clients who are familiar with stick shift transmissions for automobiles, it can be useful to describe push starting a car and popping the clutch to rev up and get the engine started. The effort-driven reward circuit represents a system very much like one that can be revved up through extra effort that can result in rewards, lifting depression. Not only does it represent the brain-based infrastructure for the behavior activation technique promoted in CBT, but the effort-driven reward circuit also results in systemic positive effects that help drive people out of depression.

SOCIAL LIFT

Lloyd Lindford, the former director of the Best Practices programs in Kaiser Permanente Medical Centers, examined the electronic charts of over 1,000 people who had been seen by both a therapist and a psychiatrist to determine the diagnostic preferences of each practitioner. Therapists were three times as likely as psychiatrists to see the issue as a relationship problem. Setting aside the Pax Medica tendency to pathologize, the point is that relationship problems are strongly associated with depression. Loneliness has been studied throughout the world, and there is a consistent association with depression.

For example, a study of depression among Portuguese adolescent immigrants to Switzerland over age 65 found that loneliness was the single most important predictor of depression (Neto, & Barrios 2001). Similarly, a study in London assessed 2,600 people over 65; more than 15% who were at risk for social isolation also suffered from depression (Iliffe et al., 2007).

Many clients need more information to motivate them to engage in social activities, especially when they feel like withdrawing from people. To this end, it can be useful to describe how the SEEDS formula (discussed in Chapter 2) represents one of the five brain-healthy factors. You can describe what is occurring in the brain when a person suffers from loneliness. A brain-based approach to helping people with depression includes a description of the social brain networks and how loneliness can shut down these systems and result in a systemic crisis. In the long run, loneliness is as detrimental to longevity as smoking (Cacioppo, & Patrick, 2008). In addition to all the social brain networks that become deactivated when people are lonely, including the temporoparietal junction (TPJ), can atrophy. This decrease in the capacity for cognitive empathy results in a downward spiral so that clients become socially isolated, and what few social experiences they do allow themselves are less successful, because clients do not practice; consequently, they become less confident and even less successful socially if they withdraw further.

CLIENT EDUCATION

Although you may feel like withdrawing from family and friends, doing so will only make you more depressed. Your social brain networks will starve, and they are key to your physical and mental health.

Limited social experiences result in less activity in the VTA, which releases less DA, and the nucleus accumbens, which thrives on DA. As a result, clients feel a reduced sense of pleasure and increased anhedonia.

Interpersonal psychotherapy (IPT) is a therapeutic approach that has gained evidence-based support for its efficacy in alleviation of depression. IPT explores the interpersonal context of clients, and depressive symptoms are linked to recent interpersonal events. Depending on the situation, the focus of therapy may be on complicated bereavement, interpersonal conflict, role transition, and interpersonal deficits (Van Schaik et al., 2006). The focus on the interpersonal aspects of mental health is consistent with the social brain network that, when not kindled, leads to depression. Originally conceived of as a distinct approach, behavior activation involves teaching clients techniques to monitor mood and daily activities, especially social activities, and then grasping the connection between them (Lewinsohn et al., 1976). Three other therapeutic behavioral approaches were folded into and subsumed by the larger family of CBT: self-control therapy (SCT), problem-solving therapy (PST), and social skills therapy (SST) (see Cuijpers et al., 2012, for a review). In SCT, there is an emphasis on self-monitoring aimed at changing the selective attention of depressed persons from negative events that follow their behavior. The self-evaluation aspect of SCT is aimed at changing the inclination to set unrealistic, perfectionist, global standards for themselves, making success improbable. Finally, the self-reinforcement component is aimed at increasing self-rewarding and decreasing self-punishment. In PST, the therapist helps clients systematically identify problems, generate alternative solutions for each problem, develop and conduct a plan, and evaluate success. SCT also emphasizes assertiveness.

The English guidelines of the National Institute for Health and Excellence recommends IPT for moderately to severely depressed patients in primary care after CBT for the initial approach (NICE, 2004). The Royal Australian and New Zealand College of Psychiatrists Clinical Guidelines Team for Depression (2004) state that IPT is equally effective compared to antidepressant medication.

The social factor, therefore, can play a significant role in the alleviation and prevention of depression. Mothers who would later be diagnosed with postpartum depression pull back from social contact, even contact with their babies. They have been observed touching their bodies less than mothers without postpartum depression the second day after delivery (Ferber, 2004). Women who felt social isolation during their pregnancy are more likely to experience postpartum depression (Nielsen Forman, Videbech, Hedegaard, Dalby Salvig, & Secher, 2000). Thus, kindling the social brain networks by increasing social support during pregnancy helps protect women from later depression and infants from the negative effects of the mothers' depression.

DEFAULT MODE AND RUMINATION

As described in Chapter 1, we spend roughly 30% of our waking hours dreaming, ruminating, and spacing off from the present moment. From a brain-based perspective, this has been called the default mode network (DMN). Particular patterns of the DMN have been identified with depression. Rumination occurring during the DMN activity appears to be one of the salient factors with depression.

For those of us fortunate not to suffer from depression, it is hard enough to stay present all the time. Our mental activity associated with the DMN may involve reflecting on what occurred earlier in the day and what we imagine might occur later. Unless we are particularly stressed about a situation, the DMN can be a source of creativity. This is not necessarily the case for clients with depression. They may spend a great deal of time ruminating with regret, remorse, and self-pity.

Helping clients with depressive DMNs involves strengthening their attention skills to orient to the present moment. The DMN increases when the DLPFC is not engaged, typically when clients are stressed, bored, or tired, or when they experience no novelty, at which time their minds are flooded with obsessive ruminations over negative experiences that occurred in the past. Because breaking out of a depressive DMN spiral can be difficult, you can encourage clients to work toward making the ruminations fade with exercise, social activities, and mindfulness. These activities disrupt the DMN because they demand a here-and-now focus. For example, if clients are jogging or briskly walking in an environment that requires attention, lest they trip and fall, it is less likely that they will drift into the DMN. When engaged in conversation, clients can inhibit the DMN to meet the here-and-now demands of sharing the moment with other people.

NEUROSCIENCE

Berman and colleagues (2011) found that patients with major depression show more functional connectivity between the PFC and the subgenual ACC than healthy individuals during rest periods. This abnormal degree of connectivity in the DMN highlights the tendency toward rumination and brooding.

Consistent with these findings, Sheline and colleagues (1999) propose that depression is characterized by both stimulus-induced heightened activity and failure to normally down-regulate activity broadly within DMN. Greicius and colleagues (2007) found abnormally increased resting-state connectivity of the subgenual ACC. Thus, it appears that dysregulation of autonomic processing points to the importance of the DMN in depression and inability to turn it off when goal-directed tasks and motivation are required.

Mindfulness has been in vogue for the last several years for good reason. The practice of nonjudgmental attention to the present moment helps pull people out of the past. Quieting ruminations through observation of what clients are doing in the present moment converges with their here-and-now focus along with deliberate and practical behavior. This concept underlies the meaning of the Zen saying "Zen is not like chopping wood. Zen *is* chopping wood."

CLIENT EDUCATION

When you find yourself drifting into ruminations, bring yourself back to the present moment. By getting out of the rumination stew and into the now, you will help yourself climb out of depression.

Mindfulness by its nature is a be-here-now activity that attempts to maximize attention to novelty in each moment. Its emphasis on the nonjudgmental observation provides an antidote to negativistic rumination. For these reasons, there has been a surge of interest in applying mindfulness to therapeutic approaches to depression since the late 1990s. Mindfulness targets depression by neutralizing specific depressive symptoms, such as monotony, by attention to novelty, and cultivation of curiosity. The ruminations so prevalent in depression can be neutralized through a wide range of nonjudgmental observation and detachment. Through mindfulness-based CBT, thinking errors can be neutralized by affective labeling. For example, clients can be taught to say "That's a depressing thought" rather than "That's depressing." This slight shift in labeling allows clients to detach the thought from the feeling. The fixation on imperfections can be addressed through acceptance, as is well articulated in ACT.

Whether you use the term "mindfulness" with clients is of little importance. What is helpful is building the capacity for nonjudgmental attention to the present moment, including decentering thoughts and feelings so that they can be understood as momentary events and not realities. Since depressed people are often on autopilot, teaching them to behave with intentionality helps establish here-and-now focus and thereby helps them break out of depressive automatic thoughts and behaviors. The intentional behavior and acceptance focus helps clients let go of the past. Consistent with kindling the L-PFC, which involves intentionally reducing avoidance, the client turns toward difficulties to resolve them.

CLIENT EDUCATION

The more you can train yourself to focus on the present moment, the more you pull yourself out of the black hole of depression.

ORCHESTRATING A BROAD APPROACH

Because clients can become depressed by multiple factors, it is advisable to help them appreciate that they must do multiple things simultaneously to rise out of depression. Therapy for clients who are depressed, therefore, involves

a concerted effort to orchestrate multiple interventions while utilizing alli-
ance-building therapeutic approaches that activate the social brain networks.
These networks are kindled through culturally positive relationships, the
synthesis of the psychodynamic, client-centered, and interpersonal therapy
approaches. Additionally, cognitive restructuring can be combined with the
co-construction of new narratives that enhance self-efficacy. Behavioral activation, through its kindling of the L-PFC, leads to enhanced affect regulation
and resilience.

You can tell clients that a well-orchestrated brain tune-up will simultaneously charge up the social brain network through relationship building, if they
engage in psychotherapy, groups, and cultivating positive relationships with
family and friends. The activity reward circuit can be kindled through behavior
activation, essentially engaging in productive behaviors. The overall health of
the hippocampus can be enhanced by cognitive and aerobic exercise that maximizes BDNF. Also, sleep hygiene techniques can protect the hippocampus from
the corrosive effects of elevated cortisol, glutamate, and epinephrine associated
with poor or not enough sleep. The frontal lobes, specifically the PFC, can be
enhanced by attention training, such as mindfulness.

Promoting the functions of the L-PFC cortex by encouraging active behaviors
instead of the avoidant and withdrawal tendencies of the R-PFC help balance
out the set point. Because many depressed clients are also anxious, teach them to
calm their amygdala and the HPA axis through mindfulness, exercise, and new
coping skills. Because negativistic and self-deprecating rumination is often part
of the cognitive set of depressed clients, you can help them switch off the depression switch in the ACC confronting their self-criticism.

CLIENT EDUCATION

Because many factors can contribute to your depression, you'll need to do
all the things we talk about doing at once to climb out of depression.

Brain-based therapy for depression must involve the simultaneous orchestration of multiple systems. Because depression can result from multiple factors
and is by nature so systemic in its aversive effects, it is imperative to apply simultaneous therapeutic interventions. In fact, if you do not employ multiple and
simultaneous interventions, clients may say "I tried that and it didn't work." Then
later, when you try another intervention, they may also say "And I tried that one
too and it didn't work either!" The truth may be that this or that specific approach
by itself is not enough to lift clients out of depression.

Remembering that up to 19% of chronically depressed people experience a
reduction in the size of the hippocampus, it makes sense that part of the concerted effort should kindle the hippocampus for neuroplasticity and neurogenesis. Exercise, as noted in Chapter 2, is one of the best ways to promote the birth

of new neurons in the hippocampus through the release of BDNF. Also, exercise promotes the up-regulation of serotonin, DA, and NE, which all help alleviate depression.

Asking clients to engage in specific detail-oriented behaviors helps temper the R-PFC bias by activating the L-PFC, which orients to details. Also since the L-PFC is kindled by approach behaviors, clients can be informed that active engagement in the environment, in contrast to passive withdrawal, will help them climb out of the pit of depression. Using the phrase "You're going to have to do what you don't feel like doing" acknowledges that clients need to make an extra effort.

The importance of describing how to build the capacity for resilience and transcendence cannot be overstated. A variety of powerful role models can serve as references for resilience as they have demonstrated an inspiring degree of transcendence. Ludwig von Beethoven is one such figure. As a child, young Ludwig was tormented and physically abused by his alcoholic father, who wanted him to be the next child prodigy. Ludwig did develop amazing skills at the keyboard and was sent on a church scholarship to Vienna to study with Hayden. By this time, Beethoven was a rebellious young man. Mozart, some 15 years Ludwig's senior, had a glimpse of his talent and remarked "that young man will someday make the world stand up and listen." Soon thereafter, Beethoven received a letter announcing that his mother had died and commanding him to return to Bonn to help raise his two younger brothers, because his father was often too drunk to do so. Beethoven did return, literally kicked his father out of town, forbade his brothers to utter his name, then guided them into young adulthood. Thereupon he returned to Vienna to become the composer who transformed classical music, inventing new styles, constructing the orchestra as we know it today, and offering new pieces of music that departed dramatically from what he had written previously. Just as he became world famous, he became deaf. Depressed by this disability, he even considered suicide. Three months after writing a letter to his brothers addressing the option of suicide, he wrote the Third Symphony, which defined the size and configuration of the orchestra today. Beethoven lived for another 18 years, writing music most conductors of symphony orchestras consider to be the greatest and transformative the world has ever seen since. Yes, people experience hardship, but we can certainly transcend them. Clients need not become Beethoven to do that, but they can use him as a reference for what is possible even in the face of great adversity.

A mnemonic that can help depressed clients remember what they need to do to help lift them out of depression needs to factor in the concept that they must do multiple things simultaneously. The word "TEAM" drives home the point that one method alone will not be enough to lift depression.

T—for thinking. Clients must think to defuse negativistic thinking associated with depression.

E—for effort. Clients must make an effort to activate the approach circuits of the L-PFC and the effort-driven reward circuit.

A—for acceptance. Clients must accept that the world is not perfect and that the things that happen are not always good.

M— for mindfulness. Clients must focus on the present moment and novelty of each experience.

I opened this book by noting that clients have been needlessly confused by the many differences in the theoretical background and language used by their therapists. The 21st century offers an opportunity to not only find common denominators among therapy types. We can also offer clients information, sometimes in the form of mnemonics, that they can use to develop skills to lower their anxiety and rise out of depression.

Abbreviation Glossary

- ACT—Acceptance Commitment Therapy
- AGEs—Advanced Glycation End Products
- ACTH—Adrenocorticotropin Hormone
- ACC—Anterior Cingulate Cortex
- BE—Beta Endorphin
- BDNF—Brain-Derived Neurotrophic Factor
- CBT—Cognitive-Behavioral Therapy
- CRH—Corticotropin Releasing Hormone
- DA—Dopamine
- DLPFC—Dorsolateral Prefrontal Cortex
- DMN—Default Mode Network
- EBP—Evidence-Based Practices
- EFT—Emotionally Focused Therapy
- EMDR—Eye Movement Desensitization And Reprocessing
- EFA—Essential Fatty Acids
- FMRI—Functional Magnetic Resonance Imaging
- IL-1—InterLeukin 1
- IL-6—InterLeukin 6
- HPA—Hypothalamic-Pituitary-Adrenal Axis
- GABA—Gamma-Aminobutyric Acid
- LC—Locus Coeruleus
- LTD—Long-Term Depression
- LTP—Long-Term Potentiation
- MPFC—Medial Prefrontal Cortex
- MS—Medium Spiny Neurons
- OFC—Orbital Frontal Cortex
- NE—Norepinephrine
- NMDA—N-Methyl-D-aspartate Receptors
- NMDA—N-Methyl-D-aspartate Receptors
- PFC—Prefrontal Cortex

- PTA—Post Traumatic Amnesia
- SAMs—Situationally Accessible Memories
- SUDS—Subjective Units of Distress Scale
- TBI—Traumatic Brain Injury
- TPJ—Temporoparietal Junction
- SSRIs—Selective Serotonin Reuptake Inhibitors
- TNF-α—Tumour Necrosis Factor Alpha
- VAMs—Verbally Accessible Memories
- VTA—Ventral Tegmental Area

REFERENCES

Aleksandrowicz, A. M. C., & Levine, D. S. (2005). Neural dynamics of psychology; what modeling might tell us about us. *Neural Networks, 18*(5–6), 639–645.

Allen, J. G. (2001). *Traumatic relationships and serious mental disorders*. New York, NY: Wiley.

Allman, H. A., Erwin, J. M., Nimchimsky, E., & Hof, P. (2001). The anterior cingulate cortex: The evolution of an interface between emotion and cognition. *Annals of the New York Academy of Sciences, 935,* 107–117.

American Psychiatric Association. (2013). Diagnostic and Statistical Manual of Mental Disorders 5 edition. American Psychiatric Publishing.

Anthony, M., Roth Ledley, D., Liss, A., & Swinson, R. P. (2006). Responses to symptom induction exercises in panic disorder. *Behavioral Research and Therapy, 44,* 85–98.

Arato, M., Banki, C. M., Bissette, G., & Nemeroff, C. B. (1989). Elevated CSF CRF in suicide victims. *Biological Psychiatry, 25,* 355–359.

Arden, J. B. (2010). *Rewire your brain*. Hoboken, NJ: Wiley.

Arden, J. B. (2014). *The brain bible*. New York, NY: McGraw-Hill.

Arden, J. B., & Linford, L. (2009a). *Brain-based therapy for adults*. Hoboken, NJ: Wiley.

Arden, J. B., & Linford, L. (2009b). *Brain-based therapy for children and adolescents*. Hoboken, NJ: Wiley.

Arroll, B., MacGillivray, S., Ogston, S., Sullivan, F., Williams, B., & Crombie, I. (2005). Efficacy and tolerability of tricyclic antidepressants and SSRIs compared with placebo for treatment of depression in primary care: A meta-analysis. *Annals of Family Medicine, 3,* 449–456.

Ashman, S. B., Dawson, G., Panagiotides, H., Yamada, E., & Wilkinson, C. W. (2002). Stress hormone levels of children of depressed mothers. *Development and Psychopathology, 14:* 333–349.

Aston-Jones, G., Valentino, R. J., Van Bockstaele, E. J., & Meyerson, A. T. (1994). Locus coeruleus, stress, and PTSD: Neurobiological and clinical parallels. In M. M. Murburg (Ed.), *Catecholamine function in post-traumatic stress disorder: Emerging concepts* (pp. 17–62). Washington, DC: American Psychiatric Press.

Aubert, G., & Lansdorp, P. M. (2008). Telomeres and aging. *Physiological Reviews, 88,* 557–579.

Babyak, M., Blumenthal, J. A., Herman, S., Khatri, P., Doraiswamy, M., Moore, K., … Krishnan, K. R. (2000). Exercise treatment for major depression: Maintenance of therapeutic benefit at 10 months. *Psychosomatic Medicine, 62*(5), 633–638.

Bailey, C. H., & Kandel, E. R. (1993). Structural changes accompanying memory storage. *Annual Review of Physiology, 55,* 397–426.

Bailey, M., Engler, H., Hunzeker, J., and Sheridan, J. F. (2003). Hypothalamic-pituitary-adrenal axis and viral infection. *Viral Immunology, 16*(2), 141–157.

Baker, D. G., Ekhator, N. N., Kasckow, J. W., Hill, K. K., Zoumakis, E., Dashevsky, B. A.,... Geracioti, T. D. Jr. (2001). Plasma and cerebrospinal fluid interleukin-6 concentrations in posttraumatic stress disorder. *Neuroimmunomodulation, 9*, 209–217.

Bandura, A. (1997). *Self-efficacy: The exercise of control.* New York: W.H. Freeman.

Barlow, D., & Craske, M. (2007). *Mastery of your anxiety and panic: Workbook (Treatments That Work),* 4th ed. New York, NY: Oxford University Press.

Bassuk, S. S., Glass, T. A., & Berkman, L. F. (1999). Social disengagement and incident cognitive decline in community-dwelling elderly persons. *Annals of Internal Medicine, 131*(3), 165–173.

Batty, M., & Taylor, M. J. (2003, October). Early processing of the six basic facial emotional expressions. *Cognitive Brain Research, 17*(3), 613–620.

Baxter, L. R., Phelps, M. E., Mazziotta, J. C., Guze, B. T., Schwartz, J. M., & Selin, C. E. (1987). Local cerebral metabolism rates in obsessive compulsive disorder: A comparison with rates in unipolar depression and in normal controls. *Archives of General Psychiatry, 44*, 211–218.

Baxter, L. R. Jr., Ackermann, R. F., Swerdlow, N. R., Brody, A., Saxena, S., Schwartz, J. M.,... Phelps, M. E. (2000). In W. K. Goodman, M. V. Rudorfer, & J. D. Maser (Eds.), *Obsessive-compulsive disorder: Contemporary issues in treatment* (pp. 573–609). Mahwah, NJ: Lawrence Erlbaum.

Baxter, L. R. Jr., Schwartz, J. M., Bergman, K. S., Szuba, M. P., Guze, B. M., Mazziotta, J. C.,... Phelps, M. E. (1992). Caudate glucose metabolic rate changes with both drug and behavioral therapy of obsessive-compulsive disorder. *Archives of General Psychiatry, 49*, 681–889.

Beck, A. T., Rush, A. J., Shaw, B. F., & Emery, G. (1979) *Cognitive therapy of depression.* New York: Guilford Press.

Bellert, J. L. (1989). Humor: A therapeutic approach in oncology nursing. *Cancer Nursing, 12*(2), 65–70.

Bergmann, U. (1998). Speculations on the neurobiology of EMDR. *Traumatology, 4,* Article 2.

Berk, L. S., Tan, S. A., Nehlsen-Cannarella, S., Napier, B., Lewis, J. W., Lee, J. A., & Eby, W. C. (1988). Humor associated laughter decreases cortisol and increases spontaneous lymphocyte blastogenesis. *Clinical Research, 36*, 435A.

Berman, M. G., Peltier, S., Nee, D. E., Kross, E., Deldin, P. J., & Jonides, J. (2011). Depression, rumination and the default network. *Social Cognitive and Affective Neuroscience, 6*(5), 548–555.

Bierhaus, A., Wolf, J., Andrassy, M., Rohleder, N., Humpert, P. M., Petrov, D.,... Nawroth, P. P. (2003). A mechanism converting psychosocial stress into mononuclear cell activation. *Proceedings of the National Academy of Sciences of the United States of America, 100*, 1920–1925.

Bishop, S. J. (2007). Neurocognitive mechanisms of anxiety: An integrative account. *Trends in Cognitive Sciences, 11*(7), 307–316.

Bloom, S. L. (1998). By the crowd they have been broken, by the crowd they shall be healed: The social transformation of trauma. In R. G. Tedeschi & C. L. Calhoun (Eds.), *Posttraumatic growth: Positive changes in the aftermath of crisis* (pp. 179–213). Mahwah, NJ: Lawrence Erlbaum.

Borkovec, T. D. (2006). Applied relaxation and cognitive therapy for pathological worry and generalized anxiety disorder. In G. C. L. Davey & A. Wells (Eds.), *Worry and its psychological disorders: Theory, assessment, and treatment* (pp. 273–287). Hoboken, NJ: Wiley.

Borovikova, L. V., Ivanova, S., Zhang, M., Yang, H., Botchkina, G. I., Watkins, L. R.,... Tracey, K. J. (2000, May). Vagus nerve stimulation attenuates the systemic inflammatory response to endotoxin. *Nature, 25,* 458–462.

Botvinick, M., Jha, A. P., Bylsma, L. M., Fabian, S. A., Solomon, P. E., & Prkachin, K. M. (2005). Viewing facial expressions of pain engages cortical areas involved in the direct experience of pain. *Neuroimage, 25,* 312–319.

Bowler, R. M., Mergler, D., Huel, G., & Cone, J. E. (1994). Psychological, psychosocial, and psychophysiological sequela in a community affected by a railroad chemical disaster. *Journal of Traumatic Stress, 7,* 601–624.

Bremner, J. D. (2002). Neuroimaging studies in posttraumatic stress disorder. *Current Psychiatry Report, 4,* 254–263.

Bremner, J. D. (2005). *Does stress damage the brain? Understanding trauma-related disorders from a mind-body perspective.* New York, NY: Norton.

Bremner, J. D., Krystal, J. H., Southwick, S. M., & Charney, D. S. (1995). Functional neuroanatomical correlates of the effects of stress on memory. *Journal of Psychiatry, 156,* 360–366.

Bremner, J. D., Licinie, J., Dainell, A., Krystal, J. H., Owens, M. J., Southwick, S. M.,... Charney, D. S. (1997). Elevated CSF corticotropin-releasing factor concentrations in posttraumatic stress disorder. *American Journal of Psychiatry, 154,* 624–629.

Bremner, J. D., Staib, L. H., Kaloupek, D. G., Southwick, S. M., Soufer, R., & Charney, D. S. (1999). Neural correlates of exposure to traumatic pictures and sounds in Vietnam combat veterans with and without posttraumatic stress disorder: A positron emission tomography study. *Biological Psychiatry, 45,* 806–816.

Bremner, J. D., Vythilingam, M., Vermetten, E., Nazeer, A., Adil, J., Khan, S.,... Charney, D. S. (2002). Reduced volume of orbitofrontal cortex in major depression. *Biological Psychiatry, 51,* 273–279.

Breslau, N., Davis, G., Andreski, P., Federman, B., & Anthony, J. C. (1998). Epidemiological findings on posttraumatic stress disorder and co-morbid disorders in the general population. In B. P. Dohrenwald (Ed.), *Adversity, stress, and psychopathology* (pp. 319–330). New York, NY: Oxford University Press.

Breslau, N., Davis, G. C., Peterson, E., & Schultz, L. R. (2001). A second look at comorbidity in victims of trauma: The posttraumatic stress disorder–major depression connection. *Biological Psychiatry, 48,* 902–909.

Brewin, C. R. (2001). A cognitive neuroscience account of posttraumatic stress disorder and its treatment. *Behavioral Research Therapy, 39,* 373–393.

Brewin, C. R. (2003). *Posttraumatic stress disorder: Malady or myth?* New Haven, CT: Yale University Press.

Brewin, C. R. (2005). Encoding and retrieval of traumatic memories. In J. J. Vasterling & C. R. Brewin, *Neuropsychology of PTSD: Biological, cognitive and clinical perspectives* (pp. 131–150). New York, NY: Guilford Press.

Brown, T. (2005). *Attention deficit disorder: the unfocused mind in children and adults.* New Haven, CT: Yale University Press.

Bruder, G. E., Stewart, J. W., Mercier, M. A., Agosti, V., Leite, P., Donovan, S., & Quitkin, F. M. (1997). Outcome of cognitive-behavioral therapy for depression: Relation to hemisphere dominance for verbal processing. *Journal of Abnormal Psychology, 106,* 138–144.

Bruder, G. E., Stewart, J. W., Tenke, C. E., McGrath, J. P., Leite, P., Bhattacharya, N., & Quitkin, F. M. (2001). Electroencephalographic and perceptual asymmetry differences between responders and nonresponders to an SSRI antidepressant. *Biological Psychiatry, 49,* 416–425.

Bryant, R. A., & Harvey, A. G. (1998). Relationship of acute stress disorder and posttraumatic stress disorder following mild traumatic brain injury. *American Journal of Psychiatry, 155,* 625–629.

Brydon, L., Edwards, S., Mohamed-Ali, V., & Steptoe, A. (2004). Socioeconomic status and stress-induced increases in interleukin-6. *Brain, Behavior, and Immunity, 18*(3), 281–290.

Buchanan, T. W., Tranel, D., & Adolphs, R. (2005). Emotional autobiographical memories in amnesic patients with medial temporal lobe damage. *Journal of Neuroscience, 25*(12), 3151–3160.

Buchanan, T. W., Tranel, D., & Adolphs, R. (2009). The human amygdala in social function. In P. J. Whalen & E. A. Phelps (Eds.), *The human amygdala* (pp. 289–318). New York, NY: Guilford Press.

Buonomano, D. V., & Merzenich, M. M. (1998). Cortical plasticity: From synapses to maps. *Annual Review of Neuroscience, 21,* 149–186. doi:10.1146/annurev.neuro.21.1.149

Bush, G., Luu, P., & Posner, M. I. (2000) Cognitive and emotional influences in the anterior cingulate cortex. *Trends in Cognitive Science, 4:* 215–222.

Buzsáki, G. (1996). The hippocampo-neocortical dialogue. *Cerebral Cortex, 6,* 81–92.

Cacioppo, J. T., & Patrick, B. (2008). *Loneliness: Human nature and the need for social connection.* New York, NY: Norton.

Cadoret, R. J., Yates, W. R., Troughton, E., Woodworth, G., & Stewart, M. A. (1995). Genetic–environmental interaction in the genesis of aggressivity and conduct disorders. *Archives of General Psychiatry, 52*(11), 916–924.

Cahill, L. (1997). The neurobiology of emotionally influenced memory. Implications for understanding traumatic memory. *Annals of the New York Academy of Science, 821,* 238–246.

Cahill, S. P., Carrigan, M. H., & Frueh, B. C. (1999). Does EMDR work? And if so, why? A critical review of controlled outcome and dismantling research. *Journal of Anxiety Disorders, 13,* 5–33.

Cahn, B. R., & Polich, J. (2006). Meditation states and traits: EEG, ERP, and neuroimaging studies. *Psychological Bulletin, 132*(2), 180–211.

Candel, I., & Merckelbach, H. (2004). Peritraumatic disassociation as a predictor of posttraumatic stress disorder: A critical review. *Comprehensive Psychiatry, 45,* 44–50.

Canli, T. (2009). Individual differences in human amygdala function. In P. J. Whalen & E. A. Phelps (Eds.), *The human amygdala* (pp. 250–264). New York, NY: Guilford Press.

Carlson, L. E., Speca, M., Patel, K. D., & Goodey E. (2003). Mindfulness-based stress reduction in relation to quality of life, mood, symptoms of stress, and immune parameters in breast and prostate cancer outpatients. *Psychosomatic Medicine, 65*(4), 571–581.

Carr, J. E. (1998). Neuroendocrine and behavioral interaction in exposure treatment of phobic experience. *Clinical Psychology Review, 16*(1), 1–15.

Carr, L. M., Iacoboni, M. C., Dubeau, J. C., Mazziotta, J. C., & Lenzi, G. L. (2003). Neural mechanisms of empathy in humans: A relay from neural systems for imitation to limbic areas. *Proceedings of the National Academy of Sciences USA, 100,* 5497–5502.

Carrion, V. G., Weems, C. F., Eliez, S., Ptwardhan, A., Brown, W., Ray, R. D., et al. (2001). Attenuation of frontal asymmetry in pediatric posttraumatic stress disorders. *Journal of Consulting and Clinical Psychology, 54,* 303–308.

Casey, B. J., Tottenham, N., Liston, C., & Durston, S. (2005). Imaging the developing brain: What have we learned about cognitive development? *Trends in Cognitive Science, 9*(3), 104–110.

Ceci, S., & Bruch, M. (1993). Suggestibility of the child witness: A historical review and synthesis. *Psychological Bulletin, 113*, 403–439.

Chajut, E., & Algom, D. (2003). Selective attention improves under stress: Implications for theories of social cognition. *Journal of Personality and Social Psychology, 85,* 231–248.

Charmandari, E., Tsigos, C., & Chrousos, C. P. (2005). Endrocrinology of the stress response. *Annual Review of Physiology, 67,* 259–284.

Cherkas, L. F., Hunkin, J. L., Kato, B. S., Richards, J. B., Gardner, J. P., Surdulescu, G. L., ... Aviv, A. (2008). The association between physical activity in leisure time and leukocyte telomere length. *Archives of Internal Medicine, 168,* 154–158.

Christian, L. M., Deichert, N. T., Gouin, J. -P., Graham, J. E., & Kiecolt-Glaser, J. K. (2012). Psychological influences on neuroendocrine and immune outcomes. In G. G. Berntson & J. T. Cacioppo (Eds.), *Handbook of neuroscience for the behavioral sciences* (pp. 1260–1279; Vol. 2, pp. 1220–1235). Hoboken, NJ: Wiley.

Chrousos, G. P. (1995). The hypothalamic-pituitary-adrenal axis and immune-mediated inflammation. *New England Journal of Medicine, 332,* 1351–1362.

Cirelli, C. (2005). A molecular window on sleep: Changes in gene expression between sleep and wakefulness. *Neuroscientist, 11,* 63–74.

Clark, C. R., Geffen, G. M., & Geffen, L. B. (1987). Catecholamines and attention: II: Pharmacological studies in normal humans. *Neuroscience and Biobehavioral Review, 11*(4), 353–364.

Clark, L., Manes, F., Antoun, N., Sahakian, B. J., & Robbins, T. W. (2003). The contributions of lesion laterality and lesion volume to decision-making impairment following frontal lobe damage. *Neuropsychologia, 41,* 1474–1483. doi:10.1016/S0028–3932(03)00081–2

Cohen, S., Doyle, W. J., Turner, R. B., MD, Alper, C. M., & Skoner, D. P. (2003). Emotional style and susceptibility to the common cold. *Psychosomatic Medicine, 65,* 652–657.

Constans, J. I. (2005). Information-processing bias in PTSD. In J. J. Vasterling & C. R. Brewin, (Eds.)*Neuropsychology of PTSD: Biological, cognitive and clinical perspectives* (pp. 105–130). New York, NY: Guilford Press.

Corcoran, K. A., & Maren, S. (2001). Hippocampal inactivation disrupts contextual retrieval of fear memory after extinction. *Journal of Neuroscience, 21,* 1720–1726.

Costanzo, E. S., Lutgendorf, S. K., Sood, A. K., Anderson, B., Sorosky, J., & Lubaroff, D. M. (2005). Psychosocial factors and interleukin-6 among women with advanced ovarian cancer. *Cancer, 104*(2), 305–313.

Cozolino, L. (2010). *The neuroscience of psychotherapy. Healing the social brain,* 2nd ed. New York, NY: Norton.

Critchley, H. D., Wiens, S., Rothstein, P., Ohman, A., & Dolan, R. J. (2004). Neural systems supporting interoceptive awareness. *Nature Neuroscience, 7,* 189–195.

Cuijpers, P., van Straten, A., Driessen, E., van Oppen, P., Bockting, C., & Andersson, G. (2012). Depression and dysthymic disorders. In P. Sturmey & M. Hersen (Eds.), *Handbook of evidence-based practice in clinical psychology. Vol. 2: Adult disorders* (pp. 243–284). Hoboken, NJ: Wiley.

Cumberland-Li, A., Eisenberg, N., Champion, C., Gershoff, E., & Fabes, R. A. (2003). The relation of parental emotionality and related dispositional traits to parental expression of emotion and children's social functioning. *Motivation and Emotion, 27,* 27–56.

Dantzer, R., & Kelley, K. W. (2007). Twenty years of research on cytokine-induced sickness behavior. *Brain, Behavior, and Immunity, 21*, 153–160.

Davidson, P. R., & Parker, K. C. K. (2001). Eye movement desensitization and reprocessing (EMDR): A meta-analysis. *Journal of Consulting and Clinical Psychology, 69*, 305–316.

Davidson, R. J., & Irwin, W. (1999). The functional neuroanatomy of emotion and affective style. *Trends in Cognitive Neuroscience, 3*, 11–21.

Davidson, R. J., Pizzagalli, D., Nitschke, J. B., & Putnam, K. (2002). Depression: Perspectives from affective neuroscience. *Annual Review of Psychology, 53*, 545–574.

Davis, M., Ressler, K., Rothbaum, B. O., & Richardson, R. (2006). Effects of D-cycloserine on extinction: Translation from preclinical to clinical work. *Biological Psychiatry, 60*(4), 369–375.

Deaner, S. L., & McConatha, J. T. (1993). The relationship of humor to depression and personality. *Psychological Reports, 72*, 755–763.

De Bellis, M. D., Hooper, S. R., & Sapia, J. L. (2005). Early trauma exposure and the brain. In J. J. Vasterling & C. R. Brewin (Eds.), *Neuropsychology of PTSD: Biological, cognitive and clinical perspectives* (pp. 131–150). New York, NY: Guilford Press.

De Bellis, M. D., Keshavan, M. S., Clark, D. B., Casey, B. J., Giedd, J. N., Borring, A. M., … Ryan, N. D. (1999). A. E. Bennett Research Award. Developmental traumatology. Part 11. Brain Development. *Biological Psychiatry, 45*, 1271–1284.

De Bellis, M. D., Keshavan, M. S., Shifflett, H., Iyengar, S., Beers, S. R., Hall, J., & Moritz, G. (2002a). Brain structures in pediatric maltreatment-related posttraumatic stress disorder: A sociodemographically matched study. *Biological Psychiatry, 52*, 1066–1078.

De Bellis, M. D., Keshavan, M. S., Shifflett, H., Iyengar, S., Dahl, R. E., Axelson, D. A., … Ryan, N. D. (2002b). Superior temporal gyrus volumes in pediatric generalized anxiety disorder. *Biological Psychiatry, 51*(7), 553–562.

De Bellis, M. D., Keshavan, M. S., Spencer, S., & Hall, J. (2000). N-acetylaspartate concentration in the anterior cingulates of maltreated children and adolescents with PTSD. *American Journal of Psychiatry, 157*, 1175–1177.

Debiec, J., & LeDoux, J. E. (2004). Disruption of reconsolidation but not consolidation of auditory fear conditioning by noradrenergic blockage in the amygdala. *Neuroscience, 129*, 269–272.

DeCosta, J. M. (1871). On irritable heart: A clinical study of a form of functional cardiac disorder and its consequences. *American Journal of Medical Science, 161*, 17–52.

de Decker, A., Hermans, D., Raes, F., & Eelen, P. (2003). Autobiographical memory specificity and trauma in inpatient adolescents. *Journal of Clinical Child and Adolescent Psychology, 32*, 22–31.

Delahanty, D. L., Raimonde, A. J., & Spoonster, E. (2000). Initial posttraumatic urinary cortisol levels predict PTSD symptoms in motor vehicle accident victims. *Biological Psychiatry, 48*, 940–947.

Delgado, P. L. (2000). Depression: The case for a monoamine deficiency. *Journal of Clinical Psychiatry, 61*, 7–11.

Depue, R. A., & Morrone-Strupinsky, J. V. (2005). A neurobehavioral model of affiliative bonding: Implications for conceptualizing a human trait of affiliation. *Behavioral and Brain Sciences, 28*, 313–350. doi:10.1017/S0140525×05000063

Devinsky, O., Morrell, M. J., & Vogt, B. A. (1995). Contributions of anterior cingulate cortex to behavior. *Brain, 118*, 279–306.

Dimburg, U., & Ohman, A. (1996). Behold the wrath: Psychophysiological responses to facial stimuli. *Motivation and Emotion, 20*, 149–182.

Dimidijian, S., Hollon, S. D., Dobson, K. S., Schmaling, K. B., Kohlenberg, R. J., Addis, M. E., … Jacobson, N. S. (2006). Randomized trial of behavioral activation, cognitive therapy, and antidepressant medication in the acute treatment of adults with major depression. *Journal of Consulting and Clinical Psychology, 74,* 658–670.

Ding, J., Gip, P., Franken, P., Lomas, L., & O'Hara, B. (2004). A proteomic analysis in brain following sleep deprivation suggests a generalized decrease in abundance for many proteins. *Sleep, 27,* A391.

Dobbs, D. (2006). Antidepressants: Good drugs or good marketing? In L. Pope, C. Linsmeier, & K. Feyen (Eds.), *Scientific American readings in clinical neuroscience* (pp. 88–91). New York, NY: Worth.

Dong, Y., Green, T., Saal, D., Marie, H., Neve, R., Neslter, E. J., & Malenka, R. C. (2006). CREB modulates excitability of nucleus accumbens neurons. *Nature Neuroscience, 9*(4), 475–477.

Draganski, B., Gaser, C., Busch, V., Schuierer, G., Bogdahn, U., & May, A. (2004). Neuroplasticity: Changes in grey matter induced by training. *Nature, 427,* 311–312.

Drevets, W. C. (2001). Neuroimaging and neuropathological studies of depression: Implications for cognitive-emotional features of mood disorders. *Current Opinion in Neurobiology, 11,* 240–249.

Drevets, W. C., & Raiche, M. E. (1998). Reciprocal suppression of regional cerebral blood flow during emotional versus higher cognitive processes: Implications for interactions between emotion and cognition. *Cognition and Emotion, 12,* 353–385.

Dunlap, B. H., & Nemeroff, C. B. (2009). Depression. In G. G. Berntson & J. T. Cacioppo (Eds.), *Handbook of neuroscience for the behavioral sciences* (pp. 1060–1090). Hoboken, NJ: Wiley.

Dunlop, S. A., Archer, M. A., Quinlivan, J. A., Beazley, L. D., & Newnham, J. P. (1997). Repeated prenatal corticosteroids deymyelination in the ovine central nervous system. *Journal of Maternal-Fetal Medicine, 6,* 309–313.

Ehlers, A., & Clark, D. M. (2000). A cognitive model of posttraumatic stress disorder. *Behaviour Research and Therapy,* 38:319–345.

Eisenberger, N., & Lieberman, M. (2004). Why rejection hurts: A common neural alarm system for physical and social pain. *Science, 87,* 294–300.

Ekman, P., Davidson, R. J., & Friesen, W. V. (1990). The Duchenne smile: Emotional expression and brain physiology II. *Journal of Personality and Social Psychology, 58*(2), 342–353.

Ekman, P. (2007). *Emotions revealed, second edition: Recognizing faces and feelings to improve communication and emotional life.* New York: Holt.

Elenkov, I. J., Iezzoni, D. G., Daly, A., Harris, A. G., & Chrousos, G. P. (2005). Cytokine dysregulation, inflammation, and well-being. *Neuroimmunomodulation, 12,* 255–269.

Epel, E. (2009). Telomeres in a life-span perspective: A new "psychobiomarker"? *Current Directions in Psychological Science, 18,* 6.

Epel, E. S., Blackburn, E. H., Lin, J., Dhabhar, F. S., Adler, N. E., Morrow, J. D., & Cawthon, R. M. (2004). Accelerated telomere shortening in response to life stress. *Proceedings of the National Academy of Sciences USA, 101*(49), 17312–17315.

Etcoff, N. L. (1989). Asymmetries on recognition of emotions. In F. Boller & J. Grafman (Eds.), *Handbook of neuropsychology* (Vol. 3, pp. 363–382). Amsterdam, the Netherlands: Elsevier.

Etcoff, N. L., Ekman, P., Frank, M., Magee, J., & Torreano, L. (1992, August). *Detecting deception: Do aphasics have an advantage?* Paper presented at conference of International Society for Research on Emotions, Carnegie Mellon University, Pittsburgh, PA.

Evans, D. L., Charney, D. S., Lewis, L., Golden, R. N., Gorman, J. M., Krishnan, K. R., . . . Valvo, W. J. (2005). Mood disorders in the medically ill: Scientific review and recommendations. *Biological Psychiatry, 58*(3), 175–189.

Expert Consensus Guidelines Series Treatment of Posttraumatic Stress Disorder. (1999). Treatment of posttraumatic stress disorder. *Journal of Clinical Psychiatry, 60* (Suppl. 16).

Eysenck, H. J. (1952). The effects of psychotherapy: An evaluation. *Journal of Consulting Psychology, 16,* 319–324.

Eysenck, H. J., & Eysneck, M. W. (1985). *Personality and individual differences: A natural science approach.* New York, NY: Plenum Press.

Fanselow, M. S. (2000). Contextual fear, gestalt, memories, and the hippocampus, *Behavioral Brain Research, 110,* 73–81.

Felitti, V. J., Anda, R. F., Nordenberg, D., Williamson, D. F., Spitz, A. M., Edwards, V., . . . Marks, J. S. (1998). Relationship of childhood dysfunction to many of the leading causes of death in adults: The Adverse Childhood Experiences (ACE) study. *American Journal of Prevention Medicine, 14,* 245–258.

Felmingham, K., Kemp, A., Williams, L., Das, P., Hughes, G., Peduto, A., & Bryant, R. (2007). Changes in anterior cingulate and amygdala after cognitive behavior therapy of posttraumatic stress disorder. *Psychological Sciences, 18*(2), 127–129.

Ferber, S. G. (2004). The nature of touch in mothers experiencing maternity blues: The contribution of parity. *Early Human Development, 79,* 65–75.

Ferber, S. G., & Makhoul, I. R. (2004). The effect of skin-to-skin contact (kangaroo care) shortly after birth on the neurobehavioral responses of the term newborn: A randomized, controlled trial. *Pediatrics, 113*(4), 858–865.

Festinger, L. (1957). *A theory of cognitive dissonance.* Stanford, CA: Stanford University Press.

Field, T. (1995). Massage therapy for infants and children. *Journal of Developmental and Behavioral Pediatrics, 6*(2), 105–111.

Field T., & Diego, M. (2008). Vagal activity, early growth, and emotional development. *Infant Behavior and Development; 31,* 361–373.

Fitzgerald, K., Moore, G., Paulson, L., Stewart, C., & Rosenberg, D. (2000). Proton spectroscopic imaging of the thalamus in treatment-naive pediatric obsessive-compulsive disorder. *Biological Psychiatry, 47,* 174–182.

Fivush, R. (1998). Children's recollections of traumatic and nontraumatic events. *Development and Psychopathology, 10,* 699–716.

Foa, E. B., Kozak, M. J., Goodman, W. K., Hollander, E., Jenike, M. A., & Rasmussen, S. A. (1995). *DSM-IV* field trial: Obsessive-compulsive disorder. *American Journal of Psychiatry, 152*(1), 90–96.

Foa, E. B., & Rothbaum, B. O. (1998). *Treating the trauma of rape: Cognitive behavioral therapy for PTSD.* New York, NY: Guilford Press.

Foa, E. B., Keane, T. M., Friedman, M. J., & Cohen, J. A. (2009). *Effective treatments for PTSD: Practice guidelines from the International Society for Traumatic Studies Stress Studies.* New York: Guilford Press.

Fonagy, P., & Target, M. (1997). Attachment and reflective function: Their role in self-organization. *Development and Psychopathology, 9*(4), 697–700.

Frankl, V. E. (1975). Paradoxical intention and dereflection. *Psychotherapy, 12,* 226–237.

Frankl, V. (2006) *Man's search for meaning.* Beacon Press.

Fredrickson, B. L., & Levenson, R. W. (1998). Positive emotions speed recovery from the cardiovascular sequelae of negative emotions. *Cognition and Emotion, 12,* 191–220.

Freud S: On narcissism: an introduction (1914), in *Complete Psychological Works, standard ed., vol 14.* London, Hogarth Press, 1957, pp. 67–102.

Friedman, M. J. (1997). Drug treatment for PTSD: Answers and questions. *Annals of the New York Academy of Sciences, 821,* 359–468.

Frith, U., & Frith, C. D. (2001). The biological basis of social interaction. *Current Directions in Psychological Science, 10*(5), 151–155.

Frodl, T., Meisenzahl, E. M., Zetzsche, T., Born, C., Jäger, M., Groll, C., … Moller, H.J. (2003). Larger amygdala volumes in first depressive episode as compared to recurrent major depression and healthy control subjects. *Biological Psychiatry, 53*(4), 338–344.

Fuchs, E., Czeh, B., Michael, S.T., de Biruran, G., Watanabe, T., & Frahm, J. (2002). Synaptic plasticity and tianeptine: Structural regulation. *European Psychiatry, 17,* 311–317.

Furmark, T., Tillfors, M., Marteinsdottir, I., Fischer, H., Pissiota, A., Långström, B., & Fredrikson, M. (2002). Common changes in cerebral blood flow in patients with social phobia treated with citalopram or cognitive-behavioral therapy. *Archives of General Psychiatry, 59*(5), 425–433.

Gauthier, I., Skudlarski, P., Gore, J. C., & Anderson, A. W. (2000). Expertise for cats and birds recruits brain areas involved in face recognition. *Nature Neuroscience, 3,* 191–197.

Gianaros, P. J., Jennings J. R., Sheu, L. K., Greer, P. J., Kuller, L. H., & Matthews, K. A. (2007). Prospective reports of chronic life stress predict decreased grey matter volume in the hippocampus. *NeuroImage, 35,* 795–802.

Gilbertson, M. W., Shenton, M. E., Cszewski, A., Kasai, K., Lasko, N. B., Orr, S. P., & Pittman, R. K. (2002). Smaller hippocampal volume predicts pathologic vulnerability to psychological traumatic. *Nature Neuroscience, 5,* 1242–1247.

Glaubman, H., Mikulincer, M., Porat, A., Wasserman, O., & Birger, M. (1990). Sleep of chronic posttraumatic patients. *Journal of Traumatic Stress, 3,* 255–263.

Gold, P. W., Gabry, K. E., Yasuda, M. R., & Chrousos, G. P. (2002). Divergent endocrine abnormalities in melancholic and atypical depression: Clinical and pathophysiologic implications. *Endocrinology and Metabolism Clinics of North America, 31,* 37–62.

Goldapple, K., Segal, Z., Garson, D., Lau, M., Bieling, P., Kennedy, S., & Mayberg, H. (2004). Modulation of the cortical limbic pathways in major depression: Treatment specific effects of cognitive behavioral therapy. *Archives of General Psychiatry, 61,* 34–41.

Gould, E., McEwen, B. S., Tanapat, P., Galea, L. A., & Fuchs, E. (1997). Adrenal steroids suppress granule cell death in the developing dentate gyrus through an NMDA receptor-dependent mechanism. *Developmental Brain Research, 103,* 91–93.

Grawe, K. (2007). *Neuropsychotherapy: How the neurosciences inform effective psychotherapy.* Mahwah, NJ: Lawrence Erlbaum.

Gray, J. A., & McNaughton, N. (2000). *The neuropsychology of anxiety: An enquiry into the functions of the septo-hippocampal system* (2nd ed.). Oxford, UK: Oxford University Press.

Graybiel, A. M., & Rauch, S. L. (2000). Toward a neurobiology of obsessive-compulsive disorder. *Neuron, 28,* 343–347.

Greicius, M. D., Flores B. H., Menon V., Glover G. H., Solvason H. B., Kenna H., Reiss A. L., & Schatzberg A. F. (2007). Resting-state functional connectivity in major depression: Abnormally increased contributions from subgenual cingulate cortex and thalamus. *Biol Psychiatry.* Sep 1; 62(5):429-437.

Gunnar, M. R., & Vazquez, D. M. (2001). Low cortisol and flattening of expected daytime rhythm: Potential indices of risk in human development. *Development and Psychopathology, 13,* 515–538.

Hamann, S. (2009). The human amygdala and memory. In P. J. Whalen & E. A. Phelps (Eds.), *The human amygdala* (pp. 177–203). New York, NY: Guilford Press.

Harvey, A. G., & Bryant, R. A. (1998a). Acute stress disorder following mild traumatic brain injury. *Journal of Nervous and Mental Disease, 186,* 133–337.

Harvey, A. G., & Bryant, R. A. (1998b). The relationship between acute stress disorder and posttraumatic stress disorder: A perspective evaluation of motor vehicle accident survivors. *Journal of Counseling and Clinical Psychology, 66,* 507–512.

Harvey, A. G., & Bryant, R. A. (1999). A qualitative investigation of the organization of traumatic memories. *British Journal of Clinical Psychologiy, 38,* 401–405.

Hayashi, T., Urayama, O., Kawai, K., Hayashi, K., Iwanaga, S., Ohta, M.,... Murakami, K. (2006). Laughter regulates gene expression in 28 patients with Type 2 diabetes. *Psychotherapy and Psychosomatics, 75* (1), 62–65.

Hayes, S. C., Strosahl, K., & Wilson, K. G. (1999). *Acceptance and commitment therapy: An experiential approach to behavior change.* New York, NY: Guilford Press.

Henry, J. (1992). Biological basis of the stress response. *Integrative Physiological and Behavioral Science, 27,* 66–83.

Hibbeln, J. R., & Salem, N. Jr. (1995). Dietary polyunsaturated fatty acids and depression: When cholesterol does not satisfy. *American Journal of Clinical Nutrition, 62*(1), 1–9.

Hobson, J. A., Stickgold, R., & Pace-Schott, E. F. (1998). The neuropsychology of REM sleep dreaming. *NeuroReport, 9,* R1–R14.

Hoebel, B. G., Rada, P. V., Mark, G. P., & Pothos, E. N. (1999). Neural systems for reinforcement and inhibition of behavior: Relevance to eating, addiction, and depression. In D. Kahneman, E. Diener, & N.Schwarz (Eds.), *Well-being: The foundations of hedonic psychology* (pp. 558–572). New York, NY: Russell Sage Foundation.

Holland, P., & Lewis, P. A. (2007). Emotional memory: Selective enhancement by sleep. *Current Biology, 17*(5), R179–R181.

Hull, A. M. (2002). Neuroimaging findings in post-traumatic stress disorder. Systematic review. *British Journal of Psychiatry, 181,* 102–110.

Iacoboni, M. (2003). Understanding intentions through imitations. In S. Johnson (Ed.), *Taking action: Cognitive neuroscience perspectives or intentional acts* (pp. 107–138). Cambridge, MA: MIT Press.

Iacoboni, M., & Lenzi, G. L. (2002). Mirror neurons, the insula, and empathy. *Behavioral and Brain Sciences, 25,* 107–138.

Iliffe, S., Kharicha, K., Harari, D., Swift, C., Gillmann, G., & Stuck, A. E. (2007). Health risk appraisal in older people. 2: The implications for clinicians and commissioners of social isolation risk in older people. *British Journal of General Practice, 57*(537), 277–282.

Jacobson, N. S., Martell, C. R., & Dimidjian, S. (2001). Behavioral activation treatment for depression: Returning to contextual roots. *Clinical Psychology: Science and Practice, 8*(3), 255–270.

James, W. (1890). *The principles of psychology.* New York: Holt. doi: 10.1037/11059-000

Ji, J., & Maren, S. (2007). Hippocampal involvement in contextual modulation of fear extinction. *Hippocampus, 17,* 749–758.

Jones, C., Harvey, A. G., & Brewin, C. R. (2005). Traumatic brain injury, dissociation, and posttraumatic stress disorder in road traffic accident survivors. *Journal of Traumatic Stress, 18,* 181–191.

Joseph, S., & Masterson, J. (1999). Posttraumatic stress disorder and traumatic brain injury: Are they mutually exclusive? *Journal of Traumatic Stress, 12,* 437–453. doi:10.1023/A:1024762919372.

Kabat-Zinn, J. (2003). Mindfulness-based interventions in context: Past, present, and future. *Clinical Psychology: Science and Practice, 10*, 144–156.

Kametani, H., & Kawamura, H. (1990). Alterations in acetylcholine release in the rat hippocampus during sleep-wakefulness detected by intracerebral dialysis. *Life Sciences, 47*(5), 421–426.

Karl, A., Malta, L., & Maercker, L. (2006). Meta-analytic review of event related potential studies in post-traumatic stress disorder. *Biological Psychology, 71*, 123–147.

Karl, A., Schaefer, M., Malta, L. S., Dorfel, D., Rohleder, N., & Werner, A. (2006). A meta-analysis of structural brain abnormalities in PTSD. *Neuroscience Biobehavioral Reviews, 30*, 1004–1031.

Kent, J. M., Coplan, J. D., Mawlawi, O., Martinez, J. M., & Browne, J. M. (2005). Prediction of panic response to a respiratory stimulant by reduced orbital frontal cerebral blood flow in panic disorder. *American Journal of Psychiatry, 162*(7), 1379–1381.

Kessler, R. C., Chiu, W. T., Demler, O., & Walters, E. E. (2005). Prevalence, severity, and comorbidity of 12-month *DSM-IV* disorders in the National Comorbidity Survey Replication. *Archives of General Psychiatry, 62*, 617–627.

Kessler, R. C., Chiu, W. T., Ruscio, A. M., Shear, K., & Walters, E. E. (2006). The epidemiology of panic attacks, panic disorder, and agoraphobia in the National Comorbidity Survey Replication. *Archives of General Psychiatry, 63*, 415–424.

Kessler, R. C., Sonnega, A., Bromet, E., Hughes, M., & Nelson, C. B. (1995). Posttraumatic stress disorder in the National Comorbidity Survey. *Archives of General Psychiatry, 52*, 1048–1060.

Kiecolt-Glaser, J. K., Preacher, K, J., MacCallum, R. C., Atkinson, C., Malarkey, W. B., & Glaser, R. (2003). Chronic stress and age-related increases in the proinflammatory cytokine IL-6. *Proceedings of the National Academy of Sciences USA, 100*, 9090–9095.

Kiecolt-Glaser, J. K., Ricker, D., George, J., Messick, G., Speicher, C. E., Garner, W., & Glaser, R. (1984). Urinary cortisol levels, cellular immunocompetency, and loneliness in psychiatric inpatients. *Psychosomatic Medicine, 46*(1), 15–23.

Kilts, C. D., Egan, G., Gideon, D. A., Ely, T. D., & Hoffman, J. M. (2003). Dissociable neural pathways are involved in the recognition of emotion in static and dynamic facial expressions. *Neuroimage, 18*(1), 156–168.

Kim, H., Somerville, L. H., Johnstone, T., Alexander, A., & Whalen, P. J. (2003). Inverse amygdala and medial prefrontal cortex responses to surprised faces. *NeuroReport, 14*, 2317–2322.

Kim, M. J., & Whalen, P. J. (2009). The structural integrity of an amygdala-prefrontal pathway predicts trait anxiety. *Journal of Neuroscience, 29*(37), 11614–11618.

Kirsch, I., Scoboria, A., & Moore, T. J. (2002). The emperor's new drugs. An analysis of antidepressant medication data submitted to the US Food and Drug Administration. *Prevention and Treatment, 5*, Article 33.

Knutson, K. L., Van Cauter, E., Rathouz, P. J., Yan, L. L., Hulley, S. B., Liu, K., & Lauderdale, D. S. (2009). Association between sleep and blood pressure in midlife: The CARDIA sleep study. *Archives of Internal Medicine, 169*(11), 1055–1061.

Koechlin, E., & Hyafil, A. (2007). Anterior prefrontal function and the limits of human decision-making. *Science, 318*, 594–598.

Kolb, B., & Whishaw, I. Q. (2009). *Fundamentals of human neuropsychology, 6th ed.* New York, NY: Worth.

Konen, K., Keltikaga-Jarinen, H., Addercreutz, H., & Hautenen, A. (1996). Psychosocial stress and the insulin resistance syndrome. *Metabolism, 45*, 1533–1538.

Konsman, J. P., Parnet, P., & Dantzer, R. (2002). Cytokine-induced sickness behavior: Mechanisms and implications. *Trends in Neuroscience, 25*(3), 154–159.

Kornstein, S. G., Schatzberg, A.F., & Thase, M. E. (2000). Gender differences in presentation of chronic major and double depression. *Journal of Affective Disorders, 60*, 1–11.

Kradin, R. (2008). *The placebo response and the power of unconscious healing.* New York, NY: Routledge.

Kuhn, C. (1994). The stages of laughter. *Journal of Nursing Jocularity, 4*(2), 34–35.

Kuhn, C. M., & Schanberg, S. M. (1998). Responses to maternal separation: Mechanisms and mediators. *International Journal of Developmental Neuroscience, 16*(3–4), 261–270.

LaBar, K. S., & Cabeza, R. (2006). Cognitive neuroscience of emotional memory. *Nature Reviews Neuroscience, 7*(1), 54–64.

Lambert, K. (2008). *Lifting depression: A neuroscientist's hands-on approach to activating your brain's healing power.* New York, NY: Basic Books.

Lambert, M. J., & Ogles, B. (2004). The efficacy and effectiveness of psychotherapy. In M. J. Lambert (Ed.), *Bergin and Garfield's handbook of psychotherapy and behavior change*, 5th ed. (pp. 139–193). Hoboken, NJ: Wiley.

Lazar, S. W., Kerr, C. E., Wasserman, R. H., Gray, J. R., Greve, D. N.,... Fischl, B. (2005). Meditation experience is associated with increased cortical thickness. *NeuroReport, 16*(17): 1893–1897.

Ledgerwood, L., Richardson, R., & Cranney, J. (2003). Effects of D-cycloserine on extinction of conditioned freezing. *Behavioral Neuroscience, 117*, 341–349.

LeDoux, J. E., & Gorman, J. M. (2001). A call to action: Overcoming anxiety through active coping. *American Journal of Psychiatry, 158*, 1953–1955.

LeDoux, J. E., & Schiller, D. (2009). The human amygdala: Insights from other animals. In P. J. Whalen & E. A. Phelps (Eds.), *The human amygdala* (pp. 42–60). New York, NY: Guilford Press.

Leibenluft, M. D. (Ed.). (1999). *Gender differences in mood and anxiety: From bench to bedside.* Washington, DC: American Psychological Association.

Lieberman, M. D., Eisenberger, N. I., Crockett, M. J., Tom, S. M., Pfeifer, J. H., & Way, B. M. (2007). Putting feelings into words: Affect labeling disrupts amygdala activity in response to affective stimuli. *Psychological Science, 18*, 421–428. doi:10.1111/j.1467-9280.2007.01916.x

Lepore, S. J., Allen, K. A. M., and Evans, G. W. (1993). Social support lowers cardiovascular reactivity to an acute stressor. *Psychosomatic Medicine, 55*, 518–524.

Lesch, K. P., Bengel, D., Heils, A., Sabol, S. Z., Greenberg, B. D., Petri, S.,... Murphy, D. L. (1996). Association of anxiety-related traits with a polymorphism in the serotonin transporter gene regulatory region. *Science, 274*, 1527–1531.

Levin, P., Lazrove, S., & van der Kolk, B. (1999). What psychological testing and neuroimaging tell us about the treatment of posttraumatic stress disorder by eye movement desensitization and reprocessing. *Journal of Anxiety Disorder, 13*, 159–172.

Levine, P. A. (2010). *In an unspoken voice: How the body releases trauma and restores goodness.* Berkeley, CA: North Atlantic Books.

Lewinsohn, P. M., Biglan, A., & Zeiss, A. M. (1976). Behavioral treatment of depression. In P. O. Davidson (Ed.), *The behavioral management of anxiety, depression and pain* (pp. 91–146). New York: Brunner/Mazel.

Linden, D. E. J. (2006). How psychotherapy changes the brain—The contribution of functional neuroimaging. *Molecular Psychiatry, 11*, 528–538.

Linehan, M. (1993). *Cognitive-behavioral treatment of borderline personality disorder.* New York, NY: Guilford Press.

Linford, L., & Arden, J. B. (2009). Brain-based therapy and the Pax Medica. *Psychotherapy in Australia. 15*, 16–23.

Littrell, J. (1998). Is the reexperience of painful emotion therapeutic? *Clinical Psychological Review, 8*, 71–102.

Lutgendorf, S. K., Logan, H., Costanzo, E., & Lubaroff, D. (2004). Effects of acute stress, relaxation, and a neurogenic inflammatory stimulus on interleukin-6 in humans. *Brain, Behavior, and Immunity, 18*, 55–64.

MacQueen, G. M., Campbell, S., McEwen, B. S., Macdonald, K., Amano, S., Joffe, R.T.,… Young, L. T. (2003). Course of illness, hippocampal function, and hippocampal volume in major depression. *Proceedings of the National Academy of Sciences USA, 100*(3), 1387–1392.

Maes, M., Lin, A. H., Delmeire, L., Van Gastel, A., Kenis, G., DeJong, L. R., & Bosmans, E. (1999). Elevated serum interleukin-6 (IL-6) and IL-6 receptor concentrations in posttraumatic stress disorder following accidental man-made traumatic events. *Biological Psychiatry, 45*, 833–839.

Maguire, E. A., Gadian, D. G., Johnsrude, I. S., Good, C. D., Ashburner, J., Frackowiak, R. S., & Frith, C. D. (2000). Navigation-related structural change in the hippocampi of taxi drivers. *Proceedings of the National Academy of Sciences USA, 97*, 4398–4403.

Marinelli, M., & Piazza, P. V. (2002). Interaction between glucocorticoid hormones, stress and psychostimulant drugs. *European Journal of Neuroscience, 16*(3), 387–394.

Marmot, M. (1994). Work and other factors influencing coronary health and sickness absence. *Work & Stress, 8*:191-201.

Martin, R. A., Kuiper, N. A., Olinger, L. J., & Dance, K. A. (1993). Humor, coping with stress, self-concept, and psychological well-being. *Humor: International Journal of Humor Research, 6*, 89–104.

Mathers, C. D., & Loncar, D. (2006, November 28). Projections of global mortality and burden of disease from 2002 to 2030. *PLoS Medicine, 3*(11), e442.

Mathews, A. M., & Mackintosh, B. (2000). Induced emotional interpretation bias and anxiety. *Journal of Abnormal Psychology, 109*, 602–615.

Mayberg, H. S. (1997). Limbic-cortical dysregulation: A proposed model of depression. *Journal of Neuropsychiatry and Clinical Neuroscience, 9*, 471–481.

Mayberg, H. S., Liotti, M., Brannan, S. K., McGinnis, S., Mahurin, R. K., Jerabek, P. A.,… Fox, P. T. (1999). Reciprocal limbic-cortical function and negative mood: Converging PET findings in depression and normal sadness. *American Journal of Psychiatry, 156*, 675–682.

Mayberg, H. S., Lozano, A. M., Voon, V., McNeely, H. E., Seminowicz, D., Hamani, C.,… Kennedy, S. H. (2005). Deep brain stimulation for treatment-resistant depression. *Neuron, 45*(5), 651–660.

McDade, T. W., Hawkley, L. C., & Cacioppo, J. T. (2006). Psychosocial and behavioral predictors of inflammation in middle-aged and older adults: The Chicago Health, Aging, and Social Relations Study. *Psychosomatic Medicine, 68*(3), 376–381.

McEwen, B. (2012). Stress and coping. In G. G. Berntson & J. T. Cacioppo (Eds.), *Handbook of neuroscience for the behavioral sciences* (Vol. 2, pp. 1220–1235). Hoboken, NJ: Wiley.

McEwen, B. S. (2006). Sleep deprivation as a neurobiologic and physiological stressor: Allostasis and allostatic load. *Metabolism, 55,* 520–523.

McEwen, B. S., & Chattarji, S. (2007). Neuroendrocrinology of stress. In *Handbook of neurochemistry and molecular neurobiology* (3rd ed., pp. 572–593). New York, NY: Springer-Verlag.

McEwen, B. S., & Stellar, E. (1993). Stress and the individual mechanisms leading to disease. *Archives of Internal Medicine, 153,* 2093–2101.

McGaugh, J. L. (2004). The amygdala modulates the consolidation of memories of emotionally arousing experience. *Annual Review of Neuroscience, 27,* 1–28.

McNaughton, N., & Corr, P. J. (2004). A two-dimensional neuropsychology of defense: Fear, anxiety and defense distance. *Neuroscience and Biobehavioral Reviews, 28,* 285–305.

Meaney, M. J., Aitken, D. H., Viau, V., Sharma, S., & Sarrieau, A. (1989). Neonatal handling alters adrenocortical negative feedback sensitivity and hippocampal type II glucocorticoid receptor binding in the rat. *Neuroendocrinology, 50,* 597–604.

Mellman, T. A. (1997). Psychobiology of sleep disturbances in posttraumatic stress disorder. *Annals of the New York Academy of Sciences, 821,* 142–149.

Metzger, L. J., Gilbertson, M. W., & Orr, S. P. (2005). Electophysiology of PTSD. In J. J. Vaserling & C. R. Brewin (Eds.), *Neuropsychology of PTSD: Biological, cognitive, and clinical perspectives* (pp. 83–102). New York, NY: Guilford Press.

Meuret, A. E., Wilhelm, F. H., Ritz, T., & Roth, W. T. (2003). Breathing training in panic disorder treatment: Useful intervention or impediment to therapy? *Behavior Modification, 27,* 731–754.

Michelson, D., Stratakis, C., Reynolds, J., Galliven, E., Chrousos, G., & Gold, P. (1996). Bone mineral density in women with depression. *New England Journal of Medicine, 335,* 1176–1181.

Miller, G. A. (1956). The magical number seven, plus or minus two: Some limits on our capacity for processing information. *Psychological Review 63* (2): 81–97.

Miller, G. (2005). Reflecting on another's mind. *Science, 308,* 945–947.

Miller, G. E., Chen, E., & Zhou, E. S. (2007). If it goes up, must it come down? Chronic stress and the hypothalamic-pituitary-adrenocortical axis in humans. *Psychological Bulletin, 133*(1), 25–45.

Miller, W. R., & Rollnick, S. (2002). *Motivational interviewing: Preparing people for change* (2nd ed.). New York, NY: Guilford Press.

Mobbs, D., Greicius, M. D., Abdel-Azim, E., Menon, V., & Reiss, A. L. (2003). Humor modulates the mesolimbic reward centers. *Neuron, 40*(5), 1041–1048.

Morgan, C. A. III, Krystal, J. H., & Southwick, S. M. (2008). Toward early pharmacological posttraumatic stress intervention. *Biological Psychiatry, 53*(9), 834–843.

Murburg, M. (1997). The psychobiology of posttraumatic stress disorder. In R. Yehuda & A. C. McFarlane (Eds.), *Psychobiology of posttraumatic stress disorder* (pp. 352–358). New York, NY: Annals of the New York Academy of Sciences.

Nachmias, M., Gunnar, M., Mangelsdorf, S., Parritz, R. H., & Buss, K. (1996). Behavioral inhibition and stress reactivity: The moderating role of attachment security. *Child Development, 67,* 508–522.

Nader, K., Schafe, G. E., & LeDoux, J. E. (2000). Fear memories require protein synthesis in the amygdala for reconsolidation after retrieval. *Nature, 406,* 722–726.

National Institute for Clinical Excellence (2004). *Depression: Management of depression in primary and secondary care.* London, UK: Author. (Clinical Guideline 23.)

Neto, F., & Barrios, J. (2001). Predictors of loneliness among adolescents from Portuguese immigrant families in Switzerland. *Social Behavior and Personality, 28*, 193-206.

Newport, D., Stowe, Z. N., & Nemeroff, C. B. (2002). Parental depression: Animal models of an adverse life event. *American Journal of Psychiatry, 159*, 1265–1283.

Nielsen Forman, D., Videbech, P., Hedegaard, M., Dalby Salvig, J., & Secher, N. J. (2000). Postpartum depression: Identification of women at risk. *British Journal of Obstetrics and Gynecology, 107*, 1210–1217.

Nitschke, J. B., Sarinopoulos, I., Oathes, D. J., Johnstone, T., Whalen, P. J., Davidson, R. J., & Kalin, N. H. (2009). Anticipatory activation in the amygdala and anterior cingulate in generalized anxiety disorder and prediction of treatment response. *American Journal of Psychiatry, 166*, 302–310.

Norcross, J. D. (2002). Empirically supported therapy relationships. In J. D. Norcross (Ed.), *Psychotherapy relationships that work: Therapist contributions and responsiveness to patients.* New York, NY: Oxford University Press.

Northrup, C. (2001). *The wisdom of menopause.* New York, NY: Bantam.

Nutt, J. D., & Malizia, A. L. (2004). Structural and functional brain changes in posttraumatic stress disorder. *Journal of Clinical Psychiatry, 65*(Suppl.), 11–17.

O'Doherty, J., Kringelbach, M. L., Rolls, E. T., Hornak, J., & Andrews, C. (2001). Abstract reward and punishment representations in the human orbital frontal cortex. *National Neuroscience, 4*, 95–102.

O'Donnell, T. O., Hegadoren, K. M., & Coupland, N. C. (2004). Noradrenergic mechanisms in the pathophysiology of post-traumatic stress disorder. *Neuropsychobiology, 50*, 273–283.

Ouimette, P., Moos, R. H., & Brown, P. J. (2003). Substance use disorder–posttraumatic stress disorder comorbidity: A survey of treatments and proposed practice guidelines. In P. Ouimette & P. J. Brown (Eds.), *Trauma and substance abuse: Causes, consequences, and treatment of comorbid disorders* (pp. 91–110). Washington, DC: American Psychological Association.

Ozer, E. J., Best, S. R., Lipsey, T. L., & Weiss, D. S. (2003). Predictors of posttraumatic stress disorder and symptoms in adults: A meta-analysis. *Psychological Bulletin, 129*, 52–73.

Pace, T. W., Mletzko, T. C., Alagbe, O., Musselman, D. L., Nemeroff, C. B., Miller, A. H., & Heim, C. M. (2006). Increased stress-induced inflammatory responses in male patients with major depression and increased early life stress. *American Journal of Psychiatry, 163*(9), 1630–1633.

Pack, A. I., & Pien, G. W. (2011). Update on sleep and its disorders. *Annual Review of Medicine, 62*, 447–460. doi:10.1146/annurevmed-050409-104056

Pantev, C., Roberts, L. E., Schulz, M., Engelien, A., & Ross, B. (2001). Timbre-specific enhancement of auditory cortical representations in musicians. *NeuroReport, 12*, 169–174.

Papanicolaou, D. A., Wilder, R., Manolagas, S., & Chrousos, G. P. (2005). Roles of interleukin-6 in human disease. *Annals of Internal Medicine, 128*, 127–137.

Paré, D. (2003). Role of basolateral amygdala in memory consolidation. *Progress in Neurobiology, 70*(5), 409–420.

Parham, P. (2005). *The immune system,* 2nd ed. New York, NY: Garland Science.

Parker, K. J., Buckmaster, C. L., Sundlass, K., Schatzberg, A., & Lyons, D.M. (2006). Maternal mediation, stress inoculation, and the development of neuroendrocrine stress resistance in primates. *Proceedings of the National Academy of Sciences, 103*, 3000–3005.

Pascual-Leone, A., & Torres, F. (1993). Plasticity of the sensorimotor cortex representation of the reading finger in Braille readers. *Brain, 116*, 39–52.

Pearce, J. M. (2004). Some neurological aspects of laughter. *European Neurology*, 52(3), 169–171.

Peres, J. F. P., McFarlane, A., Nasello, A. G., & Moores, K. A. (2008). Traumatic memories: Bridging the gap between functional neuroimaging and psychotherapy. *Australia and New Zealand Journal of Psychiatry*, 42, 478–488.

Peres, J. T. P., Newberg, A. B., Mercante, J. P., Simão, M., Albuquerque, V. E., Peres, M. J., & Nasello, A. G. (2007). Cerebral blood flow changes during retrieval of traumatic memories before and after psychotherapy: A SPECT study. *Psychological Medicine*, 37, 1481–1491.

Perls, F., Hefferine, R., & Goodwin, P. (1951). *Gestalt therapy*. New York, NY: Penguin.

Peterson, M. J., & Benca, R. M. (2006). Sleep in mood disorders. *Psychiatric Clinics of North America*, 29, 1009–1032.

Phelps, E. A. (2009). The human amygdala and the control of fear. In P. J. Whalen & E. A. Phelps (Eds.), *The human amygdala* (pp. 204–219). New York, NY: Guilford Press.

Pissiota, A., Frans, O., Fernandez, M., von Knorring, L., Fischer, H., & Fredrickson, M. (2002). Neurofunctional correlates of posttraumatic stress disorder: A PET symptom provocation study. *European Archives of Psychiatry Clinical Neuroscience*, 252, 68–75.

Plihal, W., & Born J. (1997). Effects of early and late nocturnal sleep on declarative and procedural memory. *Journal of Cognitive Neuroscience*, 9 (4), 534–547.

Porges, S. (2011). *The polyvagal theory: Neurophysiologial foundations of emotions, attachment, communication, and self-regulation*. New York, NY: Norton.

Portas, C. M., Bjorvatn, B., Fagerland, S., Gronli, J., Mundal, V., Soresen, E., & Ursin, R. (1998). On-line detection of extracellular levels of serotonin in dorsal raphe nucleus and frontal cortex over sleep/wake cycle in the freely moving rat. *Neuroscience*, 83, 807–814.

Prasko, J., Horácek, J., Zálesky, R., Kopecek, M., Novák, T., Pasková, B.,... Höschl, C. (2004). The change of regional brain metabolism (18FDG PET) in panic disorder during the treatment with cognitive behavioral therapy or antidepressants. *Neuroendocrinology Letters*, 25(5), 340–348.

Pruessner, J. C., Baldwin, M. W., Dedovic, K., Renwick, R., Mahani, N. K., Lord, C.,... Lupien S. (2005). Self-esteem, locus of control, hippocampal volume, and cortisol regulation in young and old adulthood. *Neuroimage*, 28(4), 815–826.

Pruessner, J. C., Champagne, F., Meaney, M. J., & Dagher A. (2004). Dopamine release in response to a psychological stress in humans and its relationship to early life maternal care: A positron emission tomography study using [11C]raclopride. *Journal of Neuroscience*, 24(11), 2825–2831.

Quirk, G. L., & Beer, J. S. (2006). Prefrontal involvement in the regulation of emotion: Convergence of rat and human studies. *Current Opinion in Neurobiology*, 16, 723–727.

Quirk, G. L., Likhtik, F., Pelletier, J. G., & Paré, D. (2003). Stimulation of medial prefrontal cortex decreases the responsiveness of central amygdala output neurons. *Journal of Neuroscience*, 23, 8800–8807.

Quirk, G. L., Russo, G. K., Barron, J. L., & Lebron, K. (2000). The role of ventromedial prefrontal cortex in the recovery of extinguished fear. *Journal of Neuroscience*, 20, 6225–6231.

Raison, C. L., Capuron, L., & Miller, A. H. (2006). Cytokines sing the blues: Inflammation and the pathogenesis of depression. *Trends in Immunology*, 27(1), 24–31.

Ramnani, N., & Owen, A. M. (2004). Anterior prefrontal cortex: Insights into function from anatomy and neuroimaging. *Nature Reviews Neuroscience*, 5, 184–194.

Rao, U., Dahl, R. E., Ryan, N. D., Birmaher, B., Williamson, D. E., Roa, R., & Kaufman, J. (2002). Heterogeneity in EEG sleep findings in adolescent depression: Unipolar versus bipolar clinical course. *Journal of Affective Disorders*, 70, 273–280.

Ratey, J. (2008). *Spark: The revolutionary new science of exercise and the brain*. New York, NY: Little, Brown.

Rauch, S. L., Shin, L. M., Whalen, P. J., & Pitman, R. K. (1998). Neuroimaging and the neuroanatomy of PTSD. *CNS Spectrums, 3*(Suppl.), 30–41.

Rizzolatti, G., & Arbib, M. A. (1998). Language within our grasp. *Trends in Neuroscience, 21*, 188–194.

Robbins, T. W., & Everitt, B. J. (1995). Arousal systems and attention. In M. Gazzaniga (Ed.), *The cognitive neurosciences* (pp. 703–720). Cambridge, MA: MIT Press.

Roemer, L., & Orsillo, S. M. (2005). An acceptance-based behavior therapy for generalized anxiety disorder. In S. M. Orsillo & L. Roemer (Eds.), *Acceptance and mindfulness-based approaches to anxiety: Conceptualization and treatment* (pp. 213–240). New York, NY: Springer Science.

Rohleder, N., Joksimovic, L., Wolf, J. M., & Kirschbaum, C. (2004). Hypocortisolism and increased glucocorticoid sensitivity of proinflammatory cytokine production in Bosnian war refugees with posttraumatic stress disorder. *Biological Psychiatry, 55*, 745–751.

Rosenkranz, J. A., Moore, H., & Grace, A. A. (2003). The prefrontal cortex regulates lateral amygdala neuronal plasticity and responses to previously conditioned stimuli. *Journal of Neuroscience, 23*, 11054–11064.

Rothbaum, B. O., Astin, M. C., & Marsteller, F. (2005). Prolonged exposure versus eye movement desensitization and reprocessing (EMDR) for PTSD rape victims. *Journal of Traumatic Stress, 18*(6), 607–616.

Rovzendaal, B., McReynolds, J. R., & McGaugh, J. L. (2004). The basolateral amygdala interacts with the medial prefrontal cortex in regulating glucocorticoid effects on working memory impairment. *Journal of Neuroscience, 24*(6), 1385–1392.

Royal Australian and New Zealand College of Psychiatrists Clinical Practice Guidelines. (2004). Australian and New Zealand clinical practice guidelines for the treatment of depression. *Australian and New Zealand Journal of Psychiatry, 38*, 389–407.

Ruscio, A. M., Stein, D. J., Chiu, W. T., & Kessler, R. C. (2010). The epidemiology of obsessive-compulsive disorder in the National Comorbidity Survey Replication. *Molecular Psychiatry, 15*, 53–63.

Russell, D. W., & Cutrona, C. E. (1991). Social support, stress, and depressive symptoms among the elderly: Test of a process model. *Psychology and Aging, 6*, 190–201.

Saavedra, J. M., Benicky, J., & Zhou, J. (2006). Angiotensin II: Multitasking in the brain. *Journal of the International Society of Hypertension, 24*(1, Supple.), S131–S137.

Sabbagh, M. A. (2004). Understanding orbitofrontal contributions to theory-of-mind reasoning: Implications for autism. *Brain Cognition, 55*, 209–219.

Sapolsky, R. M. (2003). Stress and plasticity in the limbic system. *Neurochemical Research, 28*, 1735–1742.

Saxena, S., Gorbis, E., O'Neil, J., Baker, S. K., Mandikern, M. A., Maidment, K. M.,… London, E. D. (2009). Rapid effects of brief intensive cognitive-behavioral therapy on brain glucose metabolism in obsessive-compulsive disorder. *Molecular Psychiatry, 14*, 197–205.

Schacter, D. (1996). *Searching for memory: The brain, the mind, and the past*. New York, NY: Basic Books.

Schacter, S., & Singer, J. E. (1962). Cognitive, social, and physiological determinants of emotional state. *Psychological Review, 69*, 379–399.

Schiepers, O. J. G., Wichers, M. C., & Maes, M. (2005). Cytokines and major depression. *Progress in Neuro-psychopharmacology and Biological Psychiatry, 29*, 201–217.

Schmidt, N. B., & Woolaway-Bickel, K. (2006). Cognitive vulnerability to panic disorder. In L. Alloy & J. H. Riskind (Eds.), *Cognitive vulnerability to emotional disorders* (pp. 207–234). Mahwah, NJ: Lawrence Erlbaum.

Schmidt, N. B., Woolaway-Bickel, K., Trakowski, J., Santiago, H., Storey, J., Koselka, M., & Cook, J. (2000). Dismantling cognitive-behavioral treatment for panic disorder: Questioning the utility of breathing retraining. *Journal of Consulting and Clinical Psychology, 68*(3), 417–424.

Schuff, N., Neylan, T., Lonoci, M., Du, A., Weiss, D., Marmar, C., & Weiner, M. (2001). Decreased hippocampal N-acetylaspartate in the absence of atrophy in posttraumatic stress disorder. *Biological Psychiatry, 50*, 952–959.

Semple, W. E., Goyer, P. F., McCormick, R., Donovan, B., Muzic, R. F. Jr., Rugle, L., . . . Schulz, S. C. (2000). Higher blood flow at amygdala and lower frontal cortex blood flow in PTSD patients with comorbid cocaine and alcohol abuse compared with normals. *Psychiatry: Interpersonal and Biological Processes, 63*, 65–74.

Shapiro, F. (1995). *Eye movement desensitization and reprocessing: Basic principles, protocols, and procedures.* New York, NY: Guilford Press.

Shapiro, F. (2001). *Eye movement desensitization and reprocessing: Basic principles, protocols and procedures,* 2nd ed. New York, NY: Guilford Press.

Sharot, T., Riccardi, A. M., Raio, C. M., & Phelps, E. A. (2007). Neural mechanisms mediating optimism bias. *Nature, 450*, 102–106.

Sheikh, J. I., Leskin, G.A., & Klein, D. F. (2002). Several epidemiological studies have demonstrated a higher prevalence of panic disorder: Findings from the National Comorbidity Survey. *American Journal of Psychiatry, 159* (1), 55–58.

Sheline, Y. I. (2003). Neuroimaging studies of mood disorder effects on the brain. *Biological Psychiatry, 54*, 338–352.

Sheline, Y. I., Sanghavi, M., & Mintun, M. A. (1999). Depression duration but not age predicts hippocampal volume loss in medically healthy women with recurrent major depression. *Journal of Neuroscience, 19*, 5034–5043.

Shin, L. M., Rauch, S. L., & Pitman, R. K. (2005). Structural and functional anatomy of PTSD. In J. J. Vasterling & C. R. Brewin (Eds.), *Neuropsychology of PTSD: Biological, cognitive and clinical perspectives.* New York, NY: Guilford Press.

Shin, L. M., Whalen, P. J., Pitman, R. K., Bush, G., MacKlin, M. L., Lasko, N. B., . . . Rauch, S.L. (2001). An fMRI study of anterior cingulate function in posttraumatic stress disorder. *Biological Psychiatry, 50*, 932–942.

Shores, E. A., Marosszeky, J. E., Sandanam, J., & Batchelor, J. (1998). Preliminary validation of a clinical scale for measuring the duration of posttraumatic amnesia. *Medical Journal of Australia, 144*, 569–572.

Siegal, M., & Varley, R. (2002). Neural systems involved in "theory of mind." *National Review of Neuroscience, 3*(6), 463–471.

Siegle, G. L., Steinhauer, S. R., Thase, M. E., Stenger, V. A., & Carter, C. S. (2002). Can't shake that feeling: Event-related amygdala activity in response to emotional information in depressed individuals. *Biological Psychiatry, 51*(9), 693–707.

Simantov, R., Blinder, E., Ratovitski, T., Tauber, M., Gabbay, M., & Porat, S. (1996). Dopamine-induced apoptosis in human neuronal cells: Inhibition by nucleic acids antisense to dopamine transporter. *Neuroscience, 74*, 39–50.

Sledjeski, E. M., Speisman, B., & Dierker, L. C. (2008). Does number of lifetime traumas explain the relationship between PTSD and chronic medical conditions? Answers from the National Comorbidity Survey—Replication (NCS-R). *Journal of Behavioral Medicine, 31*, 341–349.

Smith, M., Glass, G., & Miller, T. (1980). *The benefit of psychotherapy*. Baltimore, MD: Johns Hopkins University Press.

Smits, J. A. J., Powers, M. B., Berry, A. C., & Otto, M. W. (2007). Translating empirically-supported strategies into accessible interventions: The potential utility of exercise for the treatment of panic disorder. *Cognitive and Behavioral Practice, 14*, 364–374.

Smits, J. A. J., Powers, M. B., Cho, Y. C., & Telch, M. J. (2004). Mechanism of change in cognitive–behavioral treatment of panic disorder: Evidence for the fear of fear mediational hypothesis. *Journal of Consulting & Clinical Psychology, 72*, 646–652.

Snowdon, D. A. (1997). Aging and Alzheimer's disease: Lessons from the Nun Study. *Gerontologist, 37*, 150-156.

Sohlberg, M. M., & Mateer, C. A. (1989). *Introduction to cognitive rehabilitation: Theory and practice*. New York, NY: Guilford Press.

Sokolov, E. N. (1990). The orienting response, and future directions of its development. *Pavlovian Journal of Biological Science, 25*, 142–150.

Solomon, Z., Mikulincer, M., & Avitzur, E. (1998). Coping, locus of control, social support, and combat-related posttraumatic stress disorder: A prospective study. *Journal of Personality and Social Psychology, 55*, 279–285.

Sorrells, S. F., & Sapolsky, R. M. (2007). An inflammatory review of glucocorticoid actions in the CNS. *Brain, Behavior, and Immunity, 21*(3), 259–272.

Southwick, S. W., Rasmusson, A., Barron, J., & Arnsten, A. (2005). Neurobiological and neurocognitive alterations in PTSD: A focus on norepinephrine, serotonin, and the hypothalamic-pituitary-adrenal axis. In J. D. Vasteling & C. R. Brewin (Eds.), *The neuropsychology of PTSD*. New York, NY: Guilford Press.

Spates, C. R., Koch, E. I., Pagoto, S., Cusack, K., & Waller, S. (2009). Eye movement desensitization and reprocessing for adults, children and adolescents. In E. B. Foa, T. M. Keane, M. J. Friedman, & J. Cohen (Eds.), *Effective treatments for PTSD: Practice guidelines from the International Society for Traumatic Stress Studies*, 2nd ed. New York, NY: Guilford Press.

Spitzer, S. B., Llabre, M. M., Ironson, G. H., Gellman, M. D., & Schneiderman, N. (1992). The influence of social situations on ambulatory blood pressure. *Psychosomatic Medicine, 54*, 79–86.

Steptoe, A., Hamer, M., & Chida, Y. (2007). The effects of acute psychological stress on circulating inflammatory factors in humans: A review and meta-analysis. *Brain, Behavior, and Immunity, 21*, 901–912.

Steptoe, A., Willemsen, G., Owen, N., Flower, L., & Mohamed-Ali, V. (2001). Acute mental stress elicits delayed increases in circulating inflammatory cytokine levels. *Clinical Science (London), 101*(2), 185–192.

Stern, D. (1985). *The interpersonal world of the infant*. New York, NY: Basic Books.

Stickgold, R. (2002). EMDR: A putative neurobiological mechanism in action. *Journal of Clinical Psychology, 58* (1), 61–75.

Stickgold, R., Hobson, J. A., Fosse, R., & Fosse, M. (2001). Sleep, learning and dreams: Off-line memory reprocessing. *Science, 294*, 1052–1057.

Straube, T., Glauer, M., Dilger, S., Mentzel, H. J., & Miltner, W. H. R. (2006). Effects of cognitive-behavioral therapy on brain activation in specific phobia. *Neuroimage, 29*, 125–135.

Sullivan, R. M., & Gratton, A. (2002). Prefrontal cortical regulation of hypothalamic–pituitary–adrenal function in the rat and implications for psychopathology: Size matters. *Psychoneuroendocrinology, 27*, 99–114.

Swedo, S., Leonard, H., Garvey, M., Mittleman, B., Allen, A., Perlmutter, S.,... Dubbert, B. (1998). Pediatric autoimmune neuropsychiatric disorders associated with streptococcal infections: Clinical description of the first 50 cases. *American Journal of Psychiatry, 155*, 264–271.

Swedo, S. E., Pietrini, P., Leonard, H. M., Schapiro, M. B., Rettew, D. C., Goldberger, E. C.,... Grady, E. L. (1992). Cerebral glucose metabolism in childhood-onset obsessive-compulsive disorder: Revisualization during pharmacotherapy. *Archives of General Psychiatry, 49*, 690–694.

Taishi, P., Sanchez, C., Wang, Y., Fang, J., Harding, J. W., & Krueger, J. M. (2001). Conditions that affect sleep alter the expression of molecules associated with synaptic plasticity. *American Journal of Physiology—Regulatory, Integrative and Comparative Physiology, 281*, R839–R845.

Takahashi, K., Miyake, S., Kondo, T., Terao, K., Hatakenaka, M., Hashimoto, S., & Yamamura, T. (2001). Natural killer type 2 bias in remission of multiple sclerosis. *Journal of Clinical Investigation, 107*, R23–29.

Taylor, M. J., Freemantle, N., Geddes, J. R., & Bhagwagar, Z. (2006). Early onset of selective serotonin reuptake inhibitor antidepressant action. *Archives of General Psychiatry, 63*, 1217–1223.

Taylor, S. (2004). Efficacy and outcome predictors for three PTSD treatments: Exposure therapy, EMDR, and relaxation training. In S. Taylor (Ed.), *Advances in the treatment of posttraumatic stress disorder: Cognitive-behavioral perspectives* (pp. 13–37). New York, NY: Springer.

Teasdale, J., Moore, R., Hayhurst, H., Pope, M., Williams, S., & Segal, Z. (2002). Metacognitive awareness and prevention of relapse in depression: Empirical evidence. *Journal of Consulting and Clinical Psychology, 70*(2), 275–287.

Tedeschi, R. G. (1999). Violence transformed: Posttraumatic growth in survivors and their societies. *Aggression and Violent Behavior, 4*, 319–341.

Tedeschi, R. G., & Calhoun, L. G. (1995). *Trauma and transformation: Growing in the aftermath of suffering.* Thousand Oaks, CA: Sage.

Teicher, M. H., Andersen, S. L., Polcari, A., Anderson, C. M., Navalta, C. P., & Kim, D. M. (2003). The neurobiological consequences of early stress and childhood maltreatment. *Neuroscience and Biobehavioral Reviews, 27*(1–2), 33–44.

Tennen, H., & Affleck, G. (1998). Personality and transformation in the face of adversity. In R. Tedeschi, C. L. Park, & L. Calhoun (Eds.), *Posttraumatic growth: Positive changes in the aftermath of crisis* (pp. 65–98). Mahwah, NJ: Lawrence Erlbaum.

Thomas, L. A., & De Bellis, M. D. (2004). Pituitary volumes in pediatric maltreatment related to PTSD. *Biological Psychiatry, 55*, 752–758.

Thomas, P. D., Goodwin, J. M., & Goodwin, J. S. (1985). Effect of social support on stress-related changes in cholesterol level, uric acid level, and immune function in an elderly sample. *American Journal of Psychiatry, 142*, 735–737.

Todd, R. D. (1992). Neural development is regulated by classic neurotransmitter: Dopamine D2 receptor stimulation enhances neurite outgrowth. *Biological Psychiatry, 31*, 794–807.

Tottenham, N., Hare, T. A., & Casey, B. J. (2009). A developmental perspective on amygdala function. In P. J. Whalen & E. A. Phelps (Eds.), *The human amygdala* (pp. 107–117). New York, NY: Guilford Press.

Trafton, J. A., & Gifford, E. V. (2008). Behavioral reactivity and addiction: The adaptation of behavioral response to reward opportunities. *Journal of Neuropsychiatry and Clinical Neuroscience, 20* (1): 23–25.

Tronick, E. (2007). *The neurobehavioral and social-emotional development of infants and children.* New York, NY: Norton.

Tulving, E., Kapur, S., Creik, F. I. M., Moscovitch, M., & Houle, S. (1994). Hemispheric encoding/retrieval asymmetry in episodic memory: Positron emission tomography finding. *Proceedings of the National Academy of Sciences USA, 91*, 2016–2020.

Turner, E. H., Matthews, A. M., Linardatos, B. S., Tell, R. A., & Rosenthal, R. (2008). Selective publication of antidepressant trials and its influence on apparent efficacy. *New England Journal of Medicine, 358*, 3, 252–260.

Updegraff, J. A., & Taylor, S. E. (2000). From vulnerability to growth: Positive and negative effects of stressful life events. In J. H. Harvey & E. D. Miller (Eds.), *Loss and trauma: General and close relationship perspectives* (pp. 3–28). New York, NY: Routledge.

van der Kolk, B. A., Burbridge, J. A., & Suzuki, J. (1997). The psychobiology of traumatic memory. Clinical implications of neuroimaging studies. In R. Yehuda & A. C. McFarlane (Eds.), *Psychobiology of posttraumatic stress disorder* (pp. 99–113). New York, NY: Annals of the New York Academy of Sciences.

van der Kolk, B. A., McFarlane, A. C., & Weisaeth, L. (Eds.). (1996). *Traumatic stress: The effects of overwhelming experience on mind, body, and society.* New York, NY: Guilford Press.

van Elst, L. T., Woermann, F., Lemieux, L., & Trimble, M. R. (2000). Increased amygdala volumes in female and depressed humans. A quantitative magnetic resonance imaging study. *Neuroscience Letters, 281*, 103–106.

van Ijzendoorn, M. H., & Bakermans-Kranenburg, M. J. (1996). Attachment representations in mothers, fathers, adolescents and clinical groups: A meta-analytic search for normative data. *Journal of Consulting and Clinical Psychology, 64*, 8–21.

Van Schaik A., van Marwijk H., Ader H., Van Dyck R., de Haan M., Penninx B., vander K. K., van Hout H., & Beekman A. (2006) Interpersonal psychotherapy for elderly patients in primary care. *Am. J. Geriatr. Psychiatry., 14*: 777–786.

Viamontes, G. I., & Beitman, B. D. (2006). Normal substrates of psychotherapeutic change. Part 1: The default brain. *Psychiatric Annals, 36*(4), 225–236.

von Economo, C., & Koskinas, G. N. (1929). *The cytoarchitectonics of the human cerebral cortex.* London: Oxford University Press.

Vuilleumier, P. (2009). The role of the human amygdala in perception and attention. In P. J. Whalen & E. A. Phelps (Eds.), *The human amygdala* (pp. 220–249). New York, NY: Guilford Press.

Vyas, A., Bernal, S., & Chattarji, S. (2003). Effects of chronic stress on dendritic aborization in the central and extended amygdala. *Brain Research, 965*, 290–294.

Vyas, A., Mitra, R., Rao, B. S. S., & Chattarji, S. (2002). Chronic stress induces contrasting patterns of dendritic remodeling in hippocampal and amygdaloid neurons. *Journal of Neuroscience, 22*, 6810–6818.

Wen, L., & Zinbarg, R. E. (2007). Anxiety sensitivity and panic attacks: A 1-year longitudinal study. *Behavior Modification, 31*, 145–161.

Whalen, P. J., Kim, M. J., Neta, M., & Davis, F. C. (2013). Emotion. In R. J. Nelson & S. J. Y. Mizumori (Eds.), *Handbook of psychology. Vol. 3, Behavioral neuroscience,* 2nd ed. (pp. 422–439). Hoboken, NJ: Wiley.

Wheeler, M. A., Stuss, D. T., & Tulving, E. (1997). Toward a theory of episodic memory: The frontal lobes and autonomic consciousness. *Psychological Bulletin, 121*, 331–354.

Whitaker, R. (2010). *Anatomy of an epidemic: Magic bullets, psychiatric drugs, and the astonishing rise of mental illness in America*. New York, NY: Crown.

Williams, M., Powers, M. B., & Foa, E. B. (2012). Obsessive compulsive disorder. In P. Sturmey & M. Hersen (Eds.), *Handbook of evidence-based practice in clinical psychology. Vol. 2, Adult disorders* (pp. 313–335). Hoboken, NJ: Wiley.

Wolfe, J., Schnurr, P. P., Brown, P. J., & Furey, J. (1994). Posttraumatic stress disorder and war-zone exposure as correlates of perceived health in female Vietnam War veterans. *Journal of Consulting and Clinical Psychology, 62*, 1235–1240.

Woon, F. L., & Hedges, D. W. (2008). Hippocampal and amygdala volumes in children and adults with childhood maltreatment-related posttraumatic stress disorder: A meta-analysis. *Hippocampus, 18*, 729–736.

Wooten, P. (1996). Humor: An antidote for stress. *Holistic Nursing Practice, 10*(2), 49–55.

Yehuda, R., Boisoneau, D., Lowy, M. T., & Giller, E. L. Jr. (1995). Dose response changes in plasma cortisol and lymphocyte glucocorticoid receptors following dexamethasone administration in combat veterans with and without posttraumatic stress disorder. *Archives of General Psychiatry, 52*, 583–593.

Yehuda, R., Resnick, H. S., Schmeidler, J., Yang, R. K., & Pitman, R. K. (1998). Predictors of cortisol and 3-Methoxy-4-Hydroxyphenylglycol responses in the acute aftermath of rape. *Biological Psychiatry, 43*, 855–859.

Yoder, M. A., & Haude, R. H. (1995). Sense of humour and longevity: Older adults' self-ratings compared with ratings for deceased siblings. *Psychological Reports, 76*, 945–946.

Yovetich, N. A. J., Alexander, D., & Hudak, M. A. (1990). Benefits of humor in reduction of threat-induced anxiety. *Psychological Reports, 66*, 51–58.

Zobel, A. W., Nickel, T., Künzel, H. E., Ackl, N., Sonntag, A., Ising, M., & Holsboer, F. (2000). Effects of the high-affinity corticotropin-releasing hormone receptor 1 antagonist R121919 in major depression: The first 20 patients treated. *Journal of Psychiatric Research, 34*(3), 171–181.

Zoellner, L. A., Fitzgibbons, L. A., & Foa, E. B. (2001). Cognitive-behavioral approaches to PTSD. In J. P. Wilson, M. J. Friedman, & J. D. Lindy (Eds.), *Treating psychological trauma and PTSD* (pp. 159–182). New York, NY: Guilford Press.

Zlotnick, C., Mattia, J. I., & Zimmerman, M. (1999). Clinical correlates of self-mutilation in a sample of general psychiatric patients. *Journal of Nervous and Mental Disease, 187*, 296–301.

AUTHOR INDEX

SUBJECT INDEX

Acceptance and commitment therapy (ACT), 120, 124–125, 127, 220, 221
Addiction, 18–19. *See also* Substance use/abuse
Adrenaline. *See* Epinephrine or adrenaline
Adult Attachment Interview (AAI), 83–84
Aging:
  brain health importance during, 34–35, 36, 38, 39, 40, 42, 45–46
  dementia associated with (*see* Dementia)
  diet and nutrition during, 40, 42, 45–46
  memory development based on, 65
  social support/relationships impacting effects of, 34–35
  stress accelerating, 110
Ainsworth, Mary, 82
Alcohol abuse. *See* Substance use/abuse
Allostasis, 99–100, 102–108, 109–111
Amygdala:
  in anxiety and anxiety disorders, xv, 12, 70–71, 73–74, 93–96, 100–102, 103–106, 114, 118, 121–123, 129, 132–133, 135–136, 137–140, 145, 153–157, 161, 163, 166–167, 169, 170–171, 182, 186, 188–190, 194, 196, 205, 207
  in autostress disorders, 93–96, 100–102, 103–106
  brain hemispheres of, 12, 118
  in depression and depressive disorders, 205, 207, 215
  diet and nutrition impacting, 43, 114
  emotions activating, 11, 94
  fight, flight, or freeze response through, 70, 73
  in focalized anxiety and anxiety disorders, 129, 132–133, 135–136, 137–140, 145
  in generalized anxiety and anxiety disorders, 114, 118, 121–123
  genetic variances related to, 94–95
  hippocampus relationship to, 72, 86
  memory activity in, 64, 70–71, 72–74, 77–79, 85–88, 157, 159, 161, 166–167, 170–171

neuroplasticity in, 70
  in OCD, 186, 188–190, 194, 196
  orbitofrontal cortex connection to, 13–14, 71, 79, 95–96, 114, 153, 188–189
  in PTSD, 153–157, 161, 163, 166–167, 169, 170–171, 182
  social/therapeutic brain networks including, 22, 36, 79
Anterior cingulate cortex (ACC):
  in depression and depressive disorders, 208, 210–211, 219
  in focalized anxiety and anxiety disorders, 138
  in generalized anxiety and anxiety disorders, 122, 124
  in OCD, 187
  in PTSD, 154, 157, 162
  social/therapeutic brain networks including, 22, 35, 79
  stress impacting, 105
Anterior prefrontal cortex, 15
Antianxiety medication, 118–119, 155, 158, 165, 171, 198
Antidepressant medication, ix, xi–xii, 202
Anxiety and anxiety disorders:
  acceptance and commitment therapy for, 120, 124–125, 127
  acceptance concept for, 127, 128, 146, 159, 180
  amygdala role in, xv, 12, 70–71, 73–74, 93–96, 100–102, 103–106, 114, 118, 121–123, 129, 132–133, 135–136, 137–140, 145, 153–157, 161, 163, 166–167, 169, 170–171, 182, 186, 188–190, 194, 196, 205, 207
  anxiety sensitivity as risk factor for, 144–145
  attachment relationship to, 83
  autostress disorders as, 91–111
  brain-based therapy for, xv, 91–111, 113–128, 129–148, 149–182, 183–199
  breathing retraining for, 114–117, 148

brain health promotion through, 33–61
social support, 33–36
exercise, 36–39
education, 39–40
diet, 40–49
sleep, 50–61
Selective serotonin reuptake inhibitors (SSRIs),
    ix, xi–xii, 202
Self-control therapy, 218
Selye, Hans, 98
Serotonin:
    anxiety relationship to, 114
    depression relationship to, xii, 201–202, 204,
        206, 207, 222
    diet and nutrition impacting, 43, 48, 114
    exercise impacting, 37, 38
    orbitofrontal cortex relationship to, 43
    selective serotonin reuptake inhibitors, ix,
        xi–xii, 202
    sleep impacting, 52, 174–175
    stress response involving, 103
"Sickness behavior," 110, 203–204
Sleep:
    body temperature and, 56–57, 59–60
    brain health promotion through, 50–61
    cognitive-behavioral approaches to, 57–58
    depression relationship to, 52, 221
    diet and nutrition impacting, 41, 54–55
    emotion relationship to, 58
    exercise relationship to, 56
    medication for, 50, 51, 59
    melatonin and circadian clock for, 55–56,
        59–60
    memory relationship to, 51–52, 75, 173–175,
        176–177
    PTSD impacting, 153, 173–175, 176–177
    sleep hygiene techniques for, 54–61
    sleep-scheduling technique for, 60
    somatic therapy inducing similar state to,
        176–177
    stress impacting, 108
    substance use impacting, 51, 58–59
Social brain networks, 21–25, 34–36, 78–80, 97,
    141, 150–151, 217–218, 221
Social relationships:
    attachment through, 80–85, 97–98
    brain health via social support, 33–36
    depression buffered by, 33–34, 205, 216–218,
        221
    memory relationship to, 77–85
    PTSD development impacted by, 150–151,
        153, 178–179, 180–181
    social brain networks based on, 21–25, 34–36,
        78–80, 97, 141, 150–151, 217–218, 221

social phobia related to, 129, 139, 141–143
stress response in, 97, 98
therapeutic (see Therapeutic alliance)
Somatic therapies, 175–177
Spindle cells, 23–24
Still Face paradigm, 78–80, 121
Stress disorders. See Autostress disorders;
    Posttraumatic stress disorder
Striatum:
    in depression and depressive disorders, 215–216
    habit behavior relationship to, 16, 186
    memory activity in, 68
    in OCD, 186, 187, 188, 189–190, 194
Subjective Units of Distress Scale (SUDS), 8,
    172, 191
Substance use/abuse:
    anxiety effects from, 106, 119, 131, 152, 153
    brain health impacted by, 40, 41, 51, 58–59
    depression associated with, 203
    habit behavior associated with, 18–19
    memory impacted by, 40
    PTSD likelihood increased by, 152, 153
    sleep impacted by, 51, 58–59
    stress response impacting, 106
Sympathetic nervous system:
    in autostress disorders, 97, 100, 109
    in focalized anxiety and anxiety disorders,
        129, 145
    in generalized anxiety and anxiety disorders,
        113, 116–117
Synapses, 5, 7, 42

TEAM mnemonic, 223
Telomerase, 3, 35
Telomeres, 3, 35, 110
Temporal lobe, 10, 24–25
Temporoparietal junction, 24–25, 217
Thalamus, 73, 95, 167, 186, 187
Theory of mind (TOM), 25, 84–85
Therapeutic alliance, xv, xvi, 21–25, 35, 69–70,
    85
Therapeutic brain networks, 21–25, 35. See also
    Social brain networks
Tourette's disorder, 186, 187, 188
Transference, 69–70
Traumatic brain injury, 159–161
Tryptophan, 43, 54–55, 114

Vascular endothelial growth factor (VEGF), 37
Ventral tegmental area (VTA), 16–17, 156, 217
Vitamin D, 49

Water, hydration via, 49
Weight and obesity, 38, 54